Pediatric Imaging

A CORE REVIEW

SECOND EDITION

Pediatric Imaging

A CORE REVIEW

SECOND EDITION

EDITORS

Steven L. Blumer, MD, MBA, CPE, FAAP

Visiting Clinical Associate Professor of Radiology
University of Pittsburgh School of Medicine
Attending Pediatric Radiologist
UPMC Children's Hospital of Pittsburgh
Associate Medical Director of Radiology Informatics
UPMC Health System
Pittsburgh, Pennsylvania

David M. Biko, MD, FACR

Associate Professor of Radiology
University of Pennsylvania Perelman School of Medicine
Chief, Division of Body Imaging
Director, Section of Cardiovascular and Lymphatic Imaging
Children's Hospital of Philadelphia
Philadelphia, Pennsylvania

Safwan S. Halabi, MD

Associate Professor of Radiology
Northwestern University Feinberg School of Medicine
Pediatric Radiologist and Vice-Chair of Imaging Informatics
Ann & Robert H. Lurie Children's Hospital
Director of Fetal Imaging
Chicago Institute for Fetal Health
Chicago, Illinois

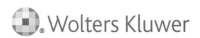 Wolters Kluwer

Philadelphia • Baltimore • New York • London
Buenos Aires • Hong Kong • Sydney • Tokyo

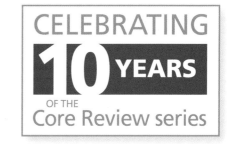
CELEBRATING 10 YEARS OF THE Core Review series

Acquisitions Editor: Nicole Dernoski
Development Editor: Eric McDermott
Editorial Coordinator: Remington Fernando
Editorial Assistant: Kristen Kardoley
Marketing Manager: Kirstin Watrud
Production Project Manager: Frances Gunning
Manager, Graphic Arts & Design: Stephen Druding
Manufacturing Coordinator: Lisa Bowling
Prepress Vendor: S4Carlisle Publishing Services

Second Edition

9 8 7 6 5 4 3 2 1

Printed in Mexico

Library of Congress Cataloging-in-Publication Data

ISBN-13: 978-1-975199-35-7

ISBN-10: 1-975199-35-9

Library of Congress Control Number: 2023916807

shop.lww.com

SERIES FOREWORD

Pediatric Imaging: A Core Review, second edition covers the vast field of pediatric radiology. This second edition builds on the success of the first edition by covering the essential aspects of pediatric imaging in a manner that serves as a guide for residents to assess their knowledge and review the material in a format that is similar to the ABR core examination. Like the prior edition, the second edition still contains 300 questions in print copy with many new questions added. References to a majority of the questions have been updated as well.

The intent of the *Core Review Series* is to provide the resident, fellow, or practicing physician a review of the important conceptual, factual, and practical aspects of a subject with multiple-choice questions written in the format like the ABR core examination. The *Core Review Series* is not intended to be exhaustive but to provide material likely to be tested on the ABR core exam and that would be required in clinical practice.

As series editor and founder of the *Core Review Series*, it has been rewarding to not only be a coeditor of one of the books in this series but to bring together and work with so many talented individuals in the profession of radiology across the country.

This series represents countless hours of work by so many individuals that would not have come together without their participation. It has been quite gratifying to receive so many comments from residents of the positive impact they feel the series has made in their board preparation. The *Core Review Series* has grown to become a trusted board exam resource for radiology residents.

I would like to commend Drs. Blumer, Biko, and Halabi for doing an outstanding job to the second edition of *Pediatric Imaging: A Core Review*. I believe this volume will serve as a valuable resource for residents during their board preparation and a useful reference for fellows and practicing radiologists.

Biren A. Shah, MD, FACR, FSBI
Section Chief, Breast Imaging,
Detroit Medical Center
Detroit, Michigan
Assistant Dean for Career Development and
Professor of Radiology
Western Michigan University Homer Stryker
M.D. School of Medicine
Kalamazoo, Michigan

PREFACE

When the American Board of Radiology (ABR) changed the radiology board certification process from the three-exam format to the current two-exam format, it not only changed the number of exams administered to radiology trainees but also fundamentally changed the way that the content was tested. The current examinations are image-rich exams that test higher-order reasoning instead of simple rote memorization of facts. In addition, the testing of practical day-to-day practice scenarios is now emphasized instead of random and obscure conditions.

In preparing the second edition of this book, we tried to keep the above guidelines in mind and improve upon the success of the first edition. We, along with our contributors Dr. Paul Clark and Dr. Kathleen Schenker, believe that we have again written a book that is full of high-quality image-rich questions about conditions commonly encountered in the daily practice of pediatric radiology. Many new questions and explanations have been added to this edition. In addition, original content has been reviewed and updated images, explanations, and references have been added where applicable. The questions are again mainly based on scenarios commonly encountered in the day-to-day practice of pediatric radiology and designed to be thought-provoking and test higher-order reasoning. We believe that this format is more interesting than old-style review books, which often tested rote memorization.

All of us have enjoyed learning about pediatric radiology from the many outstanding attending pediatric radiologists we have worked with during our training. We have also been blessed to work with many wonderful colleagues as faculty, who have served as mentors and continued to help us grow as pediatric radiologists. We would like to take the time to thank all these individuals.

In writing this book, we hope to be able to share our knowledge imparted to us with the next generation of radiology trainees. It is extremely gratifying for us to be able to help our trainees learn about pediatric radiology and to watch them succeed and progress in their careers. We hope that our trainees will use the knowledge gained in this book to provide high-quality care for pediatric patients and their respective families that they will encounter in their training and professional careers. Furthermore, this book should serve as a useful resource for radiologists at more advanced stages of their career, including current attending radiologists.

Finally, this book would not have been possible without the understanding of our families. Writing this book obviously represents a significant time commitment, and we would like to thank you for your support.

Steven L. Blumer, MD, MBA, CPE, FAAP
David M. Biko, MD, FACR
Safwan S. Halabi, MD

ACKNOWLEDGMENTS

We would like to extend our thanks to Dr. Biren Shah, the series editor, as well as Mr. Eric McDermott, Mr. Remington Fernando, and the rest of the staff at LWW for their guidance and support in preparing this book. In addition we would also like to thank Mr. Subhash Nataraj and his colleagues at S4Carlisle Publishing Services for their assistance during our revisions to this book.

CONTENTS

1 Pediatric Gastrointestinal Tract

QUESTIONS

1 Regarding intestinal malrotation, which of the following is true?

A. This entity is usually diagnosed after the first year of life.
B. Malrotation is a predisposing risk factor for the development of midgut volvulus.
C. The cecum is usually normally located in the right lower quadrant in patients who are malrotated.
D. The anatomic relationship between the SMA and SMV is usually normal in patients who are malrotated.

2 A radiograph of a 2-day-old patient with bilious vomiting is shown below. What is the next appropriate step in management?

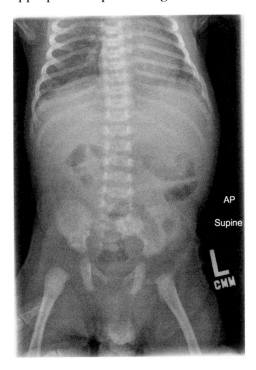

A. Contrast enema
B. Emergent upper GI series
C. Follow-up abdominal radiographs in 1 hour
D. No further workup is needed.

3 An image from an upper GI series that was subsequently performed on the same patient in Question 2 is shown below. Which of the following would be the next most appropriate step in management?

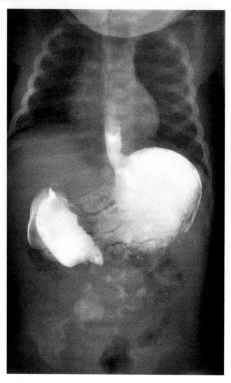

    A. Abdominal ultrasound
    B. Contrast enema
    C. Stat surgical consult
    D. CT scan of the abdomen and pelvis

4 A 6-week-old male presents to the emergency department with nonbilious projectile vomiting. Plain abdominal radiographs were obtained and are shown below. What is the next appropriate step in management?

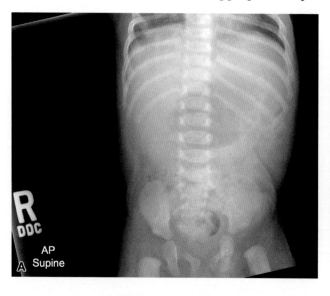 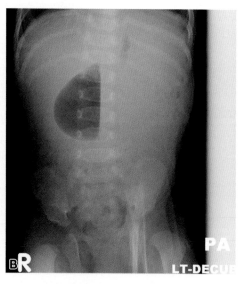

    A. Surgical consultation
    B. Nonemergent abdominal sonogram
    C. Contrast enema
    D. CT scan of the abdomen and pelvis

5 A nonemergent abdominal sonogram was subsequently performed on the same patient in Question 4, and images from the study are shown below. These images did not change over time. Regarding the entity demonstrated, which of the following is true?

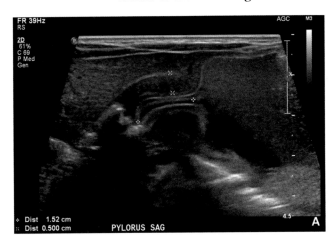 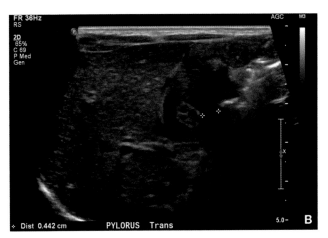

A. This condition often occurs in firstborn females.

B. The treatment of choice is medical.

C. The "double-track sign" and mucosal heaping may be seen in ultrasound exams performed for this condition.

D. Gastric contents often readily empty into the pylorus during exams performed on patients with this condition.

6 A patient presents for an MR exam of the abdomen and pelvis. Representative images from the study are shown below. Concerning the images, which of the following are true?

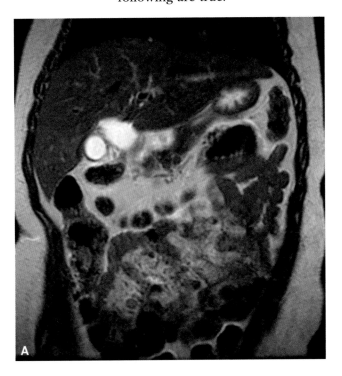 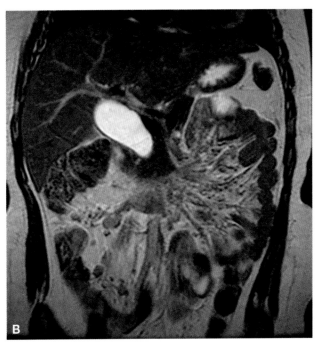

A. This lesion is the most common type of choledochal cyst.

B. This lesion is consistent with a choledochocele.

C. This lesion is consistent with Caroli disease.

D. This lesion is consistent with a type IVA choledochal cyst.

7 A radiograph from a neonate with a distended abdomen and failure to pass meconium is shown below. Which of the following is the next most appropriate step in management?

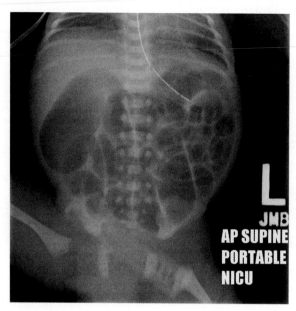

A. Upper GI series
B. Abdominal ultrasound
C. CT scan
D. Contrast enema

8 A contrast enema was subsequently performed on the patient described in Question 7. Images from the study are shown below. Which of the following is the most likely diagnosis?

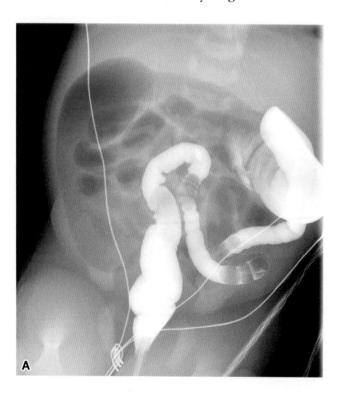
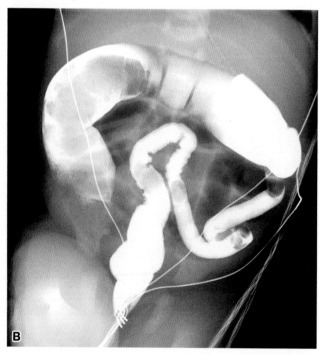

A. Hirschsprung disease
B. Functional immaturity of the colon
C. High ileal atresia
D. Low ileal atresia

9 Regarding the most likely diagnosis of the patient in Question 8, which of the following is true?

A. The initial treatment of choice is surgical.
B. Repeated enemas with water-soluble contrast do not alleviate this condition.
C. This entity is often seen in the offspring of mothers with diabetes or mothers treated with magnesium sulfate.
D. This entity is caused by a jejunal atresia.

10 Which of the following entities only occurs in patients with cystic fibrosis?

A. Functional immaturity of the colon
B. Meconium ileus
C. Ileal atresia
D. Jejunal atresia

11 Regarding microcolons, which of the following is true?

A. They are commonly seen in cases of jejunal atresia.
B. They are not seen in patients with low ileal atresia.
C. They are not often seen in meconium ileus.
D. They are seen in conditions in which there is an unused colon.

12 A CT scan is performed on a 5-year-old patient with no known medical history, and an image is shown below. Concerning the finding, which of the following is true?

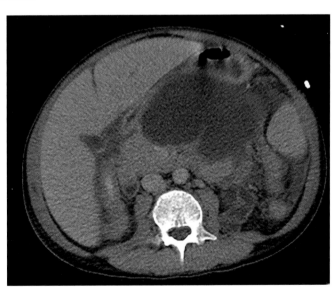

A. Nonaccidental trauma should be suspected as an etiology.
B. This is a rare complication of pediatric pancreatitis.
C. This is a known early complication of pediatric pancreatitis.
D. There are no more than two known causes of pediatric pancreatitis.

13 A babygram obtained from a neonate is shown below. Concerning the findings, which of the following is true?

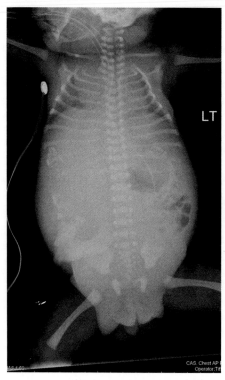

A. Most patients with this condition will require surgery.
B. Only a small minority of patients with this condition survive.
C. The findings are the result of an antenatal bowel perforation.
D. The findings are likely secondary to bowel obstruction after birth.

14 An abdominal ultrasound examination is performed in a patient who presents with neonatal jaundice and conjugated hyperbilirubinemia. A representative figure is shown below. Which of the following is the next appropriate step in management?

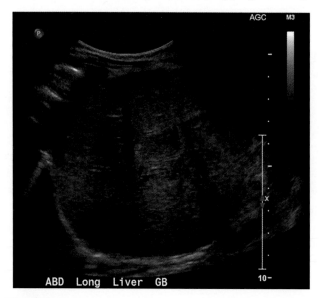

A. Upper GI series
B. Tc-99m HIDA scan
C. CT scan of the abdomen and pelvis
D. No further imaging is indicated.

15 Static images from a Tc-99m HIDA scan that was subsequently performed on the patient described in Question 14 are shown below. These images were obtained after 6 hours of imaging. Which of the following is the next appropriate step in management?

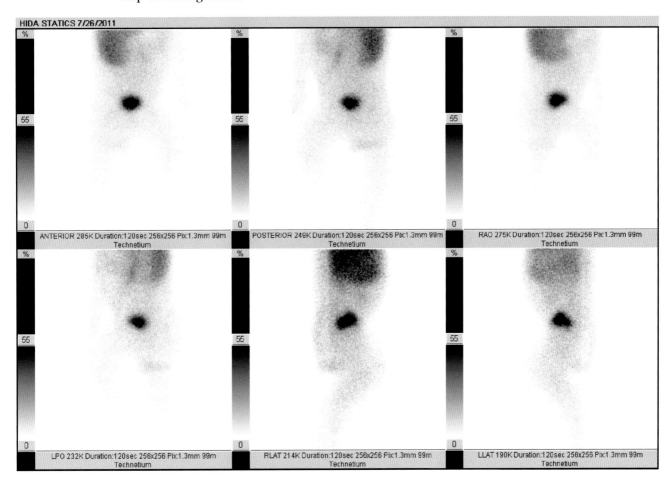

A. The study is normal and should be ended.

B. Surgery should be immediately consulted as the findings are consistent with chronic cholecystitis.

C. Delayed 24-hour images should be obtained.

D. SPECT imaging should be performed to better delineate the focus of radiotracer activity in the pelvis.

16 The decision was then made to obtain a delayed image at 24 hours after radio-tracer injection on the patient described in Questions 14 and 15. The delayed image is shown below. Concerning the findings, which of the following is true?

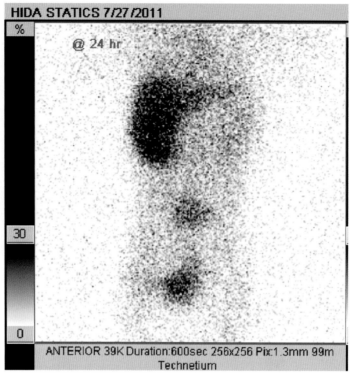

A. Neonatal hepatitis has been excluded.
B. A Kasai procedure is the treatment of choice for patients with these findings with biliary atresia.
C. The findings are not consistent with biliary atresia.
D. It is unlikely that this patient will need a liver transplant.

17 Before performing the exam depicted in Questions 15 and 16, pretreatment with which of the following agents can be used to enhance the specificity of the test?

A. Phenobarbital
B. CCK
C. Cimetidine
D. Morphine

18 Images from an ultrasound and CT scan performed in an infant with a history of GI bleeding are shown below. Regarding the findings, which of the following is true?

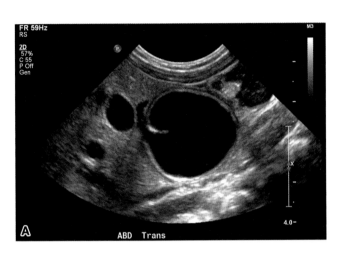
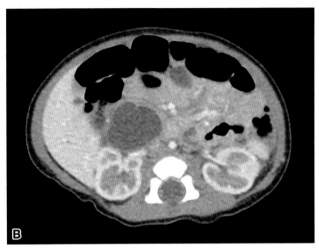

A. A Meckel (Tc-99m pertechnetate) scan can be helpful in making the diagnosis.
B. The lesion is likely adrenal in origin.
C. These findings represent the most common type of choledochal cyst.
D. The findings are suggestive of an exophytic cystic Wilms tumor.

19 An incidental abnormality is noted in the visualized portions of the abdomen on a portable chest radiograph performed on a 3-year-old patient shown below. Which of the following would be the next appropriate step in management?

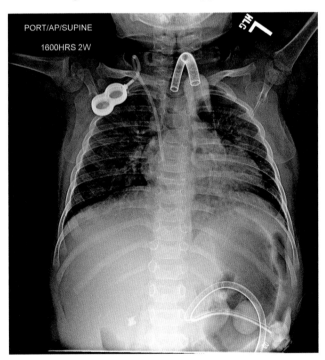

A. Notify the referring clinician of the unexpected finding and recommend an abdominal ultrasound.
B. No further workup is needed.
C. Notify the referring clinician of the unexpected finding and recommend a stat upper GI series.
D. Notify the referring clinician of the unexpected finding and recommend an IR consult to check appropriate positioning of the gastrojejunostomy tube.

20 Instead of an abdominal ultrasound, further evaluation of the patient in Question 19 was performed with a CT scan (Figure A) and MR examination (Figure B). Images from those studies are shown below. Which of the following is the most likely diagnosis?

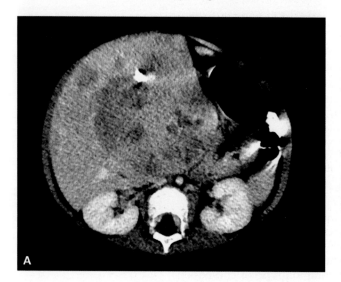
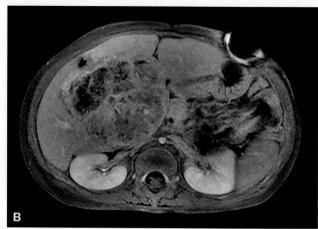

A. Mesenchymal hamartoma of the liver
B. Hepatocellular carcinoma
C. Hepatoblastoma
D. Focal nodular hyperplasia

21 Concerning hepatoblastoma, which of the following is true?

A. AFP is not typically elevated in affected patients.
B. There is a known association with Beckwith-Wiedemann syndrome.
C. There is no known association with other congenital abnormalities.
D. The bones are the most common site of metastasis.

22 An adolescent patient who is status post recent motor vehicle accident is noted to have recurrent vomiting. An upper GI series is subsequently performed and images obtained after waiting a significant amount of time after administration of oral contrast are shown below. Which of the following would be the next most appropriate step in management?

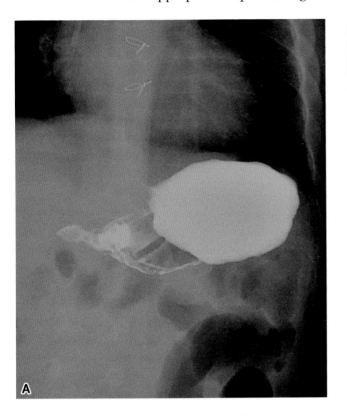
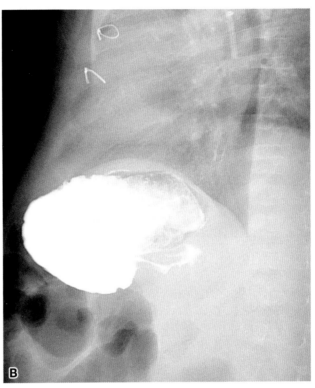

A. Abdominal plain films
B. Meckel scan
C. Contrast enema
D. Cross-sectional imaging

23 A CT scan was subsequently performed on the patient in Question 22. Representative images are shown below. Intravenous contrast was administered but oral contrast was not administered. Regarding the findings, which of the following is true?

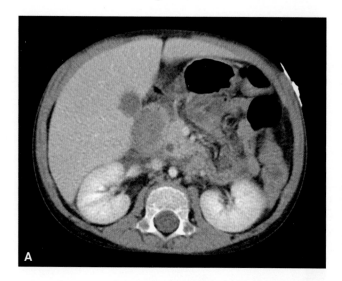 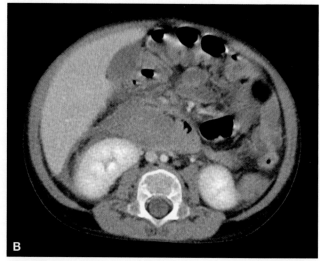

A. These lesions are often the result of penetrating abdominal trauma.
B. These lesions are almost always caused by accidental trauma.
C. Anticoagulation can often prevent these lesions from occurring.
D. These lesions can sometimes be caused by endoscopy.

24 An axial image from a CT scan is shown below. What is the most likely etiology of the appearance of the pancreas?

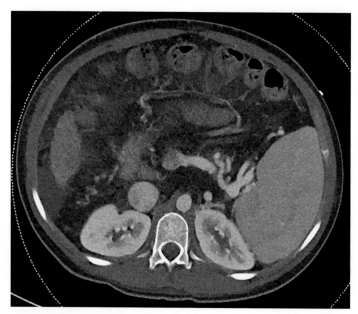

A. Tuberous sclerosis
B. von Hippel-Lindau syndrome
C. Sturge-Weber syndrome
D. Cystic fibrosis

25 Regarding the most likely etiology of the appearance of the pancreas in the patient described in Question 24, which of the following is true?

A. This entity is often suspected with the presence of echogenic bowel seen on fetal ultrasounds.

B. The inheritance pattern is autosomal dominant.

C. Bronchiectasis is rare in these patients.

D. Diagnosis usually occurs in adulthood.

26 An image from an ultrasound exam performed on a 3-year-old patient with a history of cervical lymphadenopathy, fever, a red-colored "strawberry"-appearing tongue, rash, and conjunctival injection is shown below. Regarding the most likely etiology, which of the following is true?

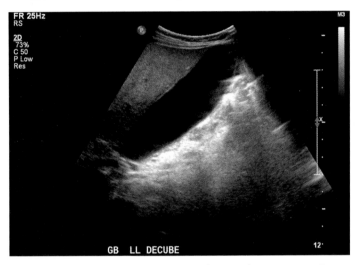

A. ECG patterns of affected patients are almost always normal.

B. Myocarditis in these patients is extremely rare.

C. There is no known therapy for this entity.

D. There is an association with coronary artery aneurysms.

27 Images obtained after a patient's nasogastric tube was injected with 10 mL of air are shown below. Regarding the findings, which of the following is true?

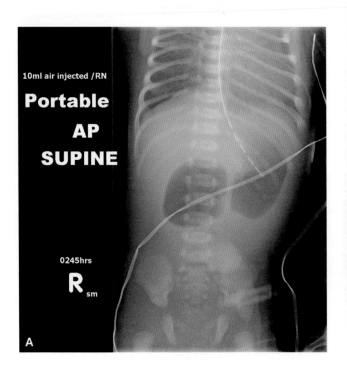
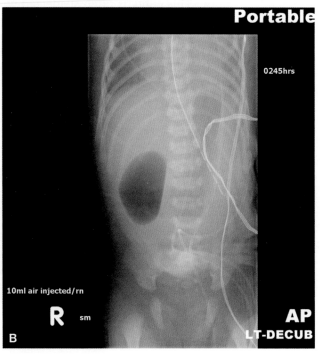

A. Further evaluation with an upper GI series is recommended.

B. The treatment of choice for this condition is medical.

C. The findings are caused by extrinsic and intrinsic conditions that lead to duodenal obstruction.

D. These findings are only seen on plain film radiographs.

28 Regarding duodenal atresia, which of the following is true?

A. The "double-bubble" sign is pathognomonic for this entity.

B. This entity usually presents with nonbilious vomiting.

C. There is a known association with Down syndrome.

D. The atretic segment is always distal to the ampulla of Vater.

29 Images from a fetal MRI are shown below. Regarding the most likely diagnosis, which of the following is true?

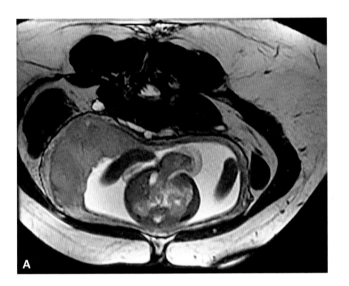
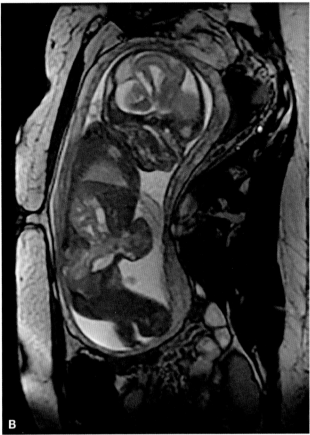

    A. Other associated anomalies are uncommon.
    B. The defect is not usually covered by a membrane.
    C. The mortality rates of this condition are low even with associated defects.
    D. The umbilical cord usually inserts into the defect.

30 Regarding gastroschisis, which of the following is true?
    A. There is usually a midline defect.
    B. There is a high association with associated anomalies.
    C. The umbilical cord usually inserts into the defect.
    D. The intrauterine mortality rate is low.

31 An abdominal radiograph from a 3-day-old premature infant with bloody stools is shown below. Which of the following would be the next most appropriate step in management?

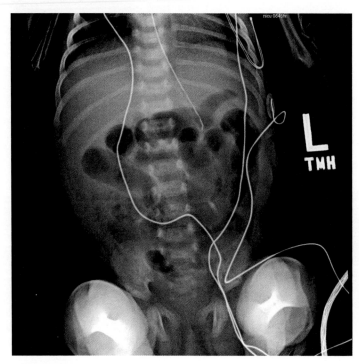

A. Stat upper GI series

B. Contrast enema

C. Emergent surgical consult

D. Bowel rest, antibiotics, and serial abdominal radiographs

32 Regarding NEC, which of the following is true?

A. The development of large bowel strictures is a known complication.

B. The disease is only treated medically.

C. It affects only premature patients.

D. Pneumatosis is an indication for surgical management.

33 Images from a study performed on a child with recurrent gastrointestinal bleeding are shown below. Regarding the abnormality, which of the following is true?

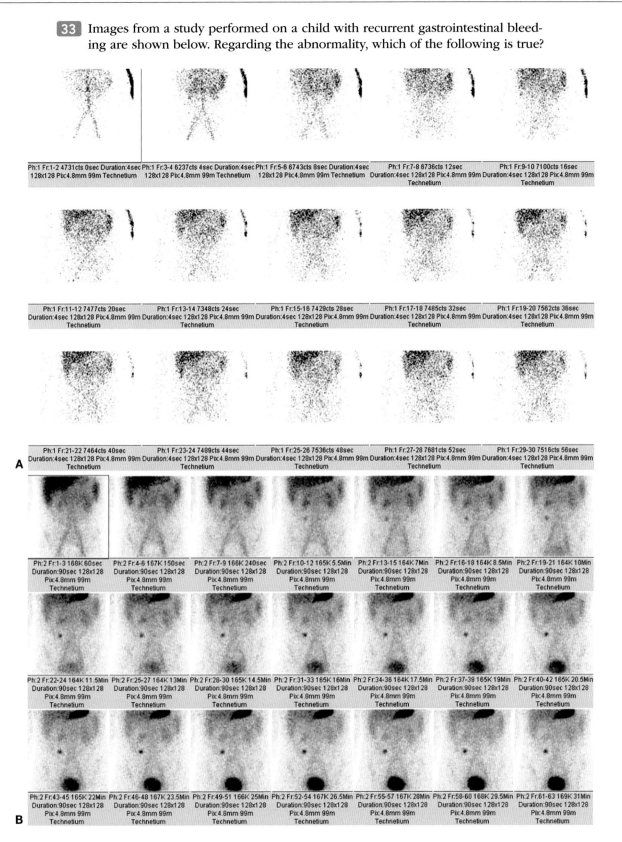

A. The finding represents a false diverticulum.
B. The abnormality is most often found in the right side of the colon.
C. These structures are frequently lined by heterotopic gastric and pancreatic mucosa.
D. No known complications of this entity have been reported.

34 Pretreating the patient before the examination performed in Question 33 with which of the following medications may help improve the sensitivity of the exam?

A. Cimetidine
B. Phenobarbital
C. CCK
D. Morphine

35 An abdominal radiograph obtained from a neonate in the NICU is shown below. Which of the following lines is not in correct position?

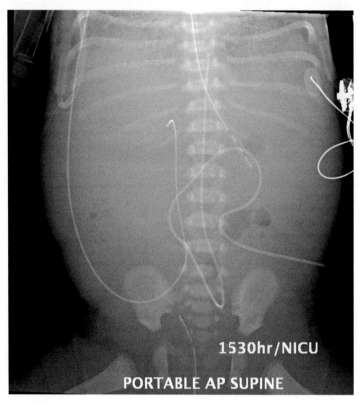

A. UA line
B. UV line
C. Bladder catheter
D. NG tube

36 Which of the following is the correct position for the tip of an umbilical venous catheter?

A. Superior cavoatrial junction
B. Inferior cavoatrial junction
C. L3 or below
D. Over the sacrum

37 An otherwise healthy 10-year-old thin patient presents with a recent onset of fever and right lower quadrant abdominal pain with guarding and rebound on physical examination. Lab results reveal an elevated white blood cell count with a left shift. A plain film of the abdomen was ordered and was unremarkable. Which of the following would be the next most appropriate step in management?

A. Contrast enema
B. Upper GI series and small bowel follow-through
C. Ultrasound of the right lower quadrant
D. CT scan of the abdomen and pelvis with IV contrast

38 A right lower quadrant ultrasound was performed on the patient from Question 37, and a representative image is shown below. Despite the findings, the clinical staff is still highly suspicious for appendicitis. Which of the following would be the next most appropriate step in management?

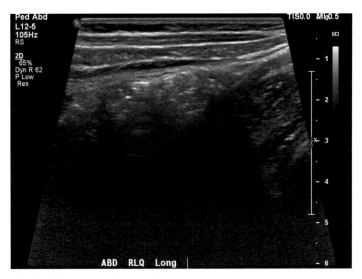

A. Meckel (Tc-99m pertechnetate) scan
B. MRI of the abdomen and pelvis
C. Upper GI and small bowel follow-through
D. CT scan of the abdomen and pelvis with intravenous contrast

39 Regarding the abnormality demonstrated in the images below from an MR of the abdomen and pelvis performed on the same patient in Questions 37 and 38, which of the following is true?

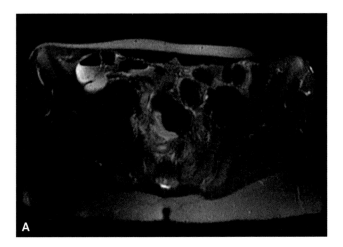
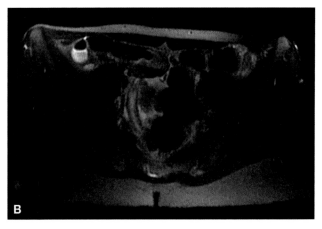

A. CT is more sensitive than MR in detecting this abnormality.
B. MR is more sensitive than CT in detecting this abnormality.
C. CT is as sensitive as MR in detecting this abnormality.
D. Ultrasound is more sensitive than CT in detecting this abnormality.

40 Images are shown below from a study performed on a 6-month-old child who has a history of wheezing. Regarding the study shown below, which is the most likely diagnosis?

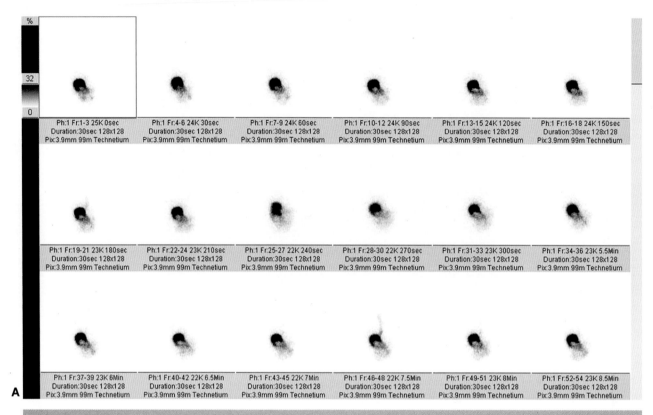

A

		Parameter	99m Technetium
Bkgd Correction	On	Emptying	1 %
Decay Correction	On	Emptying begin {T0}	0 mins
Geometric Mean	Off	Emptying end	62 mins
		T 1/2	2942 mins
		T0 -> T 1/2	2942 mins

B

    A. Normal study
    B. Gastroesophageal reflux
    C. Malrotation with midgut volvulus
    D. Duodenal atresia

41 Regarding the exam performed on the patient in Question 40, which of the following is true?

    A. The patient has rapid gastric emptying.
    B. The patient has delayed gastric emptying.
    C. The gastric emptying rate is normal.
    D. The patient likely has bilious vomiting.

42 A plain abdominal radiograph obtained from a 16-year-old patient is shown below. Regarding the patient, which of the following is true?

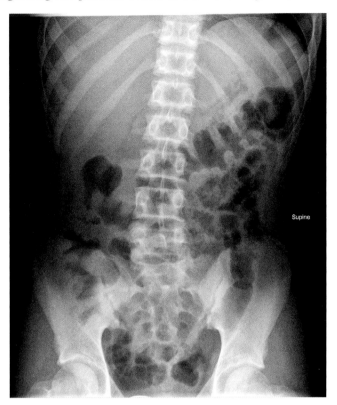

Supine

A. The radiograph is normal.
B. A pelvic ultrasound should be ordered for further evaluation.
C. The patient likely presented with abdominal pain and diarrhea.
D. An emergent upper GI should be performed.

43 A young child presents to the emergency room with abdominal pain. Abdominal radiographs obtained with the patient placed in the supine and left lateral decubitus positions are shown below. What is the next most appropriate step in management?

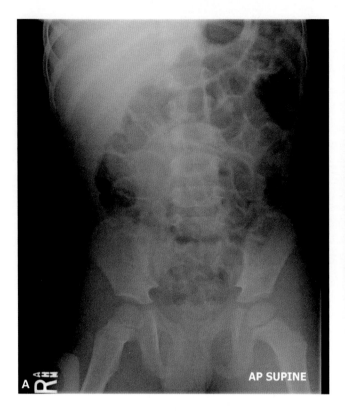

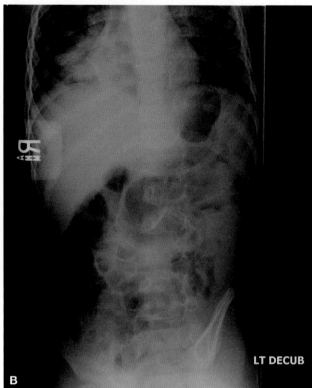

A. Emergent upper GI series
B. Abdominal ultrasound
C. Stat surgical consult
D. Treatment for pneumonia

44 An MR examination was performed on a teenage patient with a long-standing history of abdominal pain and diarrhea. Images are shown below. Which of the following is the most likely diagnosis?

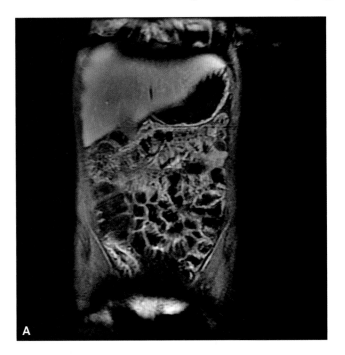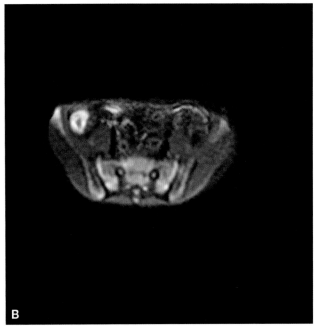

A. Crohn disease
B. Ulcerative colitis
C. Typhlitis
D. Pseudomembranous colitis

45 A 1-day-old patient presents for a CT scan of an abdominal mass and images are shown below. What is the most likely diagnosis?

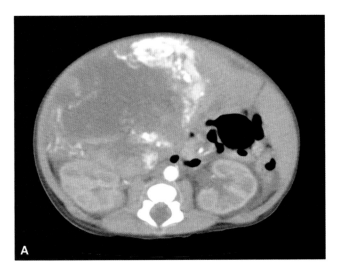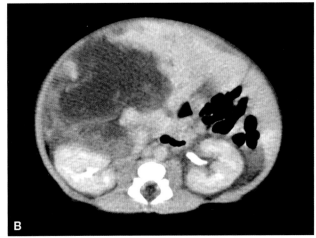

A. Focal nodular hyperplasia
B. Hepatocellular carcinoma
C. Focal fatty infiltration
D. Infantile hemangioendothelioma

46 Prior to the CT scan performed on the patient in Question 45, a babygram was obtained. Regarding the study, which of the following is true?

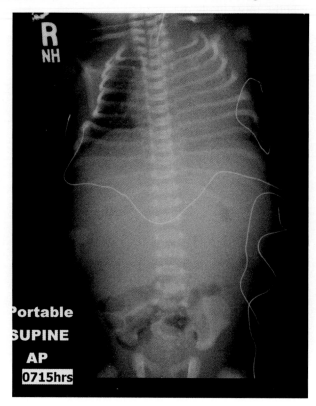

A. There is autoinfarction of the spleen.
B. There is a bowel obstruction.
C. The endotracheal tube is malpositioned.
D. There is evidence of vascular shunting.

47 The PRETEXT classification system is used to stage which of the following pediatric tumors?

A. Wilms tumor
B. Neuroblastoma
C. Hepatoblastoma
D. Osteosarcoma

48 A 2-year-old patient presents with intermittent abdominal pain and bloody stools. An abdominal radiograph was performed. Given the findings, what is the next best step in management?

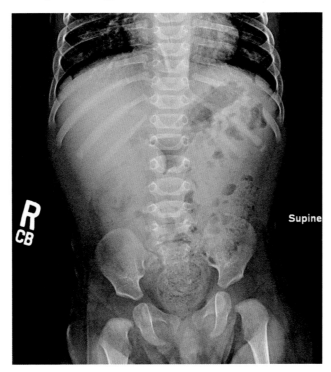

A. No further follow-up is needed.
B. Abdominal ultrasound
C. Upper GI series
D. Chest X-ray

49 An abdominal ultrasound was subsequently performed on the same patient in Question 48. Given the findings, what is the next best step in management?

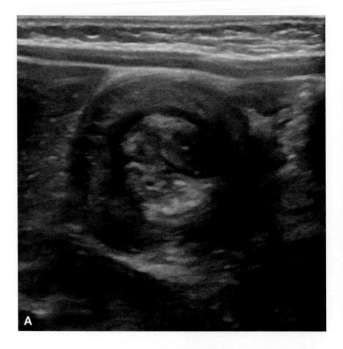
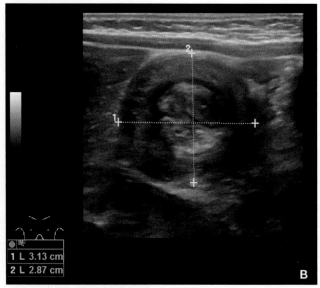

A. No further follow-up is needed.
B. Upper GI series
C. Chest X-ray
D. Air contrast enema

50 Regarding the entity demonstrated in the images from the ultrasound exam performed on the patient described in Question 48, which of the following is true?

A. There is typically a lead point in patients greater than 3 years of age.
B. Most cases in patients less than 3 months of age are idiopathic.
C. This entity is most common during the summer months.
D. A bacterial etiology is the suspected cause.

51 Regarding fluoroscopic reductions of ileocolic intussusceptions, which of the following is true?

A. There is a high perforation rate.
B. No more than one attempt should be made at reducing the intussusception.
C. Patients should be well hydrated prior to the procedure.
D. Interloop fluid is a good prognostic sign.

52 Which of the following is a common cause of small bowel obstruction in young children?

A. Meckel diverticulum
B. Appendicitis
C. Adhesions
D. All of the above

53 A radiograph obtained on a neonate after multiple attempts to place a feeding tube is shown below. Given the findings, which of the following is true?

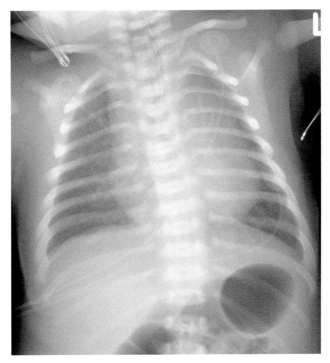

A. There are no known associations.
B. There are only two known variations of this entity.
C. An upper GI series will be needed to confirm the diagnosis.
D. Fluoroscopic exams are often not necessary to confirm the diagnosis.

54 Which of the following tests should be ordered after diagnosis of the condition affecting the patient in Question 53?

A. Renal ultrasound
B. Echocardiogram
C. A and B
D. None of the above

55 The radiographs shown below were obtained on a young child after a suspected foreign body ingestion. What is the next best step in management?

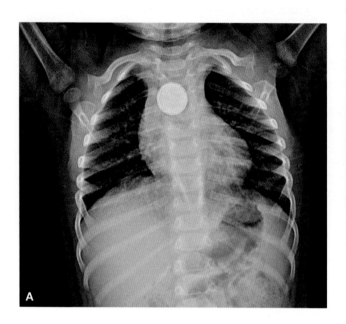

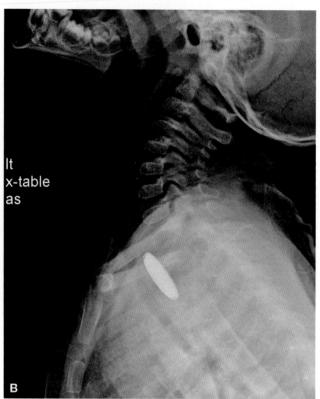

A. No further follow-up care is needed.
B. Follow-up radiographs in 1 week to ensure passage.
C. Recommend an abdominal ultrasound after the patient is made NPO for 4-6 hours.
D. Contact the referring provider as the radiographs demonstrate an emergent finding.

ANSWERS AND EXPLANATIONS

1 **Answer B.** Intestinal malrotation is a predisposing risk factor for midgut volvulus. In individuals with malrotation, the mesenteric attachment of the midgut, particularly the portion from the duodenojejunal junction (DJJ) to the cecum, is abnormally short. The gut is therefore prone to twist counterclockwise around the superior mesenteric artery (SMA) and vein (SMV), creating a volvulus. Approximately 80% of patients with malrotation have an abnormal cecal position, which a contrast enema can help demonstrate. The SMV is normally located to the right of and anterior to the SMA on axial imaging studies, but the relative positions of the vein and artery are reversed in 60% of individuals with malrotation. Malrotation is usually diagnosed in newborns and young infants; up to 75% of symptomatic cases occur in newborns, and up to 90% of symptomatic cases occur within the first year of life. The classic clinical manifestation of malrotation in newborns is bilious vomiting with or without abdominal distention associated with either duodenal obstructive bands or midgut volvulus. However, malrotation with midgut volvulus can occur at any age.

Reference: Applegate KE, Anderson JM, Klatte EC. Intestinal malrotation in children: a problem-solving approach to the upper gastrointestinal series. *Radiographics*. 2006;26(5):1485-1500.

2 **Answer B.** Bilious vomiting in a neonate is an emergency as it raises concern for intestinal malrotation with midgut volvulus. A delay in diagnosis and treatment of this entity may result in small bowel necrosis, short gut syndrome, and dependence on total parenteral nutrition (TPN). Mortality in affected newborns with malrotation and midgut volvulus ranges between 3% and 5%.

Abdominal radiographs may be normal in appearance or show distention of the stomach and proximal duodenum by air, with little distal bowel gas. The radiograph of the patient in this case does not demonstrate the abnormal findings that have been associated with volvulus or evidence of an obstruction. However, malrotation with midgut volvulus still must be excluded and repeat abdominal radiographs would not be of benefit. The most sensitive test for the diagnosis of malrotation is an upper gastrointestinal (UGI) series with sensitivities ranging from 93% to 100%. However, the sensitivity of this exam for midgut volvulus has been reported at 54%.

Even though an UGI is still considered the gold standard for documenting malrotation with midgut volvulus, these entities can also be demonstrated with an abdominal ultrasound (US) or CT scan of the abdomen and pelvis. If an US or CT scan is ordered on a neonate to assess for malrotation with or without midgut volvulus, there are three important findings that should be documented. The first is the orientation of the SMA and the SMV. Normally the SMV is larger in caliber and positioned to the right and slightly anterior in position to the SMA on axial imaging studies. The SMA is smaller in caliber and positioned to the left of the SMV. Most neonates suspected of having malrotation have an abnormal SMA/SMV relationship on CT and US. In addition, these studies when performed in neonates with malrotation accompanied by midgut volvulus may demonstrate a swirling pattern or "whirlpool sign" of bowel and mesenteric vessels about the SMA. Finally, the retroperitoneal segment of the duodenum, specifically the third portion of the duodenum (D3), should normally course between the SMA and the abdominal aorta. In neonates with malrotation, the third portion of the duodenum will not pass between these structures.

A contrast enema is often used to evaluate for the cause of a distal bowel obstruction but is not the most sensitive test to evaluate for malrotation and midgut volvulus, which can cause a proximal bowel obstruction. This exam can be helpful in assessing the location of the cecum, which is normally located in the right lower quadrant. Eighty percent of patients with malrotation have an abnormal cecal position, which a contrast enema can help demonstrate.

References: Applegate KE, Anderson JM, Klatte EC. Intestinal malrotation in children: a problem-solving approach to the upper gastrointestinal series. *Radiographics*. 2006;26(5):1485-1500.

Epelman M. The whirlpool sign. *Radiology*. 2006;240(3):910-911.

Nasser MP. Gastrointestinal. In: Donnelly LF, ed. *Fundamentals of Pediatric Imaging*. 3rd ed. Elsevier; 2022:95-138.

3   **Answer C.** The study demonstrates a "beaked" appearance of the third portion of the duodenum and only a small amount of contrast distal to the location of the beaking or obstruction (arrow in picture below). This appearance is consistent with intestinal malrotation with midgut volvulus. Other appearances of volvulus include the "corkscrew sign," which describes the spiral appearance of the distal duodenum and proximal jejunum seen in midgut volvulus. In patients with malrotation with midgut volvulus with a corkscrew sign, the duodenum and proximal jejunum do not cross the midline and instead take an inferior direction. The loops twist on a shortened small bowel mesentery, resulting in a corkscrew appearance.

The normal position of the DJJ is to the left of the left-sided pedicle of the vertebral body at the level of the duodenal bulb on frontal images obtained on an UGI. If the DJJ is located inferior or to the right of this level, malrotation should be considered. Note, however, that inferior displacement of the DJJ is a common variant seen on frontal views in infants. This finding may be due to displacement of the relatively mobile ligament of Treitz by the adjacent distended stomach or bowel.

If the diagnosis of malrotation remains in doubt or the UGI findings are equivocal, the study should be continued and delayed abdominal radiographs should be acquired to identify the position of the cecum. While the position of the colon may be normal in a child with malrotation, 80% of individuals with malrotation have an abnormal cecal position. As an alternative to delayed radiography, in an urgent situation, an enema may be administered with an water soluble contrast medium to demonstrate the position of the cecum. Generally, the shorter the distance between the DJJ and the cecum, the shorter the length of the small bowel mesentery and the greater the risk of volvulus. Therefore, if the borderline DJJ and jejunum are in the left upper quadrant and the cecum is in the right lower quadrant, the patient most likely has a long mesenteric attachment, which suggests a low risk for volvulus.

Given that the study performed in the question demonstrates findings consistent with malrotation with midgut volvulus, the patient needs to go to the operating room for further treatment. Therefore, none of the other choices are correct.

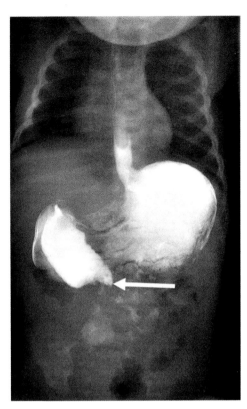

References: Applegate KE, Anderson JM, Klatte EC. Intestinal malrotation in children: a problem-solving approach to the upper gastrointestinal series. *Radiographics.* 2006;26(5):1485-1500.

Nasser MP. Gastrointestinal. In: Donnelly LF, ed. *Fundamentals of Pediatric Imaging.* 3rd ed. Elsevier; 2022:95-138.

Ortiz-Neira CL. The corkscrew sign: midgut volvulus. *Radiology.* 2007;242(1):315-316.

4 **Answer B.** The clinical history and imaging findings presented in this case are concerning for hypertrophic pyloric stenosis (HPS), a common entity in young infants. This condition is characterized by thickening of the muscular layer of the pylorus and failure of the pyloric canal to relax, resulting in gastric outlet obstruction that causes intractable nonbilious projectile vomiting. HPS has an incidence of 3 per 1,000 live births per year, although wide variations have been documented with geographic location, season, and ethnic origin. This disease usually presents between the second and sixth weeks of life and is more common in the white population, in males (male:female ratio 4:1), and typically in firstborn children. A history of an affected first-degree relative increases the risk more than fivefold. Additional common causes of nonbilious vomiting in children are pylorospasm and gastroesophageal reflux.

The radiographs of the patient demonstrate gaseous distention of the stomach with an air-fluid level on the left lateral decubitus view. There is a paucity of bowel gas beyond the stomach. These findings are suggestive of a gastric outlet obstruction as can be seen in HPS. US is the first modality of choice when there is clinical suspicion of HPS, as it is noninvasive and does not use radiation, which is a crucial advantage in children. It is also commonly available with relatively low cost. US also allows a dynamic study with direct observation of the pyloric canal morphology and behavior.

HPS is diagnosed by imaging. It should be noted that imaging to confirm or exclude the diagnosis of HPS is not considered a medical emergency. Before performing an US exam, the diagnosis of HPS is not certain. Therefore, surgical consultation is not required prior to making the diagnosis of HPS, but if the diagnosis is confirmed by US, the patient will require surgical treatment. A contrast enema of the colon would not be helpful in making the diagnosis. A CT scan of the abdomen and pelvis would also not be helpful in making the diagnosis as real-time visualization of the pylorus over an extended period is required to make the diagnosis and would expose the child unnecessarily to ionizing radiation.

References: Costa Dias S, Swinson S, Torrão H, et al. Hypertrophic pyloric stenosis: tips and tricks for ultrasound diagnosis. *Insights Imaging.* 2012;3(3):247-250.

Nasser MP. Gastrointestinal. In: Donnelly LF, ed. *Fundamentals of Pediatric Imaging.* 3rd ed. Elsevier; 2022:95-138.

5 **Answer C.** The US images shown demonstrate a thickened pyloric muscle and elongated pyloric channel, which did not change over time. These findings are consistent with HPS. As stated earlier, this condition often occurs in firstborn males. The treatment for this condition is a surgical pyloromyotomy. It is important to distinguish HPS from pylorospasm as the latter is treated medically.

On US examinations, the pyloric wall thickness should normally be <3 mm and the length of the pyloric channel should not exceed 15 mm. In the images from this case, the pyloric wall thickness measures up to 5 mm on the transverse view and the pyloric channel length measures up to 15.2 mm on the long-axis view. However, the published criteria for both measurements have varied. Most importantly, the pylorus should not open during the US examination. In pylorospasm, there is transient thickening of the pyloric muscle and elongation of the channel length.

However, the pylorus does eventually open in cases of pylorospasm. If the US examination demonstrates a closed pylorus with abnormal measurements of muscular thickness and channel length, it is important to extend the length of the examination by an extra 3 to 5 minutes to confirm that the pylorus remains closed and exclude pylorospasm.

In addition to the earlier findings, there are ancillary or secondary signs of pyloric stenosis on US including the "double-track sign." This sign is created by the abnormally thickened muscle mass that compresses the pyloric channel into two smaller channels or tracks. In addition, thickened pyloric mucosa may indent into the antrum, consistent with antral or mucosal heaping.

References: Blumer SL, Zucconi WB, Cohen HL, et al. The vomiting neonate: a review of the ACR appropriateness criteria and ultrasound's role in the work-up of such patients. *Ultrasound Q.* 2004;20(3):79-89.

Cohen HL, Blumer SL, Zucconi WB. The sonographic double-track sign: not pathognomonic for hypertrophic pyloric stenosis; can be seen in pylorospasm. *J Ultrasound Med.* 2004;23(5):641-646.

Nasser MP. Gastrointestinal. In: Donnelly LF, ed. *Fundamentals of Pediatric Imaging.* 3rd ed. Elsevier; 2022:95-138.

6 **Answer A.** The images demonstrate fusiform dilatation of the common bile duct. This is best visualized in Figure B where the long arrow points to fusiform dilatation of the common bile duct. The Todani classification system has been used to classify choledochal cysts. The imaging findings depicted on the MRI are consistent with a type I choledochal cyst. Note that in Figure A, the gallbladder (short arrow) is seen to the left (patient's right) of the common bile duct (long arrow). Type I choledochal cysts are seen in 80% to 90% of patients with choledochal cysts. Note that type I cysts can be further divided into type IA, IB, and IC cysts depending upon their morphologic characteristics. A choledochocele is a type III cyst and involves only the intraduodenal portion of the common bile duct. Caroli disease or a type V cyst involves dilatation of one or several segments of the intrahepatic bile ducts. A type IVA cyst involves dilatation of the intrahepatic and extrahepatic biliary ducts.

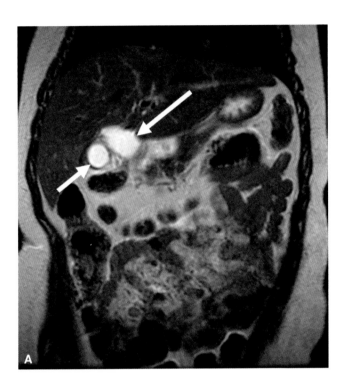

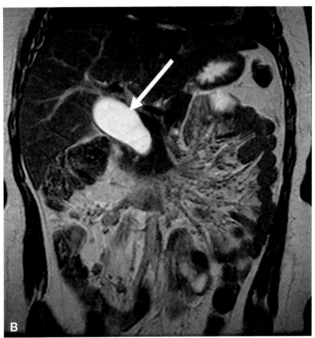

Todani Classification of Choledochal Cysts

Todani Classification	Imaging Characteristics
Type I—most common	Confined to the extrahepatic biliary ducts (EBDs). They can be further subdivided into type Ia (diffuse) cysts, which involve the entire EBD; type Ib (focal) cysts, which involve only a focal segment of the EBD; and type Ic (fusiform) cysts, which involve only the common bile duct (CBD).
Type II	True diverticula of the EBD
Type III	Choledochoceles, represent ectasia of an intramural CBD segment
Type IV	Multiple and can have both intrahepatic and extrahepatic components. They can be further subdivided into type IVa cysts, which involve both the EBD and the intrahepatic biliary duct (IBD), and type IVb cysts, which involve only the EBD with multiple saccular dilatations.
Type V	Caroli disease, which is a rare congenital cystic dilatation of the IBDs

References: Kim OH, Chung HJ, Choi BG. Imaging of the choledochal cyst. *Radiographics.* 1995;15(1):69-88.

Mortelé KJ, Rocha TC, Streeter JL, et al. Multimodality imaging of pancreatic and biliary congenital anomalies. *Radiographics.* 2006;26(3):715-731.

7 **Answer D.** The image shown in the figure demonstrates diffusely dilated loops of bowel without definite rectal bowel gas. These findings along with the patient's clinical history are concerning for an obstruction of the distal or lower GI tract. The best way to evaluate for the etiology of such lower GI tract obstructions is to perform a contrast enema. Common causes of lower tract obstructions include Hirschsprung disease, meconium plug syndrome (small left colon syndrome) (functional immaturity of the colon), ileal atresia, meconium ileus, and anal atresia or anorectal malformations. An UGI series is the test of choice to evaluate for a suspected upper or high obstruction in neonates. Common causes of upper tract obstructions include midgut volvulus/malrotation, duodenal atresia/stenosis, duodenal web, annular pancreas, and jejunal atresia. A CT scan is not an appropriate initial method to evaluate suspected distal obstructions and would needlessly expose the child to ionizing radiation. An abdominal US is not an appropriate way to evaluate a neonate with a suspected distal bowel obstruction but has been used to evaluate for malrotation with midgut volvulus, a cause of an upper or high GI tract obstruction.

References: Nasser MP. Gastrointestinal. In: Donnelly LF, ed. *Fundamentals of Pediatric Imaging*. 3rd ed. Elsevier; 2022:95-138.

Ngo AV, Stanescu AL, Phillips GS. Neonatal bowel disorders: practical imaging algorithm for trainees and general radiologists. *AJR Am J Roentgenol*. 2018;210(5):976-988.

8 **Answer B.** Figures A and B demonstrate a contrast enema examination. In contrast enemas, it is important to evaluate the rectosigmoid ratio. The rectum should have a diameter equal to or larger than the sigmoid, which is a normal rectosigmoid ratio. Patients who have Hirschsprung disease have an abnormal rectosigmoid ratio in which the sigmoid has a larger diameter than the rectum.

The study in this case demonstrates a normal rectosigmoid ratio. In addition, the left side of the colon appears small and ahaustral. The transverse and ascending colon are dilated. There are scattered filling defects seen throughout the colon likely due to meconium plugs. These findings are consistent with functional immaturity of the colon.

Patients who have a high intestinal obstruction, or an obstruction that occurs proximal to the midileum, such as a high ileal atresia, will have a normal-caliber colon. This is because there is ample proximal bowel to produce secretions that migrate distally and nourish the colon. Patients who have a low intestinal obstruction or an obstruction that occurs in the distal ileum or colon will have a microcolon or unused colon because there is not enough proximal small bowel to produce secretions to nourish the colon.

Reference: Berrocal T, Lamas M, Gutieerrez J, et al. Congenital anomalies of the small intestine, colon and rectum. *Radiographics*. 1999;19(5):1219-1236.

9 **Answer C.** The initial treatment of choice for patients with functional immaturity of the colon is a contrast enema with water-soluble contrast. Sometimes, repeated enemas are needed to flush out the meconium plugs. This condition is often seen in offspring of mothers with diabetes or mothers treated with magnesium sulfate for preeclampsia. Patients who have a jejunal atresia will have a normal-appearing colon as explained in the answer for Question 8.

Reference: Berrocal T, Lamas M, Gutieerrez J, et al. Congenital anomalies of the small intestine, colon and rectum. *Radiographics*. 1999;19(5):1219-1236.

10 **Answer B.** Meconium ileus occurs secondary to obstruction of the distal ileum due to the accumulation of abnormally tenacious meconium. It occurs exclusively in patients with cystic fibrosis and is the earliest clinical presentation of the disease.

Reference: Nasser MP. Gastrointestinal. In: Donnelly LF, ed. *Fundamentals of Pediatric Imaging*. 3rd ed. Elsevier; 2022:95-138.

11 **Answer D.** Microcolons are seen in conditions in which there is an unused colon such as distal bowel obstructions including low ileal atresia and meconium ileus. Jejunal atresias are high bowel obstructions, and there is enough proximal bowel to produce secretions to nourish the colon. Thus, a normal-caliber colon would be seen in contrast enemas performed in patients with a jejunal atresia or other more proximal bowel obstructions.

References: Dähnert W. *Radiology Review Manual*. 8th ed. Wolters Kluwer; 2017.

Nasser MP. Gastrointestinal. In: Donnelly LF, ed. *Fundamentals of Pediatric Imaging*. 3rd ed. Elsevier; 2022:95-138.

12 **Answer A.** The CT scan demonstrates a pancreatic pseudocyst, which is a known common late complication of acute pancreatitis, typically occurring 4 weeks after the development of a peripancreatic fluid collection. Pancreatic pseudocysts are the most common complication of pediatric pancreatitis. Pancreatitis in a young child should raise the suspicion of traumatic injury secondary to nonaccidental trauma (NAT). However, there are multiple other known causes of pediatric pancreatitis including pancreatitis secondary to accidental trauma, biliary anomalies, and medication-related and autoimmune etiologies.

Reference: Restrepo R, Hegerott HE, Kulkarni S, et al. Acute pancreatitis in pediatric patients: demographics, etiology and diagnostic imaging. *Am J Roentgenol*. 2016;206(3):632-644.

13 **Answer C.** The radiograph demonstrates a nonspecific bowel gas pattern with multiple calcifications throughout the abdomen (arrows). These findings are most consistent with meconium peritonitis. Meconium peritonitis is a condition that occurs following intrauterine intestinal perforation. This allows meconium to leak into the peritoneal cavity, causing an inflammatory reaction that can then calcify. Some neonates with meconium peritonitis require emergency surgery but others can be successfully managed nonsurgically. The etiology of the antenatal bowel obstruction in meconium peritonitis is variable, with the main causes being intestinal atresia, volvulus, intussusception, and meconium ileus. Mortality and morbidity rates in meconium peritonitis have been reported to vary depending on the countries and their economic resources, with a survival rate in developed countries being up to 80%.

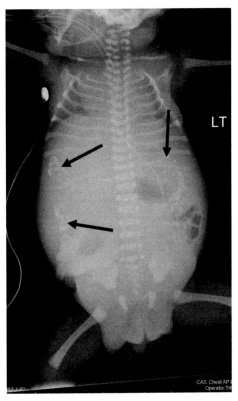

Reference: Caro-Domínguez P, Zani A, Chitayat D. et al. Meconium peritonitis: the role of postnatal radiographic and sonographic findings in predicting the need for surgery. *Pediatr Radiol*. 2018;48:1755-1762.

14 **Answer B.** The US image of the patient in the region of the gallbladder fossa fails to demonstrate the gallbladder. The clinical presentation of neonatal jaundice and absence of the gallbladder raise concern for biliary atresia. Note, however, that while some patients with biliary atresia do not have a gallbladder, some affected patients have a small gallbladder and other affected patients have a normal gallbladder. Of the answer choices listed, the next best test to evaluate for biliary atresia is with a Tc-99m hepatobiliary iminodiacetic acid (HIDA) scan. None of the other tests are helpful to make the diagnosis of biliary atresia and in the case of an UGI series and CT scan will needlessly expose the patient to ionizing radiation.

Reference: Brahee DD, Lampl BS. Neonatal diagnosis of biliary atresia: a practical review and update. *Pediatr Radiol.* 2022;52:685-692.

15 **Answer C.** The images fail to demonstrate bowel activity after 6 hours. A delayed image should then be obtained after 24 hours to evaluate for possible radiotracer excretion into bowel as biliary atresia cannot be excluded at this point in the study. This patient did not have a gallbladder and therefore could not have cholecystitis. The focus of radiotracer in the pelvis is excreted radiotracer within the urinary bladder, an expected finding.

References: Brahee DD, Lampl BS. Neonatal diagnosis of biliary atresia: a practical review and update. *Pediatr Radiol.* 2022;52:685-692.

Dähnert W. *Radiology Review Manual.* 8th ed. Wolters Kluwer; 2017.

16 **Answer B.** The image fails to demonstrate radiotracer excretion into bowel after 24 hours. Radiotracer activity is again seen in the urinary bladder, and the activity inferior to the bladder is excreted radiotracer within the diaper. Given the clinical history, the imaging findings are consistent with biliary atresia. However, these findings can also be seen in the setting of severe hepatocellular dysfunction from neonatal hepatitis, and a liver biopsy is sometimes necessary to distinguish between these two entities. The Kasai procedure (portoenterostomy) is performed in most of the patients with biliary atresia and has a greater success rate when performed in children <60 days old. Therefore, it is imperative to make the diagnosis of biliary atresia as early as possible. Note that the Kasai procedure is often a palliative procedure as most patients will eventually need a liver transplant.

References: Bijl EJ, Bharwani KD, Houwen RHJ, et al. The long-term outcome of the Kasai operation in patients with biliary atresia: a systematic review. *Neth J Med.* 2013;71(4):170-173.

Dähnert W. *Radiology Review Manual.* 8th ed. Wolters Kluwer; 2017.

17 **Answer A.** Infants with jaundice, in whom biliary atresia is suspected, phenobarbital, 5 mg/kg/d, may be given orally in two divided doses daily as pretreatment for a minimum of 3–5 days before the HIDA scan to enhance biliary excretion of the radiotracer and increase the specificity of the test. Phenobarbital stimulates biliary secretion by inducing hepatic enzymes, which increases conjugation and excretion of bilirubin. Morphine is given during HIDA scans to shorten the study time if there is nonvisualization of the gallbladder. This is typically injected 45 to 60 minutes after injection of radiotracer if activity is seen in the bowel. It causes contraction of the sphincter of Oddi, which raises intrabiliary pressure and can cause retrograde filling of the gallbladder. Cimetidine can be given before Meckel scans to decrease release of pertechnetate from the gastric mucosa. CCK is a synthetic hormone that causes gallbladder contraction, but many patients with biliary atresia do not have a gallbladder.

References: Dähnert W. *Radiology Review Manual.* 8th ed. Wolters Kluwer; 2017.

Tulchinsky M, Ciak BW, Delbeke D, et al; Society of Nuclear Medicine. SNM practice guideline for hepatobiliary scintigraphy 4.0. *J Nucl Med Technol.* 2010;38(4):210-218.

18 **Answer A.** The lesion depicted on the US images demonstrates an anechoic cystic lesion with a wall composed of two layers resembling a normal bowel wall. Classic duplication cysts have a characteristic appearance on the US: that of the double-layered wall, the so-called "gut signature," as in this case. The inner layer is hyperechoic mucosa, and the outer layer is hypoechoic muscle. Unfortunately, with inflammation, the layers may be obscured, lessening the specificity. Nonetheless, the demonstration of a cystic mass adjacent to the bowel should prompt the consideration of a duplication cyst. CT typically is not performed to evaluate a duplication cyst, but it may depict the location and extent of the cyst, as well as complications and other associated anomalies. At CT, a GI duplication cyst manifests as a fluid-filled cystic mass with a thick, slightly enhancing wall that either arises from or is extrinsic to the GI wall as in this case.

Intestinal duplications are rare congenital anomalies that can occur anywhere in the GI tract. Duplication cysts most commonly occur in the distal ileum followed by the esophagus, colon, jejunum, stomach, and duodenum. Typically, the duplication cyst is attached to the GI tract, has smooth muscle in its wall, and as stated earlier is lined with GI epithelium. Thus, these lesions are not adrenal or renal in origin. In addition, this lesion also appears separate from the kidney and right adrenal gland on the CT scan as there is no claw sign of renal or adrenal tissue. In addition, this lesion is not located in the suprarenal lesion as is typical of adrenal lesions. Because enteric duplication cysts can contain ectopic gastric mucosa, a Meckel (Tc-99m pertechnetate) scan can be helpful in making the diagnosis.

References: Di Serafino M, Mercogliano C, Vallone G. Ultrasound evaluation of the enteric duplication cyst: the gut signature. *J Ultrasound.* 2015;19(2):131-133.

Kumar R, Tripathi M, Chandrashekar N, et al. Diagnosis of ectopic gastric mucosa using 99Tcm-pertechnetate: spectrum of scintigraphic findings. *Br J Radiol.* 2005;78(932):714-720.

19 **Answer A.** Although the image presented below is a chest radiograph, there is a coarse calcification seen in the right upper quadrant (arrow). Although there are many common and incidental sources of calcifications in adult patients (e.g., arterial calcification, phleboliths, and cholelithiasis), the same cannot be said for pediatric patients. As such, the search for abnormal calcifications on radiographs is particularly important when assessing radiographs of infants and children, in whom etiological factors of calcifications range from benign renal calculi to tumoral calcifications. An UGI examination would not help to elucidate the etiology of the calcification. Although there is a gastrojejunostomy tube seen on the radiograph, the tip has been excluded from the film, and therefore, it cannot be determined whether the tube is in its appropriate position. The next most appropriate step to determine whether the tube is in the appropriate position would be to get an abdominal plain radiograph.

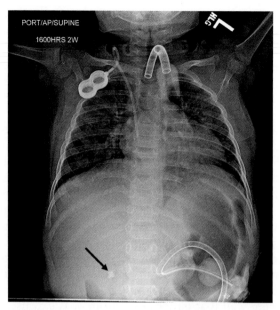

References: Menashe SJ, Iyer RS, Parisi MT, et al. Back to fundamentals: radiographic evaluation of thoracic lines and tubes in children. *AJR Am J Roentgenol.* 2019;212(5):988-996.

Nasser MP. Gastrointestinal. In: Donnelly LF, ed. *Fundamentals of Pediatric Imaging.* 3rd ed. Elsevier; 2022:95-138.

Otto RK, Weinberger E, Stanescu AL. Pediatric abdominal radiographs: common and less common errors. *AJR Am J Roentgenol.* 2017;209(2):417-429.

20 **Answer C.** Figure A is an axial image from a contrast-enhanced CT scan of the abdomen demonstrating a large heterogeneous solid mass in the liver with a large calcification (long arrow), which may represent the calcification seen on the plain film of the abdomen seen in Question 19. There are smaller satellite lesions in the periphery of the liver (short arrows). Figure B is an axial T1 fat-saturated image after contrast enhancement, which also demonstrates a heterogeneous solid enhancing mass with smaller satellite lesions in the periphery of the liver. Given the age group and constellation of imaging findings, the most likely diagnosis is hepatoblastoma, a malignant liver mass. Approximately 10% of cases of hepatoblastoma occur in children less than a year of age, with most cases occurring before age 5. Hepatocellular carcinoma, which is also a malignant solid tumor, mostly occurs in children older than 5 years. Mesenchymal hamartoma of the liver is a benign liver lesion, which often appears as a complex cystic mass and primarily affects children under 5 years of age. Focal nodular hyperplasia (FNH) is most often seen in adult women but uncommonly occurs in young children and adolescents. The presence of a central scar may aid identification of this lesion.

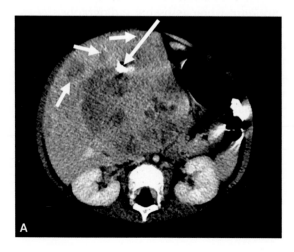

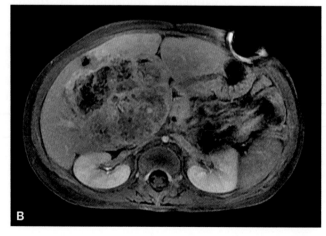

References: Dähnert W. *Radiology Review Manual*. 8th ed. Wolters Kluwer; 2017.

Nasser MP. Gastrointestinal. In: Donnelly LF, ed. *Fundamentals of Pediatric Imaging*. 3rd ed. Elsevier; 2022:95-138.

21 **Answer B.** Hepatoblastoma has been associated with several syndromes, including Beckwith-Wiedemann syndrome, Gardner syndrome, familial adenomatous polyposis, type 1A glycogen storage disease, and trisomy 18. Approximately 5% of cases occur in conjunction with other congenital anomalies, commonly of the genitourinary and GI systems. The most useful laboratory marker for hepatoblastoma is alpha-fetoprotein (AFP). At least 90% of patients with hepatoblastoma show abnormal elevation of AFP levels. The lungs are the most common site of metastasis.

References: Dähnert W. *Radiology Review Manual*. 8th ed. Wolters Kluwer; 2017.

Nasser MP. Gastrointestinal. In: Donnelly LF, ed. *Fundamentals of Pediatric Imaging*. 3rd ed. Elsevier; 2022:95-138.

22 **Answer D.** The images provided from an UGI series demonstrate obstruction of the proximal duodenum. In a patient involved in recent blunt trauma, a duodenal hematoma should be suspected. The next best step in management would be an additional cross-sectional imaging study to see if the cause of the duodenal obstruction is due to a duodenal hematoma or other lesion. Abdominal radiographs would not yield any further information about the cause of the obstruction. A contrast enema would not help to diagnose a duodenal hematoma as this study is used to evaluate the colon. A Meckel's scan is a nuclear medicine study that is commonly used to look for Meckel's diverticula, which are often lined by ectopic gastric mucosa. It would not help elucidate the cause of a duodenal obstruction.

Reference: Nasser MP. Gastrointestinal. In: Donnelly LF, ed. *Fundamentals of Pediatric Imaging*. 3rd ed. Elsevier; 2022:95-138.

23 **Answer D.** The axial images from a contrast-enhanced CT examination demonstrate an intramural lesion of mildly heterogeneous fluid attenuation, which is likely secondary to a hematoma within the second and third portions of the duodenum (arrows). The hematoma causes luminal narrowing. Intramural duodenal hematomas are often the result of blunt trauma that can be caused by accidental trauma as well as non-accidental trauma (NAT). Anticoagulation can also be a cause of spontaneous intramural duodenal hematomas. These lesions are also known to occur after endoscopy.

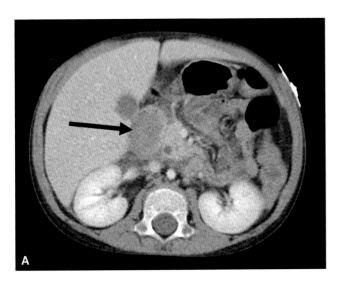 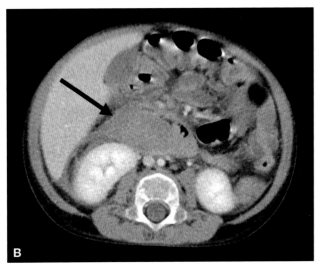

References: Dähnert W. *Radiology Review Manual*. 8th ed. Wolters Kluwer; 2017.

Nasser MP. Gastrointestinal. In: Donnelly LF, ed. *Fundamentals of Pediatric Imaging*. 3rd ed. Elsevier; 2022:95-138.

24 Answer D. The axial CT image demonstrates extensive low attenuation in the region of the pancreas so much so that it is difficult to see normal pancreatic parenchyma. These findings are compatible with fatty infiltration of the pancreas. In children, cystic fibrosis is the most common etiology of fatty replacement of the pancreas. None of the other answer choices are known causes of fatty replacement of the pancreas.

Reference: Dähnert W. *Radiology Review Manual*. 8th ed. Wolters Kluwer; 2017.

25 Answer A. Echogenic bowel detected on prenatal ultrasound exams is seen in up to 60% to 70% of patients affected with cystic fibrosis. The inheritance pattern is autosomal recessive. A sweat test is used to help make the diagnosis of cystic fibrosis, and affected patients have elevated concentrations of sodium and chloride in their sweat. There is progressive cystic and cylindrical bronchiectasis in these patients, which affects up to 100% of patients after 6 months of age. The mean age of diagnosis of cystic fibrosis is 2.9 years, and 90% of patients are diagnosed by 12 years of age.

Reference: Dähnert W. *Radiology Review Manual*. 8th ed. Wolters Kluwer; 2017.

26 Answer D. The image from the US examination demonstrates hydropic distention of the gallbladder, which along with the patient's symptoms suggests Kawasaki syndrome. The peak age of this entity is 2 to 3 years and 85% of patients are less than 5 years of age. This entity often leads to the development of coronary artery aneurysms. Myocarditis occurs in 25% of these patients and when severe can cause congestive heart failure. Atrioventricular conduction disturbances have been reported, which can cause abnormal electrocardiogram (ECG) tracings. Treatment with gamma globulins can decrease the severity of the illness and can decrease the likelihood of delayed complications such as coronary aneurysms.

Reference: Dähnert W. *Radiology Review Manual*. 8th ed. Wolters Kluwer; 2017.

27 Answer C. The radiographs demonstrate the "double-bubble" sign, which is seen in cases of duodenal obstruction caused by intrinsic as well as extrinsic causes. The intrinsic causes are duodenal atresia, duodenal stenosis, and duodenal webs; the extrinsic causes include annular pancreas, malrotation of the gut with obstruction produced by midgut volvulus or by Ladd bands, and preduodenal position of the portal vein. The two air-filled bubbles represent the stomach and proximal duodenum. The most common cause of this finding among the causes of duodenal obstruction is duodenal atresia, which is reproducible with a variety of other imaging modalities, including UGI studies and sonography. For the neonate with the classic appearance of a double bubble, additional radiologic investigation is unnecessary, and the surgeon is alerted to plan for surgery, because all congenital causes of duodenal obstruction require surgery.

Reference: Traubici J. The double bubble sign. *Radiology*. 2001;220(2):463-464.

28 Answer C. Duodenal atresia is associated with many congenital syndromes, the foremost being Down syndrome. Approximately 30% of children with duodenal atresia have trisomy 21. There is also an association with anomalies of the VACTERL (Vertebral, Anorectal, Cardiac, TracheoEsophageal, Renal, and Limb anomalies) spectrum. The atretic segment is most often just beyond or distal to the ampulla of Vater. Therefore, patients usually present with bilious vomiting. However, the atretic segment can sometimes be proximal to the ampulla of Vater, and therefore, some patients can present with nonbilious vomiting. As stated earlier, the "double-bubble" sign is seen in cases of duodenal obstruction, which can be caused by a variety of intrinsic and extrinsic causes, and therefore, this sign is not only seen in duodenal atresia.

Reference: Traubici J. The double bubble sign. *Radiology*. 2001;220(2):463-464.

29 Answer D. The fetal MR images demonstrate a midline anterior abdominal wall defect. There is herniation of the liver and bowel through the defect. The umbilical cord can be seen inserting in the defect (arrow). These are hallmarks of an omphalocele. Omphaloceles are also usually covered by a membrane. Associated abnormalities are common and can be seen in 67% to 88% of affected fetuses. The mortality rate is 80% when any associated defect is present and increases to near 100% when chromosomal or cardiovascular anomalies exist. However, if an omphalocele is found in isolation, then the mortality rate decreases to 10%.

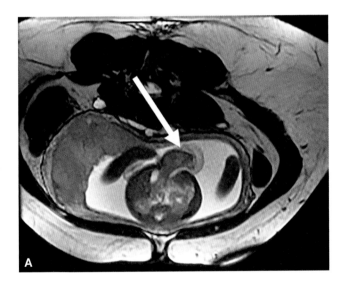
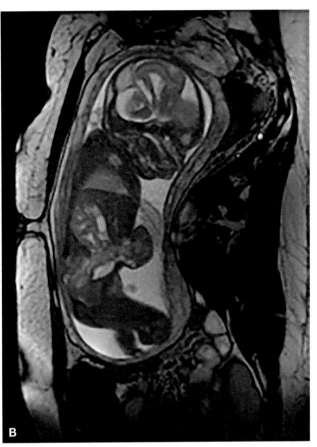

References: Daltro P, Fricke BL, Kline-Fath BM, et al. Prenatal MRI of congenital abdominal and chest wall defects. *AJR Am J Roentgenol*. 2005;184(3):1010-1016.

Revels JW, Wang SS, Nasrullah A, et al. An algorithmic approach to complex fetal abdominal wall defects. *AJR Am J Roentgenol*. 2020;214(1):218-231.

30 Answer D. Gastroschisis is the herniation of fetal bowel loops into the amniotic cavity usually through a right-sided paraumbilical abdominal wall defect. A midline defect is seen in cases of omphalocele. Herniated bowel loops in cases of gastroschisis do not have a surrounding membrane as is seen in cases of omphalocele. Associated anomalies are rare in gastroschisis. This contrasts with cases of omphalocele, which is commonly associated with other defects. The intrauterine mortality rate of gastroschisis is 10% to 15%, which is relatively low.

Comparing Gastroschisis and Omphalocele	
Gastroschisis	Omphalocele
Anterior wall defect that is lateral to midline	Midline anterior wall defect
Herniated contents (usually just bowel) are not covered by a peritoneal membrane, which allows exposure to amniotic fluid that is toxic to bowel.	Herniated contents (usually bowel and liver) are covered by a peritoneal membrane.
Associated anomalies are rare.	Up to 66% of patients have associated congenital defects (usually cardiac).

References: Daltro P, Fricke BL, Kline-Fath BM, et al. Prenatal MRI of congenital abdominal and chest wall defects. *AJR Am J Roentgenol.* 2005;184(3):1010-1016.

Revels JW, Wang SS, Nasrullah A, et al. An algorithmic approach to complex fetal abdominal wall defects. *AJR Am J Roentgenol.* 2020;214(1):218-231.

31 **Answer D.** The clinical history of a premature infant who is in the first week of life presenting with bloody stools is suggestive of necrotizing enterocolitis (NEC). The abdominal radiograph demonstrates an abnormal bowel gas pattern with fairly diffuse gaseous distention of the bowel and right lower quadrant pneumatosis intestinalis (arrow), which are findings consistent with the clinical history of NEC. On the radiographs, there is no evidence of free peritoneal air or bowel perforation which would require an emergent surgical consult. Bowel perforation is the main indication for surgical intervention in patients with NEC. A stat UGI series would not be indicated in this situation as neither the history nor the imaging findings are consistent with an upper gastrointestinal tract obstruction. A contrast enema may eventually be performed later in this patient to evaluate for colonic strictures, which can develop from NEC. However, it is not indicated at this time. The next best appropriate step in management is for the patient to be made NPO and for antibiotics to be initiated along with serial abdominal radiographs to monitor disease progression.

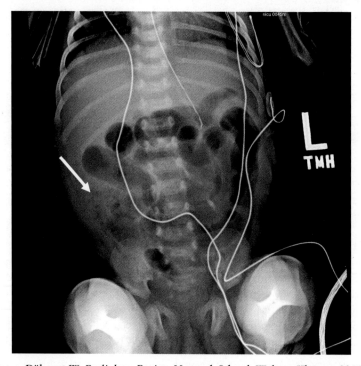

References: Dähnert W. *Radiology Review Manual.* 8th ed. Wolters Kluwer; 2017.

Nasser MP. Gastrointestinal. In: Donnelly LF, ed. *Fundamentals of Pediatric Imaging.* 3rd ed. Elsevier; 2022:95-138.

32 **Answer A.** Approximately 10% of neonates with NEC are born at term, and congenital heart disease is the main risk factor in this group. However, NEC predominantly affects premature neonates less than 32 weeks of age and very low birthweight infants weighing less than 1,500 grams. NEC is treated surgically as well as medically. Bowel perforation and free air is the main indication for surgical instead of medical therapy. Pneumatosis is not an indication for surgical treatment. In the clinical setting of NEC, the presence of intramural gas confirms the diagnosis of NEC. Portal venous gas has also been reported on plain abdominal radiographs in patients with NEC. As stated earlier, colonic strictures can develop from NEC, and contrast enemas are often performed to evaluate the bowel of patients with a history of NEC.

References: Dähnert W. *Radiology Review Manual.* 8th ed. Wolters Kluwer; 2017.

Nasser MP. Gastrointestinal. In: Donnelly LF, ed. *Fundamentals of Pediatric Imaging.* 3rd ed. Elsevier; 2022:95-138.

33 **Answer C.** The images shown are from a Meckel (Tc-99m pertechnetate) scan. The study demonstrates a tiny focus of increased radiotracer uptake in the right lower quadrant with activity in the stomach appearing at the same time, which is best seen in Figure B in the question stem which is also shown below. After intravenous (IV) injection of Tc-99m pertechnetate, a Meckel diverticulum containing gastric mucosa will manifest as a small, rounded area of increased activity in the right lower quadrant. A Meckel diverticulum is a true diverticulum, composed of all layers of the intestinal wall, and is lined by normal small intestinal mucosa. It frequently contains heterotopic gastric and pancreatic mucosa and, less commonly, duodenal, colonic, or biliary mucosa. They commonly occur in the distal ileum. Clinical symptoms arise from complications of the diverticulum such as peptic ulceration with hemorrhage; diverticulitis; intestinal obstruction from diverticular inversion, intussusception, volvulus, torsion, or inclusion of the diverticulum in a hernia; formation of enteroliths; and development of neoplasia within the diverticulum.

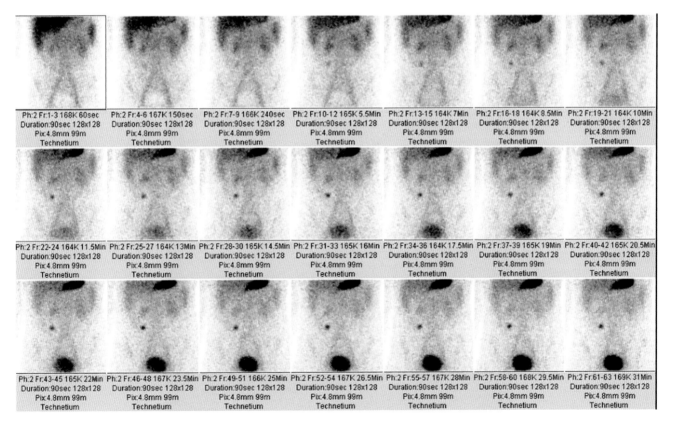

References: Elsayes KM, Menias CO, Harvin HJ, et al. Imaging manifestations of Meckel's diverticulum. *AJR Am J Roentgenol.* 2007;189(1):81-88.

Kotha VK, Khandelwal A, Saboo SS, et al. Radiologist's perspective for the Meckel's diverticulum and its complications. *Br J Radiol.* 2014;87(1037):20130743.

34 **Answer A.** Histamine H_2 blockers (cimetidine, ranitidine, famotidine) inhibit acid secretion by the parietal cells, thus limiting release of Tc-99m pertechnetate by the mucosal cells and improving the sensitivity of the Meckel scan. Phenobarbital stimulates biliary secretion by inducing hepatic enzymes, which increases conjugation and excretion of bilirubin. It is given prior to HIDA scans to evaluate for biliary atresia to increase the specificity of the test. Morphine is given during HIDA scans to shorten the study time if there is nonvisualization of the gallbladder and is typically injected 45 to 60 minutes after injection of radiotracer if activity is seen in the bowel. It causes contraction of the sphincter of Oddi, which raises intrabiliary pressure and can cause retrograde filling of the gallbladder. CCK is a synthetic hormone that causes gallbladder contraction and can be used to pretreat patients who have been fasting for a prolonged period prior to HIDA scans.

References: Dähnert W. *Radiology Review Manual*. 8th ed. Wolters Kluwer; 2017.

Kotha VK, Khandelwal A, Saboo SS, et al. Radiologist's perspective for the Meckel's diverticulum and its complications. *Br J Radiol*. 2014;87(1037):20130743.

35 **Answer B.** Note that on a single anteroposterior (AP) radiograph, it is difficult to say with certainty whether lines and tubes are within certain anatomical structures, and therefore, it is preferable to say that lines and tubes project over or within anatomical structures. The tip of the umbilical vein (UV) line projects in the right upper quadrant presumably within the portal venous system (long arrow) and is clearly in an inferior position to the inferior cavoatrial junction, which is its proper position. The tip of the umbilical artery (UA) line projects over the T8/T9 intervertebral disc space (short arrow), which is an acceptable position. The UA line should be placed in the abdominal aorta either in a high position at the T6 to T10 level or in a low position at the L3 to L5 level. If placed in either of these positions, it should avoid the mesenteric branches of the abdominal aorta where it could potentially cause end-organ damage secondary to dissections or thrombus formation. The distal tip and side ports of the nasogastric tube project over the stomach, which is in the correct position. The side port and tip of the bladder catheter are in normal position and project over the urinary bladder.

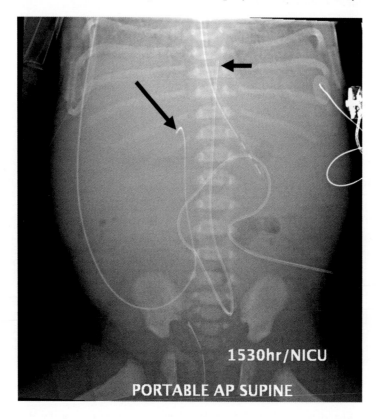

1530hr/NICU

PORTABLE AP SUPINE

References: Epelman M. Chest. In: Donnelly LF, ed. *Fundamentals of Pediatric Imaging.* 3rd ed. Elsevier; 2022:27-70.

Kim HH, Tulin-Silver S, Yu RN, et al. Common genitourinary catheters: a systematic approach for the radiologist. *Pediatr Radiol.* 2018;48(8):1155-1166.

Liszewski MC, Daltro P, Lee EY. Back to fundamentals: radiographic evaluation of thoracic lines and tubes in children. *AJR Am J Roentgenol.* 2019;212(5):988-996.

36 **Answer B.** As stated earlier, the correct placement for an umbilical venous catheter is over the inferior cavoatrial junction. The correct placement for the other major lines and tubes often used in neonates can be found in the explanation for Question 35.

References: Epelman M. Chest. In: Donnelly LF, ed. *Fundamentals of Pediatric Imaging.* 3rd ed. Elsevier; 2022:27-70.

Liszewski MC, Daltro P, Lee EY. Back to fundamentals: radiographic evaluation of thoracic lines and tubes in children. *AJR Am J Roentgenol.* 2019;212(5):988-996.

37 **Answer C.** The clinical picture is concerning for appendicitis. Of the exams listed, an US of the right lower quadrant would be the next most appropriate test to evaluate for appendicitis in this clinical setting. US is the initial imaging modality of choice for diagnosing acute appendicitis in children primarily because of its lack of ionizing radiation.

Reference: Larson DB, Trout AT, Fierke SR, et al. Improvement in diagnostic accuracy of ultrasound of the pediatric appendix through the use of equivocal interpretive categories. *Am J Roentgenol.* 2015;204(4):849-856.

38 **Answer B.** The US exam fails to visualize the appendix. In addition, there are no secondary signs of appendicitis such as echogenic fat, abscesses, or abnormal-appearing loops of bowel. However, appendicitis is still clinically suspected. Of the exams listed, an MR examination of the abdomen and pelvis is the most appropriate next test in this clinical scenario. MRI has a sensitivity of 100% and specificity of 96% for appendicitis in pediatric patients after inconclusive appendix sonography. These results are similar to published sensitivity and specificity rates of CT for appendicitis, which historically has been the preferred way to evaluate for appendicitis after an inconclusive US. However, unlike MR, CT utilizes ionizing radiation. CT is still often the preferred way to evaluate for appendicitis in younger patients or those patients who need sedation to complete an MR examination, which is significantly longer than a CT examination and requires greater patient cooperation.

References: Dillman JR, Gadepalli S, Sroufe NS, et al. Equivocal pediatric appendicitis: unenhanced MR imaging protocol for nonsedated children—a clinical effectiveness study. *Radiology.* 2016;279(1):216-225.

Herliczek TW, Swenson DW, Mayo-Smith WW. Utility of MRI after inconclusive ultrasound in pediatric patients with suspected appendicitis: retrospective review of 60 consecutive patients. *Am J Roentgenol.* 2013;200(5):969-973.

39 **Answer C.** The images shown are two axial ultrafast spin echo fat-saturated sequences from an MR of the abdomen and pelvis. They demonstrate a fluid-filled, tubular structure (arrows) with surrounding edema and inflammatory changes of the adjacent fat planes. These findings are consistent with acute appendicitis.

The reported sensitivities of MR and CT for the detection of appendicitis in children have been found to be similar in multiple publications and MR is preferred to CT in patients who do not require sedation due to its lack of ionizing radiation. CT is more sensitive than US for the detection of appendicitis in children. However, US is often utilized prior to CT or MR because it is cheaper and does not utilize ionizing radiation as in the case of CT.

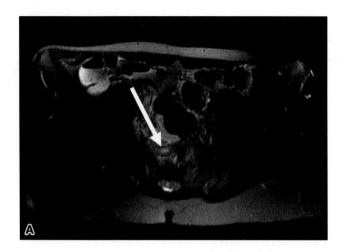
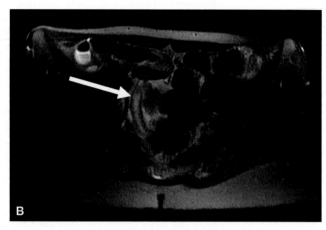

References: Dillman JR, Gadepalli S, Sroufe NS, et al. Equivocal pediatric appendicitis: unenhanced MR imaging protocol for nonsedated children—a clinical effectiveness study. *Radiology*. 2016;279(1):216-225.

Herliczek TW, Swenson DW, Mayo-Smith WW. Utility of MRI after inconclusive ultrasound in pediatric patients with suspected appendicitis: retrospective review of 60 consecutive patients. *Am J Roentgenol*. 2013;200(5):969-973.

Strouse PJ. Pediatric appendicitis: an argument for US. *Radiology*. 2010;255(1):8-13.

40 **Answer B.** Figure A in the question stem shows sequential images from a liquid gastric emptying exam, which demonstrates reflux of radiotracer from the stomach to the esophagus on several images (arrows). Therefore, the study is not normal. In these studies, Tc-99m sulfur colloid is mixed with milk or formula. Duodenal atresia is best diagnosed on a plain film with the "double-bubble" sign. Malrotation and midgut volvulus are best diagnosed on an UGI series.

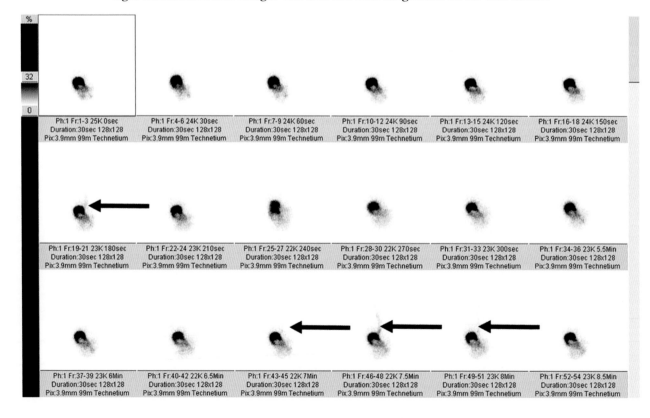

References: Applegate KE, Anderson JM, Klatte EC. Intestinal malrotation in children: a problem-solving approach to the upper gastrointestinal series. *Radiographics*. 2006;26(5):1485-1500.

Reyhan M, Yapar AF, Aydin M, et al. Gastroesophageal scintigraphy in children: a comparison of posterior and anterior imaging. *Ann Nucl Med*. 2005;19(1):17-21.

Traubici J. The double bubble sign. *Radiology*. 2001;220(2):463-464.

41 **Answer B.** Figure B in the question stem reports the percent of gastric emptying after 62 minutes is 1%. Although the published normative values for gastric emptying of liquids vary by age, 1% is delayed based on published studies. In small children <2 years of age, the published normal gastric emptying rate is 32% or greater. In children older than 2 years, the normal reported range is 44% or higher. Memorizing these numbers is not as important as realizing that 1% would be markedly low by these standards. Based on these standards, the gastric emptying rate is not normal, and the patient has markedly delayed gastric emptying, not rapid gastric emptying. Delayed gastric emptying is not a cause of bilious vomiting. Note that nonbilious vomiting as opposed to bilious vomiting is associated with gastroesophageal reflux.

Reference: Heyman S. Gastric emptying in children. *J Nucl Med*. 1998;39(5):865-869.

42 **Answer C.** The plain abdominal radiograph demonstrates thickening of the haustral folds consistent with colonic "thumbprinting" (arrows). This sign is usually indicative of submucosal edema. Classically described with ischemic colitis, it is also noted in other forms of colitis, including ulcerative and infectious colitis. Thus, the radiograph is abnormal. Abdominal pain and diarrhea are often signs of a colitis. Both an UGI series and pelvic US would not be helpful in evaluating the colon.

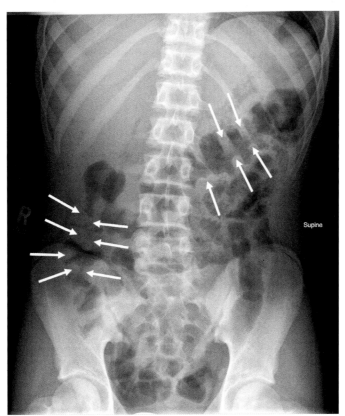

Reference: Cutinha AH, De Nazareth AG, Alla VM, et al. Clues to colitis: tracking the prints. *West J Emerg Med*. 2011;11(1):112-113.

43 **Answer D.** There is a nonobstructive bowel gas pattern seen on the abdominal radiographs. However, there is extensive air-space opacity at the right lung base on the left lateral decubitus view, which likely represents pneumonia. Therefore, this patient should be treated for pneumonia. Abdominal pain can be a presentation of pneumonia in children and that is why it is important to always look at the lung bases on pediatric abdominal radiographs. An emergent upper GI series, abdominal ultrasound and stat surgical consult would not be necessary for this patient.

Reference: Kanegaye JT, Harley JR. Pneumonia in unexpected locations: an occult cause of pediatric abdominal pain. *J Emerg Med.* 1995;13(6):773-779.

44 **Answer A.** Figure A is a coronal T1 fat-saturated contrast-enhanced MRI image, which demonstrates contrast enhancement of the terminal ileum (arrow). Figure B is an axial diffusion-weighted imaging (DWI) image that shows restricted diffusion of the terminal ileum (arrow). Although high signal on a DWI image should correspond with low signal on an apparent diffusion coefficient (ADC) map if there is true restricted diffusion, the combination of the contrast enhancement and high signal on the DWI sequence in the terminal ileum is suggestive of a terminal ileitis. Note that the remainder of the bowel including the colon appears normal on both images. Therefore, typhlitis or neutropenic colitis, which usually affects the right colon, is unlikely as is pseudomembranous colitis, which usually manifests as a pancolitis. Although there can be a "backwash ileitis" in ulcerative colitis, this usually occurs when the entire colon is affected.

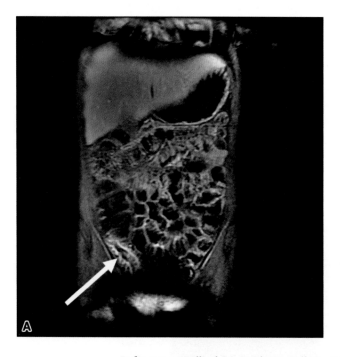
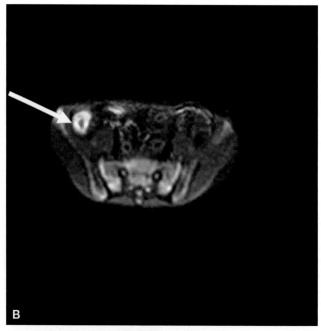

References: Mollard BJ, Smith EA, Dillman JR. Pediatric MR enterography: technique and approach to interpretation-how we do it. *Radiology.* 2015;274(1):29-43.

Nasser MP. Gastrointestinal. In: Donnelly LF, ed. *Fundamentals of Pediatric Imaging.* 3rd ed. Elsevier; 2022:95-138.

Roggeveen MJ, Tismenetsky M, Shapiro R. Best cases from the AFIP: ulcerative colitis. *Radiographics.* 2006;26(3):947-951.

Towbin AJ, Sullivan J, Denson LA, et al. CT and MR enterography in children and adolescents with inflammatory bowel disease. *Radiographics.* 2013;33(7):1843-1860.

45 **Answer D.** Figure A and B are axial images from a contrast-enhanced CT scan of the abdomen and pelvis in the early arterial (Figure A) and delayed excretory (Figure B) phases of contrast enhancement. Figure A demonstrates a heterogeneous mass with central low attenuation and early peripheral puddling of contrast (arrow). Figure B demonstrates later peripheral pooling of contrast (arrow). These findings are most consistent with an infantile hemangioendothelioma. FNH is a solid lesion that often has a central scar, which fills in on delayed imaging. Although hepatocellular carcinoma can have a varied appearance, this is not the right age group for this diagnosis. Finally, the heterogeneity of the lesion and the presence of contrast enhancement argue against focal fatty infiltration.

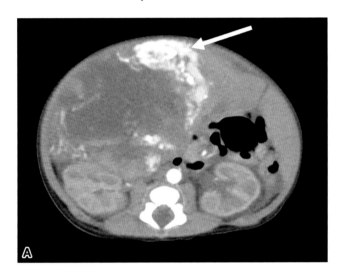
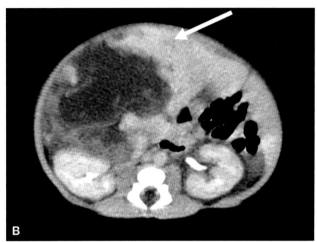

References: Chung EM, Cube R, Hall GJ, et al. From the archives of the AFIP: pediatric liver masses: radiologic-pathologic correlation part 1. Benign tumors. *Radiographics.* 2010;30(3):801-826.

Chung EM, Lattin GE Jr, Cube R, et al. From the archives of the AFIP: Pediatric liver masses: radiologic-pathologic correlation part 2. Malignant tumors. *Radiographics.* 2011;31(2):483-507.

Roos JE, Pfiffner R, Stallmach T, et al. Infantile hemangioendothelioma. *Radiographics.* 2003;23(6):1649-1655.

46 **Answer D.** Both the liver and spleen appear enlarged on this study, and thus, there is no evidence of splenic autoinfarction. Infantile hemangioendotheliomas are often large tumors and affected patients often have enlarged livers, abdominal distention, or a palpable upper abdominal mass. Note that the bowel loops are inferiorly displaced on this study because of mass effect from the liver and spleen. There may be extensive arteriovenous shunting within infantile hemangioendotheliomas, resulting in decreased peripheral vascular resistance. Thus, increased blood volume and cardiac output are required to maintain vascular bed perfusion, which may lead to high cardiac output and congestive heart failure in up to 50% to 60% of patients. This explains why the cardiothymic silhouette appears enlarged on this study. The endotracheal tube is properly positioned with its tip seen projecting over the mid-trachea. Although the bowel loops appear inferiorly displaced, they do not appear obstructed. Note that the bladder is distended on this study, which likely accounts for the lack of rectal bowel gas.

References: Liszewski MC, Daltro P, Lee EY. Back to fundamentals: radiographic evaluation of thoracic lines and tubes in children. *AJR Am J Roentgenol.* 2019;212(5):988-996.

Roos JE, Pfiffner R, Stallmach T, et al. Infantile hemangioendothelioma. *Radiographics.* 2003;23(6):1649-1655.

47   **Answer C.** Imaging is a vital step in the assessment of children with a primary hepatic tumor. Since it was first described in 1992, the PRETEXT (PRE-Treatment EXTent of tumor) system has become the primary method of risk stratification for hepatoblastoma and pediatric hepatocellular carcinoma in numerous cooperative group trials across the world. The PRETEXT system is comprised of two components, which are the PRETEXT group and the annotation factors. The PRETEXT group describes the extent of tumor in the liver while the annotation factors help to describe associated features such as vascular involvement (either portal vein or hepatic vein/inferior vena cava), extrahepatic disease, multifocality, tumor rupture, and metastatic disease (to both the lungs and lymph nodes).

Reference: Towbin AJ, Meyers RL, Woodley H, et al. 2017 PRETEXT: radiologic staging system for primary hepatic malignancies of childhood revised for the Paediatric Hepatic International Tumour Trial (PHITT). *Pediatr Radiol.* 2018;48:536-554.

48   **Answer B.** The clinical history of a 2-year-old with intermittent abdominal pain and bloody stools is concerning for an ileocolic intussusception. Abdominal radiographs are usually not sensitive in identifying ileocolic intussusceptions. However, they can be abnormal in positive cases. Abnormal findings include a paucity of bowel gas in the right hemiabdomen, the absence of an air-filled cecum, a meniscus of a soft tissue mass within the ascending or transverse colon, and small bowel obstruction. On this radiograph, almost all the findings described except for a small bowel obstruction are seen including a meniscus (long black arrow) of a soft tissue mass (short black arrows). Note that even with the presence of the abnormal findings, an abdominal US is the preferred exam to diagnose or exclude an ileocolic intussusception. The main use for abdominal radiographs is to exclude free air prior to an air enema reduction.

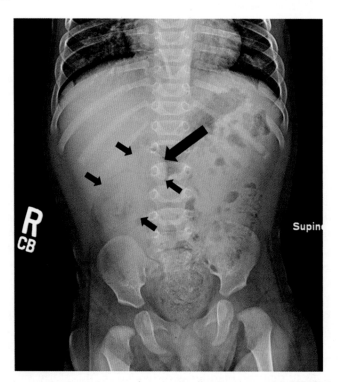

Reference: Nasser MP. Gastrointestinal. In: Donnelly LF, ed. *Fundamentals of Pediatric Imaging.* 3rd ed. Elsevier; 2022:95-138.

49 **Answer D.** The transverse US image demonstrates a mass with alternating rings of hypoechogenicity and hyperechogenicity. This is consistent with the target or donut sign. Both the imaging findings and clinical history are consistent with idiopathic ileocolic intussusception, the most common form of intussusception in children. Most patients with this entity present between the ages of 3 months and 3 years. Presenting symptoms typically include crampy abdominal pain, bloody (currant jelly) stools, emesis, and a palpable right-sided abdominal mass. US is the primary imaging modality for the evaluation of children with suspected intussusception. The benefits include a lack of radiation and high sensitivity and specificity.

Ileocolic intussusceptions will usually measure >2.5 cm in the transverse dimension as in this case. This fact can help differentiate ileocolic intussusceptions from small bowel-small bowel intussusceptions, which usually measure <2.0 cm in transverse dimension.

Small bowel-small bowel intussusceptions are predominantly transient and will usually spontaneously reduce. They are often encountered as incidental findings on abdominal US or CT examinations. Ileocolic intussusceptions do not typically self-reduce. If left untreated, they result in an obstruction that can lead to ischemia, necrosis, or bowel perforation.

There are several methods for increasing the pressure within the colon to reduce an ileocolic intussusception while using image guidance. They include air insufflation with fluoroscopic guidance (air contrast enema), contrast enema with fluoroscopic guidance, and hydrostatic reduction with US guidance. One recent analysis showed that the combined probability of successful reduction with a fluoroscopic-guided air contrast method was 81% with a perforation rate of 1%.

References: Nasser MP. Gastrointestinal. In: Donnelly LF, ed. *Fundamentals of Pediatric Imaging*. 3rd ed. Elsevier; 2022:95-138.

Plut D, Phillips GS, Johnston PR, Lee EY. Practical imaging strategies for intussusception in children. *AJR Am J Roentgenol*. 2020;215(6):1449-1463.

50 **Answer A.** A pathologic lead point should be suspected in children less than 3 months and greater than 3 years of age presenting with an ileocolic intussusception. Pathological lead points include an inflamed appendix, Meckel diverticulum, duplication cyst, intraluminal polyps, Henoch-Schönlein purpura (HSP), or lymphoma. Cases of intussusception are more common during the months when viral illnesses in children peak in the winter and spring. The mechanism causing idiopathic ileocolic intussusceptions is thought to be due to lymphoid hypertrophy in the terminal ileum secondary to a viral illness. The terminal ileum then acts as the intussusceptum, telescoping into the proximal colon (intussuscipiens).

References: Nasser MP. Gastrointestinal. In: Donnelly LF, ed. *Fundamentals of Pediatric Imaging*. 3rd ed. Elsevier; 2022:95-138.

Plut D, Phillips GS, Johnston PR, Lee EY. Practical imaging strategies for intussusception in children. *AJR Am J Roentgenol*. 2020;215(6):1449-1463.

51 **Answer C.** After the diagnosis of ileocolic intussusception is confirmed, the child should have a surgical consultation to decide on the method of treatment. Treatment of most intussusceptions is noninvasive radiologic reduction. Noninvasive radiologic reduction techniques include air insufflation with fluoroscopic guidance (air contrast enema), contrast enema with fluoroscopic guidance, and hydrostatic reduction with US guidance. If noninvasive reduction is not successful, surgery is required. Children with evidence of peritonitis, shock, or perforation are not candidates for noninvasive reduction and require immediate surgical treatment.

There are findings on US that signify that an intussusception may be difficult to reduce. Diminished or no color Doppler flow within the intussusception indicates the presence of ischemia or necrosis, which can complicate the reduction. Free intraperitoneal fluid, fluid trapped within the layers of the intussusception (interloop fluid), and the presence of a small bowel obstruction also suggest the possibility of a difficult reduction or higher chance of perforation. Contraindications for performing the procedure include peritonitis on physical exam or free intraperitoneal air on abdominal radiographs. Duration of symptoms >24 hours and lethargy are not contraindications but are associated with decreased success of the procedure.

Prior to performing the reduction, the patient should have a working IV inserted, adequately hydrated and given additional IV fluids if needed, an abdominal examination by an experienced physician, and a pediatric surgery consultation. The members of the surgical service must know that a reduction will be attempted and should have examined the patient prior to the procedure. Members of the surgical or emergency medicine team should be present for reductions performed in lethargic patients.

During air contrast enemas, the pressure generated within the colon should not exceed 120 mm Hg when the patient is at rest. Pressures will often exceed this number when the patient cries or performs the valsalva maneuver. One recent analysis showed that the combined probability of successful reduction with a fluoroscopic-guided air contrast method was 81% with a perforation rate of 1%.

A perforation during an air reduction can lead to tension pneumoperitoneum, which must be reduced immediately as it may lead to circulatory collapse. An 18-guage needle should be kept at the bedside during these procedures. When there are signs of tension pneumoperitoneum, the needle should be inserted in the midline inferior to the umbilicus, which should rapidly release the tension pneumoperitoneum. Surgery should immediately be notified.

In cases when the initial reduction procedure is not successful in reducing the intussusception, a delayed repeated attempt should be considered when partial reduction has been achieved with the first attempt and the patient is clinically stable. Sometimes additional consecutive repeated attempts are needed to fully reduce the intussusception. Such repeated attempts can be successful in reducing the intussusception in up to 50% of cases.

The risk for recurrent intussusception after a successful reduction is less than 10%, with most occurring within the first 24 hours after reduction. Recurrent intussusceptions can be treated with repeated air enemas if the patient is stable.

References: Gartner RD, Levin TL, Borenstein SH, et al. Interloop fluid in intussusception: what is its significance? *Pediatr Radiol.* 2011;41(6):727-731.

Nasser MP. Gastrointestinal. In: Donnelly LF, ed. *Fundamentals of Pediatric Imaging.* 3rd ed. Elsevier; 2022:95-138.

Plut D, Phillips GS, Johnston PR, Lee EY. Practical imaging strategies for intussusception in children. *AJR Am J Roentgenol.* 2020;215(6):1449-1463.

52 **Answer D.** The mnemonic *"AAIIMM"* is helpful to remember the common causes of small bowel obstruction in young children. Each letter in AAIIMM represents the first letter of an etiology of small bowel obstruction in young children. These include **A**ppendicitis, **A**dhesions, **I**nguinal hernia, **I**ntussusception, **M**eckel diverticulum, and **M**alrotation with midgut volvulus.

Reference: Nasser MP. Gastrointestinal. In: Donnelly LF, ed. *Fundamentals of Pediatric Imaging.* 3rd ed. Elsevier; 2022:95-138.

53 **Answer D.** The image demonstrates the tip of a nasogastric tube to project in the proximal esophagus (arrow) despite multiple attempts to pass the tube. These findings are suspicious for esophageal atresia (EA). EA can occur with or without an associated tracheoesophageal fistula (TEF). Radiographs of the chest and abdomen are often the first exam ordered in a neonate with suspected EA. If there is absence of bowel gas in the abdomen, then no TEF is suspected. If there is bowel gas present as in this case, then a TEF is suspected. There are five types of TEF but greater than 80% involve a fistula between the trachea and distal esophageal segment. Less common variations include a fistula between the trachea and the proximal or both the proximal and distal esophageal segments. A TEF can also occur in the absence of EA, which is known as an H-type fistula. Fluoroscopic imaging is rarely performed as surgical repair occurs within 1-2 days after birth. EA is often associated with other congenital anomalies.

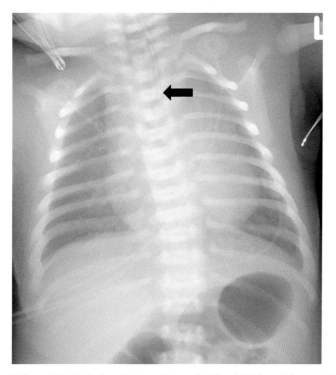

References: Dähnert W. *Radiology Review Manual*. 8th ed. Wolters Kluwer; 2017.

Kamble RS, Gupta R, Gupta A, et al. Passage of nasogastric tube through tracheo-esophageal fistula into stomach: a rare event. *World J Clin Cases*. 2014;2(7):309-310.

Nasser MP. Gastrointestinal. In: Donnelly LF, ed. *Fundamentals of Pediatric Imaging*. 3rd ed. Elsevier; 2022:95-138.

54 **Answer C.** EA is usually associated with other congenital anomalies that can be remembered by the "*VACTERL*" mnemonic. Chest and abdominal radiographs should be scrutinized for vertebral and cardiac anomalies. An echocardiogram should be ordered to evaluate for cardiac anomalies. In addition, surgery for EA is performed by a thoracotomy, which is carried out on the side of the patient contralateral to the aortic arch. Therefore, it is important to document the side of the aortic arch by an echocardiogram. A renal US should also be performed to evaluate for the presence of renal anomalies.

References: Nasser MP. Gastrointestinal. In: Donnelly LF, ed. *Fundamentals of Pediatric Imaging*. 3rd ed. Elsevier; 2022:95-138.

Scott DA. Esophageal atresia/tracheoesophageal fistula overview. In: Adam MP, Everman DB, Mirzaa GM, et al, eds. *GeneReviews® [Internet]*. University of Washington; 2009:1993-2023. Updated September 20, 2018.

55 **Answer D.** The images demonstrate a circular radiopaque foreign body in both images. On the lateral view of the neck, it is located posterior to the trachea and is likely in the upper thoracic esophagus. On the frontal view which is magnified below, there is a peripheral "double rim" or "halo sign," which is commonly seen in button batteries and which help to distinguish them from coins which are the most commonly ingested foreign bodies in children. In recent years, particular dangers, specifically from ingested button batteries, have become increasingly recognized as a public health issue. Esophageal full-thickness burns and perforation may occur within as little as 2 hours following the ingestion of button batteries. Other complications include the development of TEFs or fatal esophagoaortic fistulas within hours of ingestion. Therefore, batteries lodged in the esophagus must be removed as soon as possible, ideally within 2 hours.

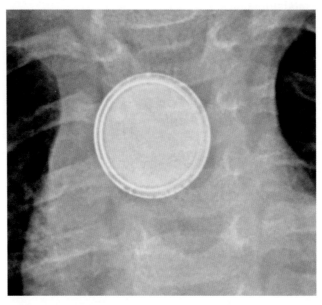

Reference: Semple T, Calder AD, Ramaswamy M, et al. Button battery ingestion in children-a potentially catastrophic event of which all radiologists must be aware. *Br J Radiol.* 2018;91(1081):20160781.

QUESTIONS

1 A 1-month-old male neonate with an abdominal mass presents for an abdominal ultrasound. Images from the examination are shown below. What is the next appropriate step in management?

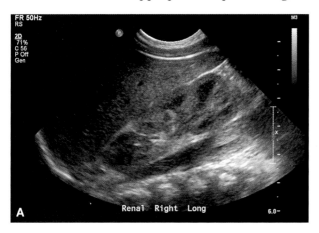 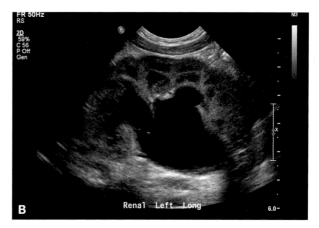

A. Plain radiographs of the abdomen
B. Voiding cystourethrogram (VCUG)
C. CT scan of the abdomen and pelvis
D. Testicular ultrasound

2 A representative image obtained from a VCUG examination subsequently performed on the same patient in Question 1 is shown below. What would be the next appropriate step in management?

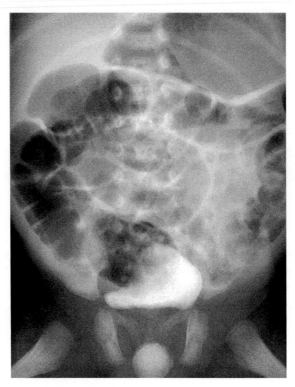

A. Tc-99m MAG3 scan
B. Tc-99m DMSA scan
C. CT scan of the abdomen and pelvis
D. Right upper quadrant ultrasound

3 A Tc-99m MAG3 scan was subsequently performed on the same patient in Questions 1 and 2. The pre-Lasix renogram for the right kidney was normal. The pre-Lasix renogram for the left kidney was abnormal. The post-Lasix renogram for the left kidney is shown below. Which of the following is *true*?

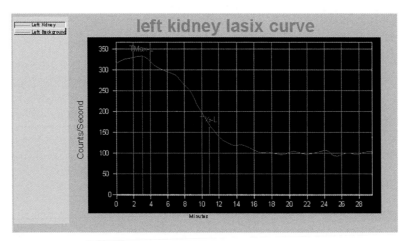

A. There is a definite obstruction.
B. The patient will require surgical intervention.
C. The patient will likely not require surgical intervention.
D. The time from max to half-max is 15 minutes.

4 Images from a renal ultrasound are demonstrated below with the patient imaged in the left lateral decubitus position. Regarding the entity demonstrated in the images of the right kidney, which of the following is *true*?

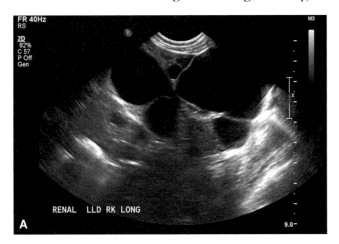 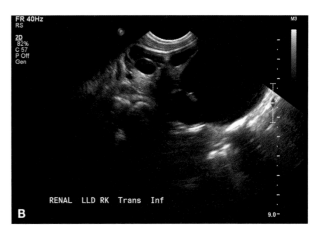

A. These lesions almost always develop into a Wilms tumor.
B. There is an association with contralateral UPJ obstructions.
C. The kidney often maintains this appearance for the rest of the patient's life.
D. There would be extensive radiotracer uptake by the right kidney on a MAG3 scan.

5 Coronal images from a contrast-enhanced CT scan of the abdomen and pelvis are demonstrated below in a 16-year-old patient who has new-onset hypertension. Concerning the entity demonstrated, which of the following is *true*?

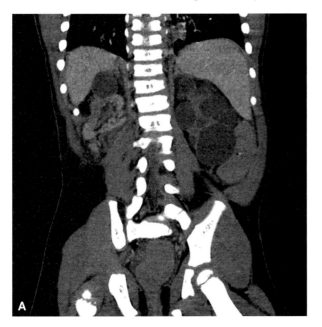 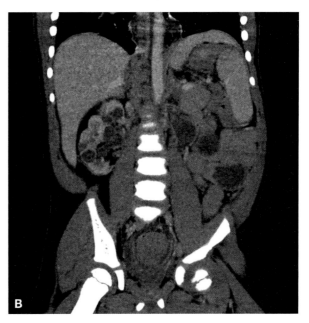

A. The inheritance pattern is likely autosomal recessive.
B. There is often an onset in early childhood.
C. There is an association with berry aneurysms.
D. There is an association with hepatic fibrosis.

6 A 3-year-old presents with left upper quadrant pain and vomiting. A supine abdominal radiograph was subsequently obtained and is shown below. What is the next most appropriate step in management?

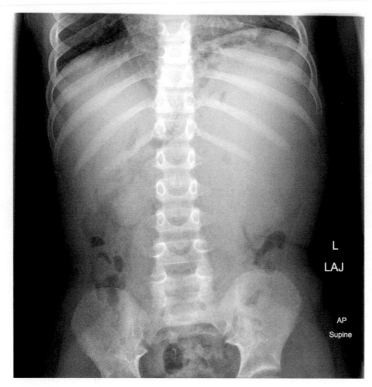

A. Tc-99m MAG3 scan
B. I-123 MIBG scan
C. Abdominal ultrasound
D. Tc-99m DMSA scan

7 An abdominal ultrasound of the patient in Question 6 was subsequently performed. Representative images are shown below. What is the next most appropriate step in management?

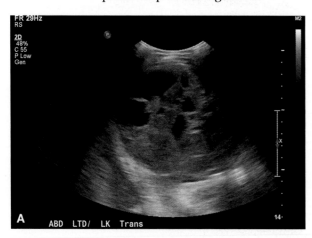
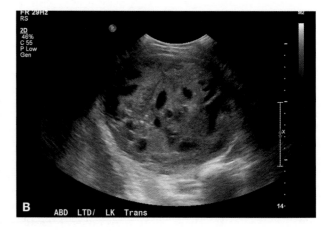

A. I-123 MIBG scan
B. Tc-99m MAG3 scan
C. VCUG
D. MRI of the abdomen

8 An MRI of the abdomen was subsequently performed on the same patient in Questions 6 and 7. Representative images are shown below. What is the most likely diagnosis?

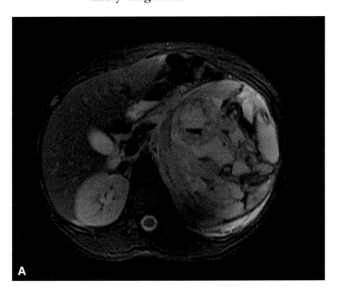
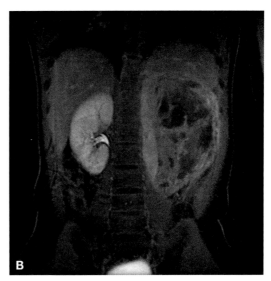

    A. Neuroblastoma
    B. Mesoblastic nephroma
    C. Wilms tumor
    D. Renal cell carcinoma

9 Which of the following additional tests would be indicated on the patient depicted in Questions 6, 7, and 8?

    A. CT scan of the chest
    B. Bone scan
    C. I-123 MIBG scan
    D. Testicular sonogram

10 Regarding Wilms tumor, which of the following is *true*?

    A. There is only one histology.
    B. Overall survival rates are around 90%.
    C. There are no known associated abnormalities.
    D. Nephroblastomatosis is a known sequela of this entity.

11 Which of the following renal tumors is associated with sickle cell trait?

    A. Renal cell carcinoma
    B. Multilocular cystic renal tumor
    C. Mesoblastic nephroma
    D. Medullary carcinoma

12 A 10-year-old male presents with right testicular pain. A testicular ultrasound was performed, and representative images are shown below. Regarding the images, which of the following is *true*?

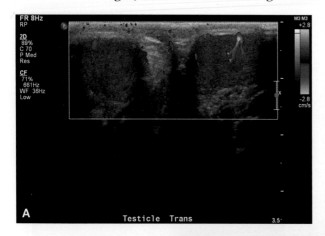

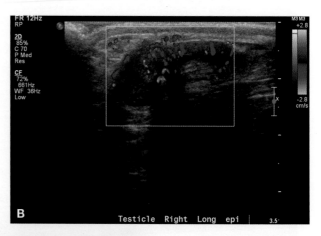

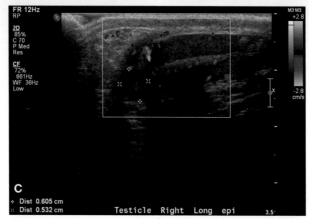

A. These findings constitute a urologic emergency and require emergent surgical exploration.

B. These findings demonstrate a testicular mass, and the patient should be referred to oncology.

C. These findings are likely secondary to infection, and the patient will need to be started on antibiotics.

D. Only supportive care is indicated.

13 A teenage female presents to the emergency department with intermittent pelvic pain. Representative images of the pelvic ultrasound that was performed are shown below. Which of the following would be the next most appropriate step in management?

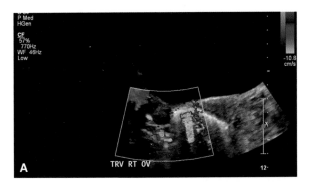
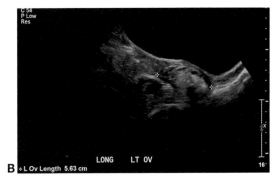
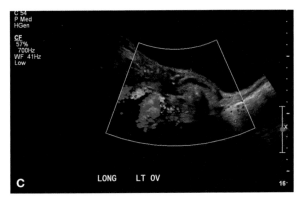

A. MRI of the pelvis

B. Abdominal plain film

C. I-123 MIBG scan

D. No further imaging is needed.

14 Because of the inability of the patient in Question 13 to tolerate an MR examination and problems with sedating the patient, a CT scan of the pelvis was performed instead of an MR study. A representative image of the study is shown below. Regarding the abnormality, which of the following is *true*?

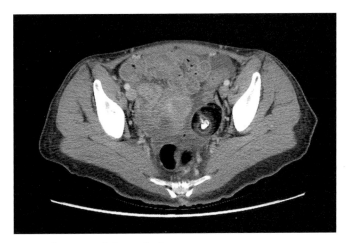

A. Approximately 90% of these lesions rupture.

B. Torsion of the affected ovary occurs in approximately 95% of cases.

C. A Rokitansky nodule is commonly seen in these lesions.

D. There is no risk of malignant transformation.

15 A 1-day-old male with a history of prenatal hydronephrosis presents for a renal ultrasound. Images from the examination are shown below. Which of the following would be the next most appropriate step in management?

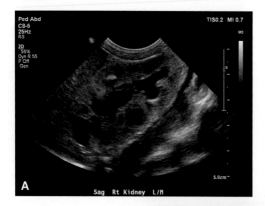

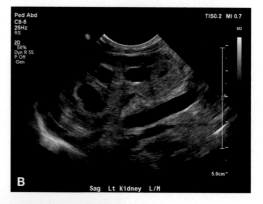

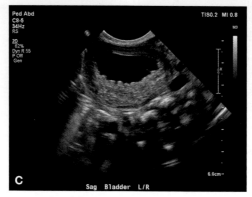

A. Emergent surgical intervention
B. VCUG
C. Tc-99m MAG3 scan
D. Tc-99m DMSA scan

16 A fluoroscopic VCUG study was subsequently performed on the patient described in Question 15. An image from the study is shown below. Regarding the entity shown, which of the following is *true*?

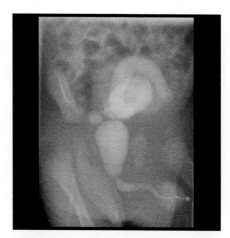

A. There is marked dilatation of the anterior urethra.
B. Urinary ascites is a good prognostic indicator.
C. This entity is found exclusively in females.
D. The definitive treatment is medical.

17 An image from a testicular ultrasound is shown below. Which of the following would be the next most appropriate step in management?

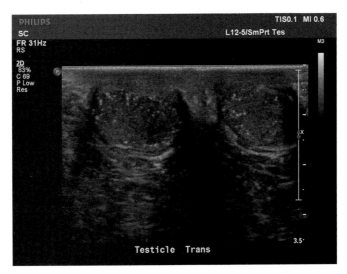

A. Urology consultation
B. CT scan of the chest, abdomen, and pelvis to look for metastatic disease
C. MRI of the pelvis to look for a source of infection
D. DMSA scan to evaluate for pyelonephritis

18 A patient presents for a VCUG examination for a history of urinary tract infections. A representative image from the study is shown below. Regarding the findings, which of the following is *true*?

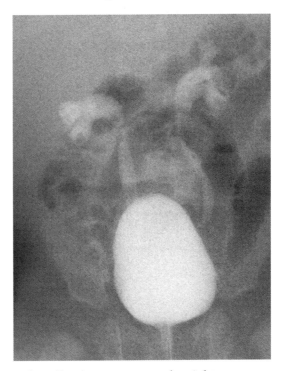

A. There is a single collecting system on the right.
B. There is a duplex collecting system on the right.
C. There is a duplex collecting system on the left.
D. There is no vesicoureteral reflux.

19 According to the Weigert-Meyer rule, which of the following is *true*?

    A. The upper pole moiety is more prone to reflux.

    B. The upper pole moiety is more prone to a UPJ obstruction.

    C. The ureter for the lower pole moiety frequently ends in a ureterocele.

    D. The ureter for the upper pole moiety has an ectopic bladder insertion and inserts inferomedially to the bladder insertion of the upper pole moiety.

20 A 5-year-old male presents for a CT scan and MR exam to better evaluate abnormal findings on an abdominal ultrasound. Images from the CT scan (Figure A) and MRI exam (Figure B) are shown below. Which of the following would be the next most appropriate step?

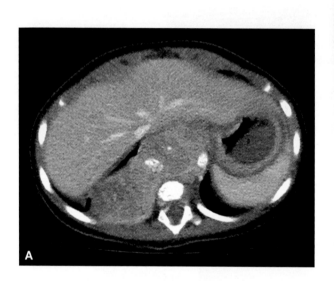 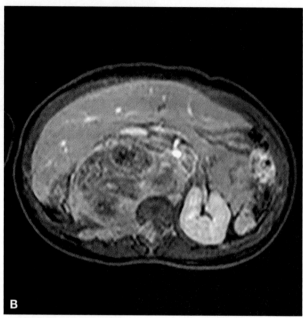

    A. I-123 MIBG scan

    B. Gallium 67 scan

    C. Tc-99m MAG3 scan

    D. Tc-99m DMSA scan

21 An I-123 MIBG scan was performed on the patient described in Question 20 and images from the examination are shown below. Which of the following features of this tumor are associated with a better prognosis?

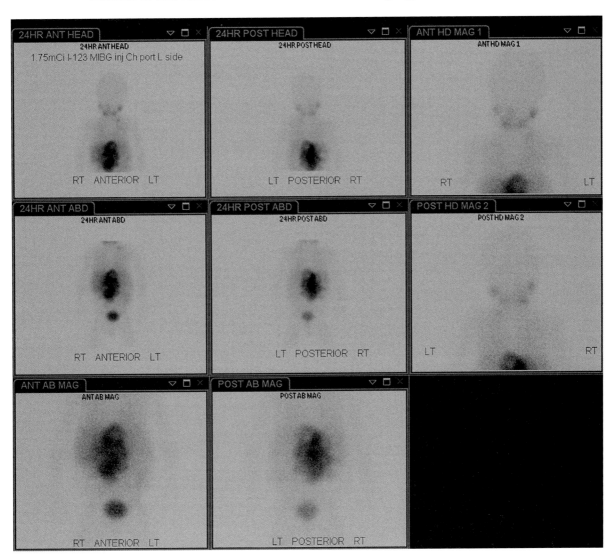

A. N-Myc amplification
B. Age of diagnosis of less than 18 months
C. Age of diagnosis greater than 18 months.
D. Elevated levels of ferritin

22 When performing an I-123 MIBG nuclear medicine examination for evaluation of this tumor, which of the following drugs should be discontinued if possible prior to the examination?

A. Imipramine
B. Potassium chloride
C. Omeprazole
D. Furosemide

23 Regarding neuroblastoma stage MS, which of the following is *true*?

  A. It is associated with a poor prognosis.
  B. It affects the skin, liver, and/or bone marrow.
  C. It is seen in children older than 2 years.
  D. There is no metastatic disease.

24 A CT scan performed on a 2-month-old patient is shown below. What is the most likely diagnosis?

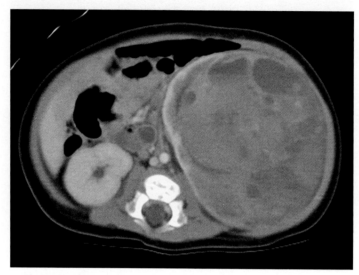

  A. Congenital neuroblastoma
  B. Wilms tumor
  C. Renal cell carcinoma
  D. Congenital mesoblastic nephroma

25 Regarding congenital mesoblastic nephroma, which of the following is *true*?

  A. There is more than one subtype.
  B. The tumor is never aggressive.
  C. It is easy to differentiate this tumor from other lesions based on imaging.
  D. It is a rare tumor in neonates.

26 An ultrasound exam was performed on a 4-year-old patient, and an image is shown below. What is the most likely diagnosis?

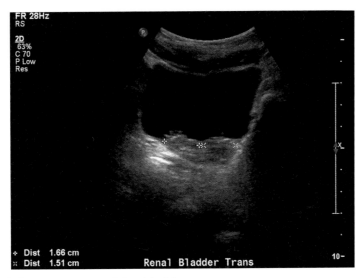

A. Rhabdomyosarcoma of the bladder
B. Distal ureteral calculi
C. Treatment of vesicoureteral reflux
D. Neurogenic bladder

27 An ultrasound examination was performed on a 1-month-old patient. Images are shown below. No kidney on the right side was able to be demonstrated after further imaging. Regarding the entity demonstrated, which of the following is *true*?

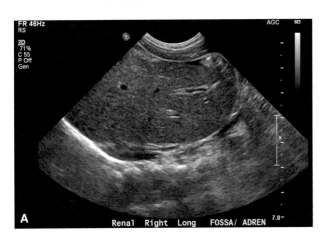
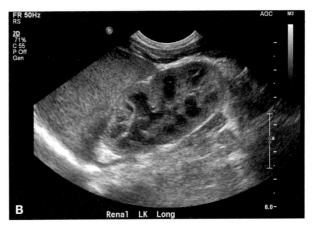

A. Seminal vesicle cysts are associated with this condition in males.
B. The contralateral solitary kidney is usually smaller in size for age in a majority of cases.
C. Only a small percentage of women with this condition have uterine anomalies.
D. This condition is more common in females.

28 A CT scan from a patient is shown below. What is the most likely diagnosis?

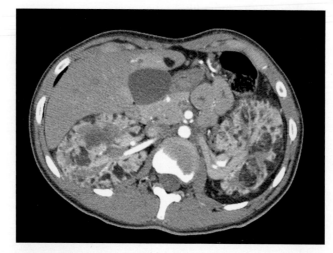

A. Tuberous sclerosis
B. Sturge-Weber syndrome
C. Prune belly syndrome
D. Multifocal pyelonephritis

29 Regarding angiomyolipomas (AMLs), which of the following is *true*?

A. They are pathognomonic of tuberous sclerosis.
B. There is an increased risk of hemorrhage with lesions greater than 4 cm in size.
C. They are malignant lesions.
D. They occur more commonly in males.

30 Concerning crossed fused renal ectopia, which of the following is *true*?

A. It occurs more commonly in females.
B. The risk of complications such as nephrolithiasis, infection, and hydrone-phrosis is low and approaches 5%.
C. Although the kidneys are fused to each other on the same side, the ureters insert in their normal location at both the right and left ureterovesical junctions.
D. Right-to-left ectopy is more common than left-to-right ectopy.

31 A pelvic ultrasound exam is performed on a 15-year-old female patient who has yet to have her first menstrual cycle. An image from the exam is shown below. Which of the following is *true*?

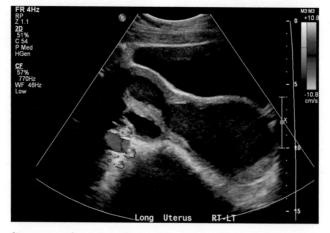

A. The findings may be secondary to an imperforate hymen.
B. There are no known associated presenting symptoms.
C. This entity cannot be cured.
D. The uterus usually expands to a greater degree than does the vagina.

32 Regarding multilocular cystic renal tumors, which of the following is *true*?

A. They usually occur in young girls and older males.

B. Different variants are easy to distinguish on a macroscopic level.

C. There is an association with pleuropulmonary blastoma.

D. No further management is needed because these tumors are almost always benign.

33 An image from a VCUG examination performed on a 4-year-old female is shown below. Which of the following is *true*?

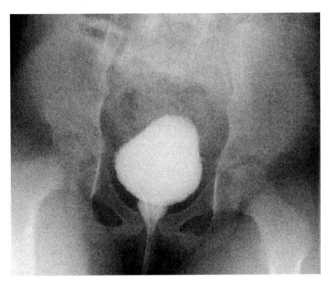

A. There are posterior urethral valves.

B. There is vesicoureteral reflux.

C. This condition is associated with dysfunctional voiding.

D. There is a ureterocele.

34 A 1-year-old female presents with vaginal discharge. An ultrasound exam is performed, and representative images are shown below. Which of the following is the next best step in management?

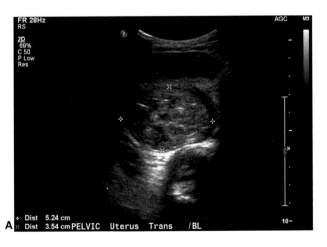
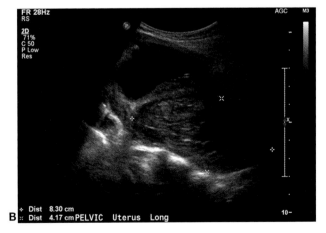

A. VCUG

B. Renal ultrasound

C. MRI of the pelvis

D. Tc-99m MAG3 scan

35 An MRI of the pelvis was subsequently performed on the patient described in Question 34, and representative images are shown below. Concerning the most likely diagnosis, which of the following is *true?*

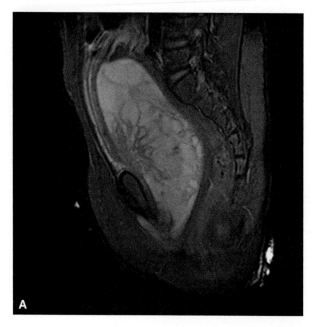
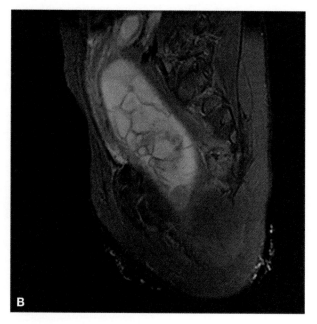

    A. This tumor is a subtype of adenocarcinoma.

    B. The "grape-like" appearance of the tumor suggests sarcoma botryoides as the etiology.

    C. The survival rate for nonmetastatic disease is approximately 5% to 10%.

    D. Recurrence is uncommon after surgery.

36 Which of the following renal tumors is most likely to demonstrate osseous metastasis?

    A. Mesoblastic nephroma

    B. Wilms tumor

    C. Clear cell sarcoma

    D. Atypical rhabdoid tumor

37 Regarding nephroblastomatosis, which of the following is *true?*

    A. There is an association with the subsequent development of Wilms tumor.

    B. There are only two histologic subtypes.

    C. There are no known associations with other diseases.

    D. Once detected, there is no need for follow-up imaging.

38 A young child presents with bacteriuria and vague abdominal pain prompting concern for pyelonephritis. Which of the following studies would be the most sensitive test for the detection of acute pyelonephritis?

    A. CT scan of the abdomen and pelvis without contrast

    B. Renal ultrasound

    C. Tc-99m DMSA scan

    D. Abdominal plain film

39 Images from a Tc-99m DMSA scan obtained on the patient described in Question 38 are shown below. Given the findings on the images, what is the likely diagnosis?

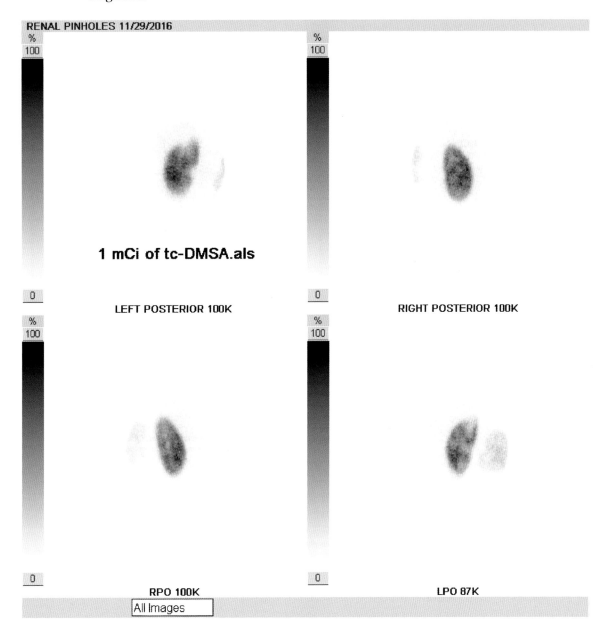

RENAL PINHOLES 11/29/2016

1 mCi of tc-DMSA.als

LEFT POSTERIOR 100K   RIGHT POSTERIOR 100K

RPO 100K   LPO 87K

All Images

A. Left-sided pyelonephritis in the mid-upper pole
B. Right-sided pyelonephritis in the upper pole
C. Normal study
D. Right-sided pyelonephritis in the lower pole

40 A 16-year-old stable female presents with a 2-hour history of acute sharp right lower quadrant pain. The patient had a negative pregnancy test. A pelvic ultrasound was performed, which was equivocal for the diagnosis of right ovarian torsion. The appendix was normal. What other examination would be the next most appropriate step in imaging?

A. Abdominal plain film
B. Emergent MRI of the pelvis with and without IV contrast
C. Repeat ultrasound in 4 hours
D. No other imaging studies would be helpful.

41 An MRI of the pelvis was performed on the patient described in Question 40. Representative images are shown below. Which of the following is *true*?

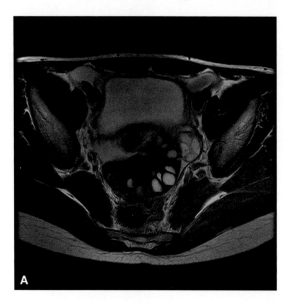 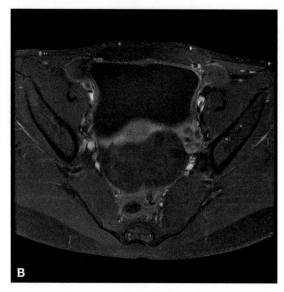

A. The right ovary is torsed and likely viable.
B. The left ovary is torsed and likely nonviable.
C. The right ovary is torsed and likely nonviable.
D. The left ovary is torsed and likely viable.

42 In ovarian torsion, what is the proper order of vascular compromise from the first affected vascular supply to the last?

A. Venous, lymphatic, arterial
B. Lymphatic, venous, arterial
C. Arterial, venous, lymphatic
D. Venous, arterial, lymphatic

43 A renal ultrasound examination was performed on a 10-year-old patient, and representative images are shown below. Concerning the study, which of the following is *true*?

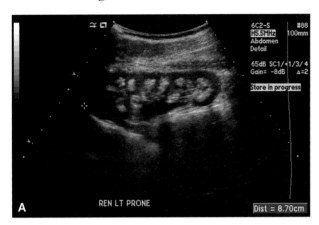 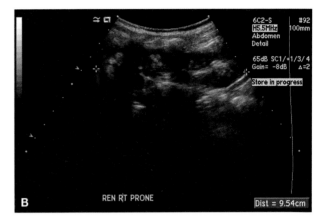

A. This condition is usually associated with proximal renal tubular acidosis.
B. This entity is uncommon among immobilized patients.
C. Most causes of this condition are associated with hypercalciuria.
D. The renal pyramids are normal appearing for the patient's age group.

44 Concerning the differences in size between the kidneys in the exam performed on the patient in Question 43, which of the following is *true*?

A. The difference in sizes of the kidneys is too large.
B. The difference in sizes of the kidneys is too small.
C. The difference in size of the kidneys is within normal limits.
D. There is compensatory hypertrophy of the left kidney.

45 A teenage male presents with acute right side testicular pain. A scrotal ultrasound was performed, and a representative image is shown below. What is the next appropriate step in management?

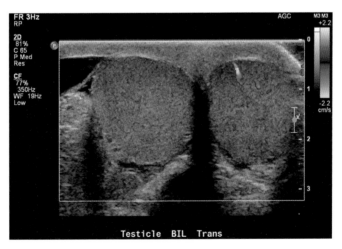

A. Antibiotics
B. Conservative treatment
C. Stat urologic consult
D. No further treatment is indicated.

46 A 1-month-old male with fluid draining from his umbilicus presents for a renal and bladder ultrasound, and a representative image is shown below. Concerning the entity demonstrated, which of the following is *true*?

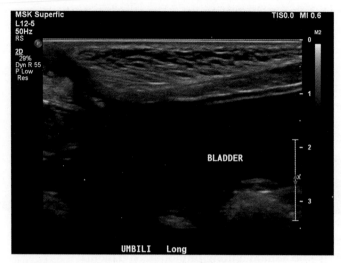

A. This entity is more common in women.
B. This structure is usually lined by columnar epithelium.
C. Later on in life, these lesions can give rise to adenocarcinoma.
D. There are only two types of this entity.

47 Regarding the abnormality seen below on the axial CT and MR images, which of the following is *true*?

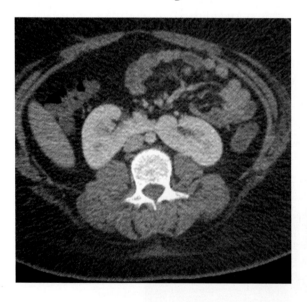
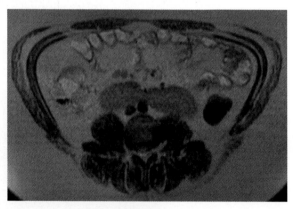

A. Renal cell carcinoma has been reported to be the most common type of renal tumor in children with this condition.
B. Fusion of the upper poles of the kidneys is usually responsible for this condition.
C. The abnormal ureteral course can result in ureteral obstruction or slow drainage of urine (or both), which can lead to hydronephrosis, infections, and stones.
D. There is no known association of this condition with extrarenal disease.

48 Which vessel prevents further superior migration of horseshoe kidneys into the abdomen?

A. Inferior mesenteric artery
B. Superior mesenteric artery
C. Celiac axis
D. Superior mesenteric vein

49 Below are images from a plain film of the pelvis, CT scan of the abdomen and pelvis, and MR examination of the pelvis. Which of the following is the most likely etiology of the radiodensity seen projecting over the left side of the pelvis on the plain film and seen within the right side of the pelvis on the CT scan?

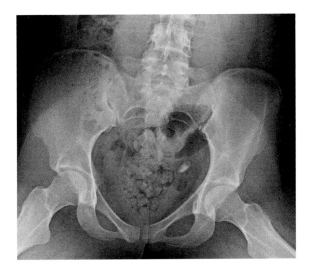
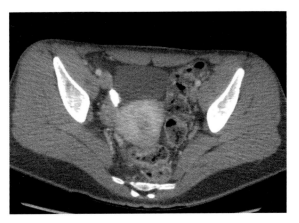

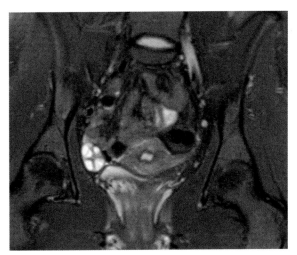

A. Normal right ovary
B. Right ovarian dermoid
C. Left ovarian dermoid
D. Necrotic left ovary

50 The images shown were obtained during an exam utilizing which of the following modalities?

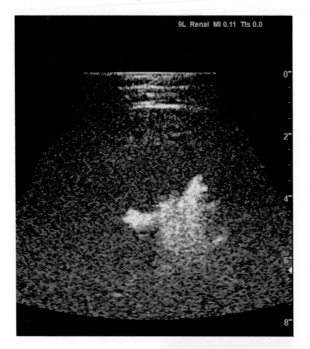

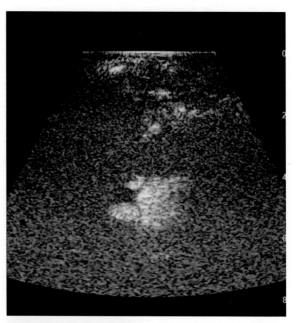

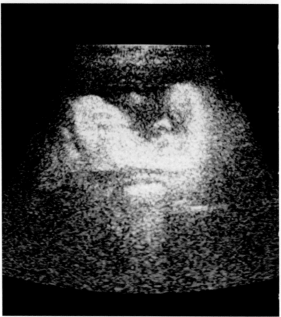

A. MR
B. Fluoroscopy
C. Nuclear medicine scintigraphy
D. Ultrasound

51 Which of the following is *true* regarding the UTD classification system?

A. It was designed to be applied only to postnatal studies.

B. The renal pelvis is not considered to be dilated when the anterior-posterior renal pelvic diameter measures less than 10 mm.

C. Distinguishing between central or central and peripheral calyceal dilatation is not necessary for proper classification.

D. The appearance of the urinary bladder has no bearing on the UTD classification.

52 A 16-year-old male presents for a testicular ultrasound after palpating a painless mass in his right testicle. Which of the following is true regarding the findings?

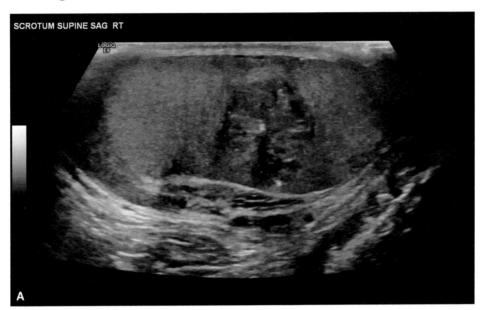

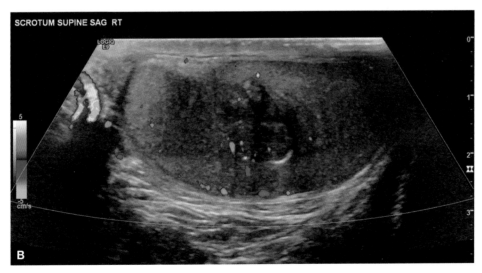

A. The most common etiology of this lesion is due to metastatic disease from leukemia or lymphoma.

B. A germ cell tumor is the most likely diagnosis.

C. A rhabdomyosarcoma is the most likely diagnosis.

D. The ultrasound appearance of the tumor can definitively determine tumor histology.

ANSWERS AND EXPLANATIONS

1 **Answer B.** The images demonstrate dilatation of the left renal pelvis and calyces without ureterectasis. The right kidney is normal. These findings are often seen in a ureteropelvic junction (UPJ) obstruction. However, vesicoureteral reflux (VUR) should be excluded as the cause of the left-sided pelvicaliectasis, which is why a voiding cystourethrogram (VCUG) would be the next best step in management. VCUG examinations can be performed under fluoroscopy or by a contrast-enhanced voiding urosonography (ceVUS) examination. Note that in a male, a VCUG would also help exclude a posterior urethral valve (PUV), which can cause bladder outlet obstruction and pelvicaliectasis. Plain radiographs of the abdomen will not be helpful in determining the cause of the pelvicaliectasis, and a CT scan of the abdomen and pelvis will also not be helpful in determining whether VUR is the cause of the pelvicaliectasis. Plain radiographs and a CT scan would needlessly expose the child to ionizing radiation. Although a testicular ultrasound (US) does not utilize ionizing information, it would not give us any information about the cause for the pelvicaliectasis.

References: Blickman JG, Parker BR, Barnes PD. *Pediatric Radiology: The Requisites.* 3rd ed. Elsevier/Saunders; 2009.

Navarro OM. Genitourinary. In: Donnelly LF, ed. *Fundamentals of Pediatric Imaging.* 3rd ed. Elsevier; 2022:139-174.

Toulia A, Aguirre Pascual E, Back SJ, et al. Contrast-enhanced voiding urosonography, part 1: vesicoureteral reflux evaluation. *Pediatr Radiol.* 2021;51(12):2351-2367.

2 **Answer A.** The image from the fluoroscopic VCUG examination fails to demonstrate VUR, which can now be excluded as a cause for the left-sided pelvicaliectasis. Based on the imaging findings, there is now a suspected left-sided UPJ obstruction, and a functional and dynamic imaging study should be ordered to determine whether surgical intervention will be necessary. A Tc-99m mercaptoacetyltriglycine (MAG3) study should provide that information as it is a dynamic test that evaluates for uptake and clearance of radiotracer by the kidneys as well as for drainage of radiotracer into the ureters and bladder. A Tc-99m dimercaptosuccinic acid (DMSA) scan is a functional but not a dynamic study used to evaluate for cortical scarring and/or pyelonephritis. This exam might be helpful if the patient had VUR, especially if it was accompanied by a urinary tract infection (UTI), but the VCUG was negative for reflux. A CT scan is not a dynamic exam. A right upper quadrant US also would not be helpful as it is not a functional or dynamic exam but could evaluate the gray-scale appearance of the right kidney. However, the right kidney was normal on the initial US exam. In addition, the left kidney is not typically imaged on RUQ ultrasound exams.

References: Blickman JG, Parker BR, Barnes PD. *Pediatric Radiology: The Requisites.* 3rd ed. Elsevier/Saunders; 2009.

Fernbach SK, Feinstein KA, Schmidt MB. Pediatric voiding cystourethrography: a pictorial guide. *Radiographics.* 2000;20(1):155-168; discussion 168-171.

Navarro OM. Genitourinary. In: Donnelly LF, ed. *Fundamentals of Pediatric Imaging.* 3rd ed. Elsevier; 2022:139-174.

3 **Answer C.** The image shown is a renogram of the left kidney obtained after Lasix administration. The time of maximum activity (Tmax) is approximately 2.5 minutes, and the time of half-maximum activity (T½max) is around 10.5 minutes. Therefore, the time from max to half-max is about 8 minutes. In addition, there is significant downsloping of the curve consistent with a good response to Lasix.

Dilated collecting systems secondary to fixed or functional obstruction may produce continuously rising renogram curves before Lasix administration, with little to no evidence of excretion or downsloping. After Lasix administration, the curve should be inspected for change. In dilated, nonobstructed systems, Lasix causes increased urine flow through the collecting system, which washes out the initial increase in activity and causes a decline of the excretion like in this case. In the case of significant mechanical obstruction, there is very little decrease in the renal collecting system activity after administration of Lasix because of the narrowed and fixed lumen of the ureter. The rising renogram curve is changed little or is unaffected. These patients are often treated with a surgical pyeloplasty.

Reference: Mettler FA, Guiberteau MJ. *Essentials of Nuclear Medicine*. 7th ed. Elsevier; 2019.

4 **Answer B.** The images demonstrate multiple noncommunicating cysts throughout the right kidney without a dilated renal pelvis. These cysts do not follow the distribution of dilated calyces, allowing differentiation from urinary tract dilatation (UTD). These findings are consistent with a multicystic dysplastic kidney (MCDK). In patients with MCDK, it is important to exclude other associated congenital abnormalities of the contralateral kidney. These lesions are associated with a contralateral UPJ obstruction in 7% to 27% of cases. There is some controversy whether these lesions have a risk of malignant transformation and because of this are usually followed by serial US exams. These lesions usually slowly decrease in size over time, and often, the remaining residual dysplastic kidney will no longer be visualized by imaging techniques. Rarely this condition can be isolated to an upper or lower pole in a duplicated kidney. There is typically no radiotracer uptake by the affected kidney on a MAG3 scan as there is no function. Because of this, the contralateral kidney will often be enlarged in size due to compensatory hypertrophy.

References: Dähnert W. *Radiology Review Manual*. 8th ed. Wolters Kluwer; 2017.

Navarro OM. Genitourinary. In: Donnelly LF, ed. *Fundamentals of Pediatric Imaging*. 3rd ed. Elsevier; 2022:139-174.

5 **Answer C.** The images are coronal images from a contrast-enhanced CT scan of the abdomen and pelvis, which demonstrate multiple round foci of low attenuation compatible with renal cysts. The cysts appear to be a few centimeters in size. These findings are most compatible with autosomal dominant polycystic kidney disease (ADPKD). This can be ascertained by the age of the patient as well as the size of the cysts. Although autosomal recessive polycystic kidney disease (ARPKD) can give renal macrocysts, most cysts are usually small and in the range of 1 to 3 mm. There is an association of ARPKD with congenital hepatic fibrosis. In addition, ARPKD usually affects children in the first decade of life, whereas ADPKD usually affects patients during the teenage to adult years. However, this condition can also be seen in younger children and even potentially neonates. If ADPKD presents in the neonatal period, the imaging findings can overlap with ARPKD. ADPKD is associated with berry aneurysms in approximately 10% of cases.

References: Dähnert W. *Radiology Review Manual*. 8th ed. Wolters Kluwer; 2017.

Navarro OM. Genitourinary. In: Donnelly LF, ed. *Fundamentals of Pediatric Imaging*. 3rd ed. Elsevier; 2022:139-174.

6 **Answer C.** The abdominal plain film demonstrates a soft tissue density in the left hemiabdomen, which is concerning for a mass lesion (arrows). The next best test would be a cross-sectional imaging study to try and identify the mass and its origin. An abdominal US would be the best way to accomplish this in an inexpensive manner without the use of ionizing radiation. A Tc-99m MAG3 scan may show some renal abnormality, but it would not be the best way to visualize the suspected tumor. An I-123 meta-iodobenzylguanidine (MIBG) scan would be helpful to see if the tumor is MIBG avid as in cases of tumors of neural crest origin such as neuroblastomas (NBs), which often originate in the adrenal region. However, at this point, we do not know the origin of the tumor. A VCUG would not be helpful to visualize the tumor as this test is usually performed to look for VUR.

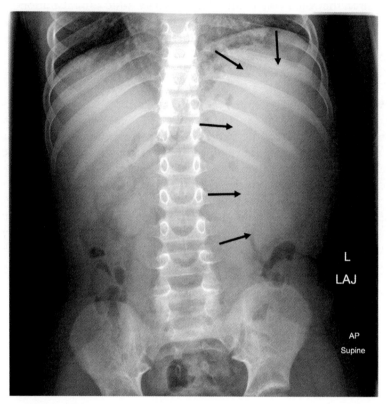

References: Dähnert W. *Radiology Review Manual.* 8th ed. Wolters Kluwer; 2017.

Navarro OM. Genitourinary. In: Donnelly LF, ed. *Fundamentals of Pediatric Imaging.* 3rd ed. Elsevier; 2022:139-174.

7 **Answer D.** The US images demonstrate a heterogeneous mass in the region of the left kidney labeled as "LK" on the US images. It is still difficult to determine the origin of the tumor. Therefore, an alternative cross-sectional imaging modality is needed to define the origin and extent of the mass lesion. An MRI of the abdomen and pelvis with and without intravenous (IV) contrast would be a good way to further image the tumor without the use of ionizing radiation although a child this young would likely need to be sedated for the exam. For similar reasons given in the explanation to Question 6, neither an I-123 MIBG scan, nor a Tc-99m MAG3 scan, nor a VCUG scan would be helpful. A contrast-enhanced CT scan of the abdomen and pelvis would also be appropriate to further image the tumor but would require the use of ionizing radiation.

References: Navarro OM. Genitourinary. In: Donnelly LF, ed. *Fundamentals of Pediatric Imaging.* 3rd ed. Elsevier; 2022:139-174.

Son J, Lee EY, Restrepo R, et al. Focal renal lesions in pediatric patients. *AJR Am J Roentgenol.* 2012;199(6):W668-W682.

8 **Answer C.** Figure A is an axial T2-weighted image with fat saturation from an MR exam, which demonstrates a heterogeneous mass arising from the left kidney. A "claw sign" of renal tissue is seen medially (arrows). Figure B is a coronal image from a T1-weighted image with fat saturation and after contrast administration, which again demonstrates a heterogeneous lesion arising from the left kidney with a medial "claw sign" of renal parenchyma (arrows). Given the patient's age group, a Wilms tumor would be the most likely tumor as the peak incidence of this tumor occurs at 3 years of age. Approximately 80% of Wilms tumor cases are detected between 1 and 5 years of age. Renal cell carcinoma (RCC) occurs in older children and the adult population, and mesoblastic nephroma, a generally benign tumor, usually occurs in neonates. NBs often arise from the adrenals and not the kidneys.

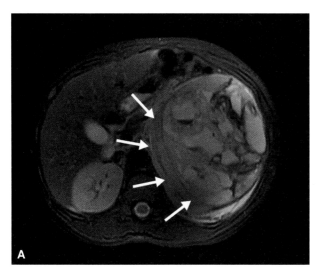
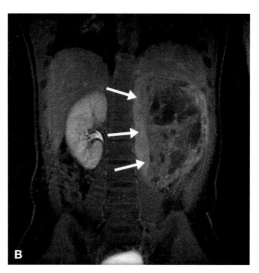

References: Navarro OM. Genitourinary. In: Donnelly LF, ed. *Fundamentals of Pediatric Imaging.* 3rd ed. Elsevier; 2022:139-174.

Son J, Lee EY, Restrepo R, et al. Focal renal lesions in pediatric patients. *AJR Am J Roentgenol.* 2012;199(6):W668-W682.

9 **Answer A.** When evaluating a suspected Wilms tumor, it is important to document the following features: lymph node involvement, liver and lung metastasis, involvement of the contralateral tumor by a synchronous tumor, the anatomic distribution of the intrarenal tumor, involvement of the renal vein or inferior vena cava, and the path of the ureters in relation to the mass. Therefore, a CT scan of the chest would be indicated. It is also important to evaluate for tumor thrombus into the right atrium, so an echocardiogram is often performed as well. If tumor thrombus is found in the right atrium, cardiothoracic surgery often becomes involved. A testicular sonogram would not be helpful to evaluate any of the above features. An I-123 MIBG scan would be helpful to evaluate the extent of a NB but is not indicated for a Wilms tumor. Because osseous metastatic disease is rare in Wilms tumor, bone scans are not required as part of the workup.

References: Carroll WL, Finlay JL. *Cancer in Children and Adolescents.* Jones and Bartlett Publishers; 2010.

Navarro OM. Genitourinary. In: Donnelly LF, ed. *Fundamentals of Pediatric Imaging.* 3rd ed. Elsevier; 2022:139-174.

Umuerri EM, Odion-Obomhense HK. Nephroblastoma with right atrial extension. *J Cardiovasc Echography.* 2021;31:107-109.

10 **Answer B.** The current overall survival rates for Wilms tumor are now around 90%. The Children's Oncology Group (COG) histological classification system separates Wilms tumor into three broad categories based on the degree of anaplasia: favorable histology (no anaplasia), focal anaplasia, and diffuse anaplasia. Although most cases of Wilms tumor occur in normal children, there is an association between the development of Wilms tumor and other overgrowth disorders (congenital hemihypertrophy, Beckwith-Wiedemann syndrome), sporadic aniridia, and other malformations. Nephroblastomatosis is a rare entity that is related to the persistence of nephrogenic rests within the renal parenchyma. These nephrogenic rests can be precursors but are not sequela of Wilms tumors.

References: Navarro OM. Genitourinary. In: Donnelly LF, ed. *Fundamentals of Pediatric Imaging*. 3rd ed. Elsevier; 2022:139-174.

Servaes SE, Hoffer FA, Smith EA et al. Imaging of Wilms tumor: an update. *Pediatr Radiol.* 2019;49:1441-1452.

11 **Answer D.** Renal medullary carcinoma is a rare aggressive renal malignancy that is strongly associated with sickle cell (SC) trait or hemoglobin SC disease. With a peak age of presentation at 20 years, this neoplasm arises predominantly from the renal medulla. None of the other tumors listed are associated with SC trait.

Reference: Son J, Lee EY, Restrepo R, et al. Focal renal lesions in pediatric patients. *AJR Am J Roentgenol.* 2012;199(6):W668-W682.

12 **Answer D.** The US images demonstrate a hypoechoic oval avascular mass located between the right testicle and epididymis (arrows). This is consistent with a torsed appendix testis. Note that torsed testicular appendages can be of varying echogenicity. Testicular appendageal torsion is a common cause of an acute scrotum in prepubertal boys. The appendages are normal remnants of embryonic tissue and are usually located adjacent to the superior testicle or epididymal head. Testicular appendages are more prevalent than epididymal appendages; however, the distinction is often difficult to make and is not important clinically. Additional findings may include scrotal edema and reactive hydroceles. Color Doppler may show hyperemia surrounding the torsed appendage. Treatment involves conservative management.

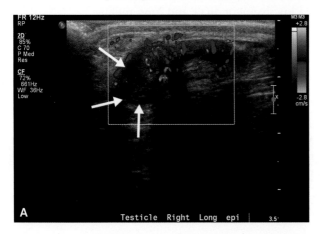 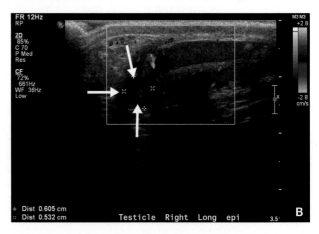

Reference: Sung EK, Setty BN, Castro-Aragon I. Sonography of the pediatric scrotum: emphasis on the Ts–torsion, trauma, and tumors. *AJR Am J Roentgenol.* 2012;198(5):996-1003.

13 **Answer A.** The US images demonstrate a lesion within the left ovary that contains echogenic foci, which appear to shadow. Thus, this lesion may contain calcium. The lesion itself appears avascular, but there does appear to be flow in the surrounding left ovarian parenchyma. An abdominal radiograph may demonstrate calcifications but a cross-sectional imaging modality is necessary to better define and characterize the lesion. An MRI would be preferred over CT because of the lack of ionizing radiation, its ability to characterize sonographically indeterminate adnexal masses of uncertain origin, and solid or complex cystic content. Although this lesion may contain calcium, it appears to arise from the left ovary and therefore is extremely unlikely to be a NB, so an MIBG scan would not be indicated.

Reference: Adusumilli S, Hussain HK, Caoili EM, et al. MRI of sonographically indeterminate adnexal masses. *AJR Am J Roentgenol.* 2006;187(3):732-740.

14 **Answer C.** The CT scan demonstrates a lesion arising from the left ovary, which contains fat and calcium as well as solid components. These findings are consistent with an ovarian dermoid or mature cystic teratoma. These lesions lead to torsion of the involved ovary in approximately 16% of cases. Approximately 1% to 4% of ovarian teratomas rupture, and approximately 1% to 2% undergo malignant transformation. It is common to see a soft tissue protuberance in a mature cystic teratoma; this is known as a Rokitansky nodule or dermoid plug. Although this protuberance may be partly solid and consist of diverse tissues, benign teratomas never show transmural growth of the protuberance. Contrast enhancement of a Rokitansky nodule raises the possibility of malignant transformation, although this finding does not always necessarily indicate malignancy.

Reference: Park SB, Kim JK, Kim KR, et al. Imaging findings of complications and unusual manifestations of ovarian teratomas. *Radiographics.* 2008;28(4):969-983.

15 **Answer B.** The images demonstrate bilateral pelvicaliectasis. In addition, the bladder wall appears irregularly thickened and trabeculated even for a partially contracted bladder. In a male, these findings raise the possibility of bladder outlet obstruction from a posterior urethral valve (PUV). A fluoroscopic VCUG or sonographic VCUG (ceVUS) exam will evaluate the urethra as well as test for VUR. None of the other tests will be able to determine if there is a PUV. Although the patient will require surgery if there is a PUV, it is necessary to determine if the patient has a PUV prior to surgical intervention.

References: Barnewolt CE, Acharya PT, Aguirre Pascual E, et al. Contrast-enhanced voiding urosonography part 2: urethral imaging. *Pediatr Radiol.* 2021;51:2368-2386.

Navarro OM. Genitourinary. In: Donnelly LF, ed. *Fundamentals of Pediatric Imaging.* 3rd ed. Elsevier; 2022:139-174.

Toulia A, Aguirre Pascual E, Back SJ, et al. Contrast-enhanced voiding urosonography, part 1: vesicoureteral reflux evaluation. *Pediatr Radiol.* 2021;51(12):2351-2367.

16 **Answer B.** The image demonstrates marked dilatation of the posterior urethra (long arrows) with a normal appearance of the anterior urethra (short arrows). These findings are consistent with a PUV, which is found exclusively in males. These lesions are treated surgically. In patients with PUVs, severe unilateral VUR is one of the three conditions associated with preservation of renal function. Others are urinary ascites or urinoma in newborns and large congenital bladder diverticula. These conditions most likely provide a pop-off mechanism preventing the development of high intravesical pressure. Only 5% of patients with PUV and an associated pop-off mechanism will develop renal failure as opposed to 40% of patients with PUV without a protective factor.

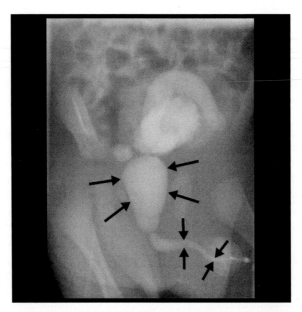

References: Goodwin OI, Ayotunde OO. Posterior urethral valves with severe unilateral vesicoureteral reflux in a 3-year-old boy. *Ann Ib Postgrad Med.* 2007;5(2):73-76.

Navarro OM. Genitourinary. In: Donnelly LF, ed. *Fundamentals of Pediatric Imaging.* 3rd ed. Elsevier; 2022:139-174.

17 **Answer A.** The US image demonstrates multiple bright echogenic nonshadowing foci throughout the testes. These findings are consistent with testicular microlithiasis (TM). There is often no posterior acoustic shadowing because of the small size of the calcifications. In children, TM has a reported incidence of 0.7% to 3.8%, is more often bilateral, and is usually an incidental finding. TM has a strong association with testicular neoplasms. Boys with TM have approximately 22 times greater odds of having a malignant germ cell tumor as compared to those without TM. However, there is controversy on the need and type of US follow-up of boys with this finding. In adults, routine surveillance with annual US follow-up is only recommended in the presence of risk factors, which include previous malignancy, maldescent of the testes, small testes, and prior orchidopexy.

This condition is not associated with active infection, and therefore an MRI of the pelvis to look for a site of infection or a DMSA scan to evaluate for pyelonephritis is not indicated. A metastatic workup is not indicated in the absence of a known testicular neoplasm.

Reference: Navarro OM. Genitourinary. In: Donnelly LF, ed. *Fundamentals of Pediatric Imaging.* 3rd ed. Elsevier; 2022:139-174.

18 **Answer B.** The image is taken from a VCUG, which demonstrates bilateral VUR. A "drooping lily" sign is seen on the right (arrows). This sign is identified in patients with a duplex collecting system. The drooping lily sign is due to inferior and lateral displacement of the lower pole moiety of a duplex kidney, rather than displacement of an entire kidney. An obstructed, poorly functioning upper pole moiety exerts a mass effect on the lower pole collecting system, which is responsible for the abnormal axis of the lower pole calices and which causes the droop of the lily. Because only the lower pole collecting system is opacified with contrast material, fewer calices are depicted, as no calices extend cephalad from the renal pelvis. No drooping lily sign is seen in the left kidney, which has a single collecting system and more opacified calices than the right kidney.

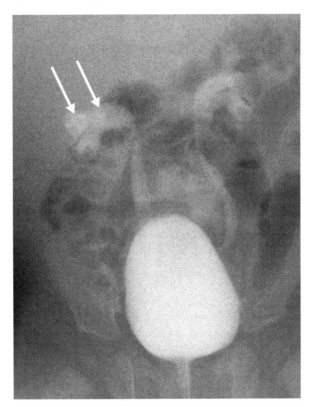

Reference: Callahan MJ. The drooping lily sign. *Radiology*. 2001;219(1):226-228.

19 **Answer D.** In patients with complete ureteropelvic duplication, the ureteral orifice of the upper pole moiety inserts more medially and inferiorly than does the orifice of the lower pole ureter. The lower pole system is more prone to VUR and UPJ obstruction. The upper pole moiety is more prone to obstruction secondary to a ureterocele. This is known as the Weigert-Meyer rule.

Reference: Navarro OM. Genitourinary. In: Donnelly LF, ed. *Fundamentals of Pediatric Imaging*. 3rd ed. Elsevier; 2022:139-174.

20 **Answer A.** The images demonstrate a large paravertebral mass, which is seen in the right lower portions of the thorax and upper retroperitoneum. There are internal calcifications seen on the CT scan (arrows in Figure A). On the MR image, there is extension of the tumor into the right spinal canal (arrow in Figure B). In a child of this age group, the most likely etiology of the lesion is a neurogenic tumor such as neuroblastoma NB or a ganglioneuroblastoma (GNB). In an older child, a ganglioneuroma (GN) could also be considered. I-123 MIBG is taken up by catecholamine-producing tumors such as NB, GNB, and GN. Although 90% to 95% of NB and GNB secrete catecholamines, only about 70% of NB and GNB are MIBG positive; one of the drawbacks of I-123 MIBG imaging is that a considerable minority of tumors (30%) are not MIBG avid.

Tc-99m MAG3 scans are used to determine renal function and evaluate for possible obstruction. Tc-99m DMSA scans are used to evaluate for pyelonephritis or renal cortical scarring. There is no evidence of the tumor involving the kidneys. Gallium 67 scans are used to evaluate for sources of chronic infection. In addition, this radiotracer is also taken up by certain neoplasms such as non-Hodgkin lymphoma, Hodgkin disease, hepatocellular carcinoma (HCC), and melanoma. Gallium 67 scans are not useful to evaluate NB.

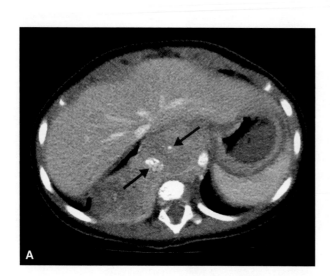

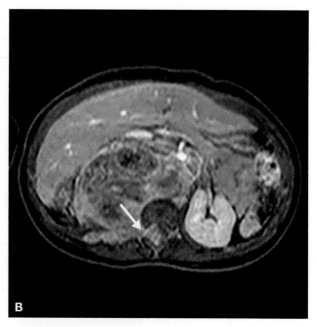

References: Dähnert W. *Radiology Review Manual.* 8th ed. Wolters Kluwer; 2017.

Lonergan GJ, Schwab CM, Suarez ES, et al. Neuroblastoma, ganglioneuroblastoma, and ganglioneuroma: radiologic-pathologic correlation. *Radiographics.* 2002;22(4):911-934.

21 **Answer B.** The tumor seen on the CT and MR images is MIBG avid and therefore likely represents a NB. Children who are diagnosed with these tumors at <18 months of age usually have a good prognosis. In these patients, the disease tends to spread to the liver and skin. In the International Neuroblastoma Risk Group Staging System there is a stage of NB known as MS that is given to patients who are diagnosed at less than 18 months of age with metastatic disease that is confined to the skin, liver, and/or rarely bone marrow. Cortical bone involvement is not considered to be part of MS. In children older than 18 months, NB tends to spread to the bone. These patients have a poorer prognosis.

Expression of the N-Myc protein has been found to correlate with poor prognosis and aggressive tumor behavior in children older than 1 year. Elevated serum levels of ferritin portend a worse prognosis.

References: Lonergan GJ, Schwab CM, Suarez ES, et al. Neuroblastoma, ganglioneuroblastoma, and ganglioneuroma: radiologic-pathologic correlation. *Radiographics.* 2002;22(4):911-934.

Navarro OM. Genitourinary. In: Donnelly LF, ed. *Fundamentals of Pediatric Imaging.* 3rd ed. Elsevier; 2022:139-174.

22 **Answer A.** Imipramine is a tricyclic antidepressant that may inhibit localization of radioiodinated MIBG. Therefore, this drug should be discontinued before imaging when practical. Other drugs that may similarly inhibit localization of radioiodinated MIBG and that should be withheld if possible prior to MIBG exams include insulin, reserpine, other tricyclic antidepressants, and amphetamine-like drugs. None of the other drugs listed need to be withheld prior to an MIBG exam.

Reference: Mettler FA, Guiberteau MJ. *Essentials of Nuclear Medicine.* 7th ed. Elsevier; 2019.

23 **Answer B.** Stage MS is assigned to patients who are diagnosed at less than 18 months of age with metastatic disease that is confined to the skin, liver, and/or bone marrow. These patients have a good prognosis. Cortical bone involvement is not considered to be part of MS.

Reference: Navarro OM. Genitourinary. In: Donnelly LF, ed. *Fundamentals of Pediatric Imaging*. 3rd ed. Elsevier; 2022:139-174.

24 **Answer D.** The CT image demonstrates a heterogeneous solid mass arising from the left kidney as evidenced by a rim of renal tissue medially (arrows) consistent with a "claw sign." In a 2-month-old patient, this lesion most likely represents a congenital mesoblastic nephroma (CMN). CMN is the most common solid renal tumor in the neonate. It is usually identified within the first 3 months of life, with 90% of cases discovered within the first year of life. Imaging studies demonstrate a large solid intrarenal mass that typically involves the renal sinus. The mass replaces a large portion of renal parenchyma and may contain cystic, hemorrhagic, and necrotic regions. CMN was first described in 1967 as a benign leiomyoma-like tumor. Current research now suggests that a spectrum of disease exists, ranging from the classic benign CMN to a more aggressive cellular CMN variant, which accounts for 42% to 63% of cases.

The peak age of Wilms tumor is 3 to 4 years. It is rare in neonates, with <0.16% of cases manifesting in this age group. RCC has been reported in patients <6 months of age. However, the tumor is rare in children, accounting for <7% of all primary renal tumors presenting in the first two decades of life. Less than 2% of all cases of RCC occur in pediatric patients, with a peak incidence in the sixth decade of life. Renal medullary carcinoma is a highly aggressive malignant tumor that occurs almost exclusively in adolescent and young adult black patients with SC trait or hemoglobin SC disease. The age range of this tumor is 10 to 39 years, with a mean age of 20 years.

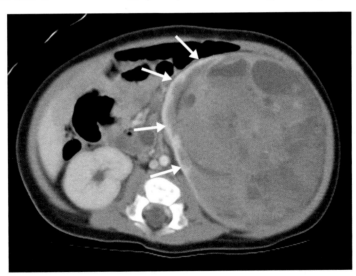

References: Lowe LH, Isuani BH, Heller RM, et al. Pediatric renal masses: Wilms tumor and beyond. *Radiographics*. 2000;20(6):1585-1603.

Sheth MM, Cai G, Goodman TR. AIRP best cases in radiologic-pathologic correlation: congenital mesoblastic nephroma. *Radiographics*. 2012;32(1):99-103.

25 **Answer A.** CMN is the most common renal tumor in neonates and in infants under 1 year of age. CMN was first described in 1967 as a benign leiomyoma-like tumor. Current research now suggests that a spectrum of disease exists, ranging from the classic benign CMN to a more aggressive cellular CMN variant, which accounts for 42% to 63% of cases. The imaging appearances of CMN vary depending on tumor composition, because classic variants are predominantly solid, whereas cellular variants are largely cystic. Unfortunately, many diverse disease processes may present as a solid, cystic, or mixed renal mass within the first year of life. The differential diagnosis is broad and includes renal and nonrenal tumors such as Wilms tumor, clear cell sarcoma, rhabdoid tumors, NB, and multilocular cystic renal tumor (MCRT). Although patient history, presentation, and associated findings can suggest a particular diagnosis, in many cases, a definitive diagnosis can be made only based on histopathologic findings.

Reference: Sheth MM, Cai G, Goodman TR. AIRP best cases in radiologic-pathologic correlation: congenital mesoblastic nephroma. *Radiographics*. 2012;32(1):99-103.

26 **Answer C.** Minimally invasive endoscopic treatment or periureteral injection is considered for the treatment of VUR when the degree of VUR is severe, if there is evidence of renal scarring, if the reflux has not resolved over a reasonable time, or if breakthrough infections occur frequently. After periureteral injection, US will show iso- or hyperechoic mounds in the bladder wall in the region of the ureteral orifices without posterior acoustic shadowing. A dextranomer-hyaluronic acid copolymer (Deflux) has been used as an injectable material in pediatric urology for 15 years. Dextranomer-hyaluronic acid copolymer is currently the most used agent and will consequently be most frequently encountered on imaging studies. Deflux mounds should not be mistaken for distal ureteral calculi. They should not be mistaken for rhabdomyosarcomas or other bladder masses based on their characteristic location and imaging features. They also should not be mistaken for bladder wall trabeculations, which are often seen in neurogenic bladders.

References: Cerwinka WH, Kaye JD, Scherz HC, et al. Radiologic features of implants after endoscopic treatment of vesicoureteral reflux in children. *AJR Am J Roentgenol*. 2010;195(1):234-240.

Navarro OM. Genitourinary. In: Donnelly LF, ed. *Fundamentals of Pediatric Imaging*. 3rd ed. Elsevier; 2022:139-174.

27 **Answer A.** The US images fail to demonstrate a kidney on the right. The findings are consistent with right-sided renal agenesis. This condition is more common in males than in females. Associated genitourinary (GU) anomalies in males include hypoplasia or agenesis of the testes and vas deferens as well as seminal vesicle cysts. Ninety percent of females with renal agenesis have uterine anomalies. There is compensatory hypertrophy of the contralateral kidney in 50% of cases.

Reference: Dähnert W. *Radiology Review Manual*. 8th ed. Wolters Kluwer; 2017.

28 **Answer A.** The image demonstrates multiple small foci of low attenuation fat-containing lesions in both kidneys that likely represent angiomyolipomas (AMLs). AMLs are an uncommon tumor that consists of a disordered arrangement of vascular, smooth muscle, and fatty elements. Its histologic composition suggests a hamartoma, but it is currently believed to represent a benign neoplasm. These tumors most often occur sporadically. However, they may occur in 40% to 80% of patients with tuberous sclerosis. AMLs are also associated with neurofibromatosis and von Hippel-Lindau syndrome. In children, AMLs are rare in the absence of tuberous sclerosis. Eighty percent of children with tuberous sclerosis may be expected to develop lesions by the age of 10 years. Multifocal pyelonephritis typically demonstrates multiple peripheral and triangular regions of decreased contrast enhancement as well as a striated nephrogram on contrast-enhanced CT scans. AMLs are not found in patients with Prune belly or Sturge-Weber syndrome.

References: Lowe LH, Isuani BH, Heller RM, et al. Pediatric renal masses: Wilms tumor and beyond. *Radiographics*. 2000;20(6):1585-1603.

Navarro OM. Genitourinary. In: Donnelly LF, ed. *Fundamentals of Pediatric Imaging*. 3rd ed. Elsevier; 2022:139-174.

29 **Answer B.** AMLs most often occur sporadically. However, they may occur in 40% to 80% of patients with tuberous sclerosis. AMLs are also associated with neurofibromatosis and von Hippel-Lindau syndrome. In children, AMLs are rare in the absence of tuberous sclerosis. AMLs larger than 4 cm in diameter often contain dysplastic arteries and aneurysms and may spontaneously hemorrhage, leading to flank or abdominal pain, hematuria, or even severe life-threatening hemorrhage. Therefore, AMLs greater than 4 cm in diameter are often treated with prophylactic embolization. There is a 4:1 female predominance of AMLs. AMLs are believed to represent a benign neoplasm.

References: Lowe LH, Isuani BH, Heller RM, et al. Pediatric renal masses: Wilms tumor and beyond. *Radiographics.* 2000;20(6):1585-1603.

Navarro OM. Genitourinary. In: Donnelly LF, ed. *Fundamentals of Pediatric Imaging.* 3rd ed. Elsevier; 2022:139-174.

30 **Answer C.** In cross-fused renal ectopia, both kidneys lie on the same side of the abdomen and are fused. The ureter from the ectopic kidney crosses the midline and enters the bladder in the expected location of the contralateral ureterovesical junction. This condition is more common in males. Approximately half of the patients manifest with complications such as hydronephrosis, infections, and nephrolithiasis. Left-to-right crossover occurs more frequently, and the upper pole of the crossed ectopic kidney is fused to the lower pole of the normally located kidney in most instances.

References: Navarro OM. Genitourinary. In: Donnelly LF, ed. *Fundamentals of Pediatric Imaging.* 3rd ed. Elsevier; 2022:139-174.

Solanki S, Bhatnagar V, Gupta AK, et al. Crossed fused renal ectopia: challenges in diagnosis and management. *J Indian Assoc Pediatr Surg.* 2013;18(1):7-10.

31 **Answer A.** The long-axis US image demonstrates distention of the vagina and uterine cavity with fluid-containing echoes that are likely secondary to blood products. Note that the vagina (long arrow) is distended to a greater degree than the uterine cavity (short arrow). In a 15-year-old patient who has not begun her menstrual cycle, these findings are most likely secondary to hematometrocolpos. This entity is often caused by an imperforate hymen that obstructs flow from the vagina. This entity is cured by relieving the obstruction. Patients with this condition often present with cyclic abdominal pain as well as a midline abdominal mass. Because the vagina is more elastic, it can distend to a greater degree than the uterus and composes the bulk of the mass.

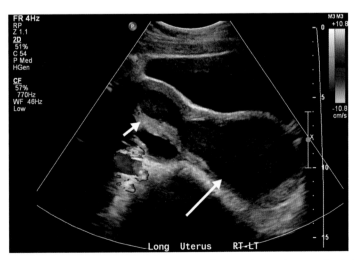

Reference: Navarro OM. Genitourinary. In: Donnelly LF, ed. *Fundamentals of Pediatric Imaging.* 3rd ed. Elsevier; 2022:139-174.

32 **Answer C.** Cystic nephroma (CN) and cystic partially differentiated nephroblastoma (CPDN) are rare histologically distinct but macroscopically indistinguishable cystic tumors of the kidney, which are collectively described by the term multilocular cystic renal tumor. Previously thought to represent developmental or hamartomatous lesions, these tumors were known by various names, including multilocular cyst and multilocular cystic nephroma. They are now recognized as neoplasms originating from metanephric tissue and are considered to represent part of a spectrum of differentiation analogous to the spectrum of neuroblastoma, ganglioneuroblastoma, and ganglioneuroma. At the benign end of the spectrum is cystic nephroma and at the malignant end is nephroblastoma (Wilms tumor). CPDN lies in between. Infants and young children ages 3 months to 4 years are affected, and there is a 2:1 male predilection. A bimodal age and sex distribution has been observed affecting young boys and middle-aged women, but it is likely that many of the tumors diagnosed as cystic nephroma in adults represent distinct clinical entities. Most patients present with an asymptomatic palpable abdominal mass, although a small number have hematuria, presumably caused by herniation of the tumor into the renal collecting system. A familial association of cystic nephroma with the cystic type of pleuropulmonary blastoma related to the DICER1 mutation has recently been described.

Reference: Chung EM, Graeber AR, Conran RM. Renal tumors of childhood: Radiologic-pathologic correlation part 1. The 1st decade: From the radiologic pathology archives. *Radiographics*. 2016 Mar-Apr;36(2):499-522.

33 **Answer C.** The image provided from a VCUG examination performed on a young female demonstrates dilatation of the posterior urethra (arrow) in the shape of a "spinning top." This configuration of the urethra is known as a "spinning top urethra." The most common mechanism for this entity is unstable bladder contractions that are resisted by a voluntary increase in distal sphincter tension to prevent leakage of urine. This entity is associated with dysfunctional voiding. PUVs are only found in males and not in females. There is no evidence of VUR or a ureterocele on the image provided.

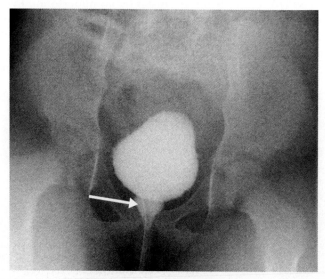

References: Dähnert W. *Radiology Review Manual*. 8th ed. Wolters Kluwer; 2017.

Ichim G, Fufezan O, Farcău M, et al. Clinical, imaging and cystometric findings of voiding dysfunction in children. *Med Ultrason*. 2011;13(4):277-282.

Saxton HM, Borzyskowski M, Mundy AR, et al. Spinning top urethra: not a normal variant. *Radiology*. 1988;168(1):147-150.

34 **Answer C.** The US images demonstrate a mass that is incompletely evaluated and that appears to involve or displace the uterus and is located posterior to the urinary bladder. MRI provides precise demonstration of anatomic features in multiple planes in cases of complex anomalies when US findings are incomplete or inconclusive. A VCUG is used to evaluate for VUR and is not indicated in this case. A Tc-99m MAG3 scan is used to evaluate renal function and potential obstruction and would not be indicated in this instance. Finally, a renal US would also not help localize or determine the etiology of the tumor that is seen in the pelvis.

References: Dähnert W. *Radiology Review Manual.* 8th ed. Wolters Kluwer; 2017.

Garel L, Dubois J, Grignon A, et al. US of the pediatric female pelvis: a clinical perspective. *Radiographics.* 2001;21(6):1393-1407.

Navarro OM. Genitourinary. In: Donnelly LF, ed. *Fundamentals of Pediatric Imaging.* 3rd ed. Elsevier; 2022:139-174.

35 **Answer B.** The sagittal T2 fat-saturated images demonstrate a large heterogeneous lesion, which arises from and markedly distends the vagina. The uterus is displaced superiorly toward the superior extent of the image as can be discerned from the linear-appearing and T2 hyperintense endometrial canal (arrows). The tumor appears as a septated high T2 signal cystic mass. Given the clinical history and imaging findings, this lesion likely represents sarcoma botryoides, a variant of embryonal rhabdomyosarcoma. This tumor is the most common malignancy arising in the GU tract of the pediatric population prior to 15 years of age. In children, rhabdomyosarcoma has a bimodal distribution pattern, the first peak occurring between 2 and 6 years and the second peak between 14 and 18 years of age. Gross pathology examination of sarcoma botryoides typically reveals an exophytic multinodular polyploid mass caused by cellular tumor growth pushing outward upon the overlying mucosal surface; hence the term "botryoid," meaning "grape like." In general, local recurrence of rhabdomyosarcoma is common with or without metastatic disease. Children presenting with nonmetastatic rhabdomyosarcoma have been shown to have an excellent survival rate. If the primary tumor completely arises from a favorable site such as the vagina and is completely excised, the overall 3-year survival rate is >90%.

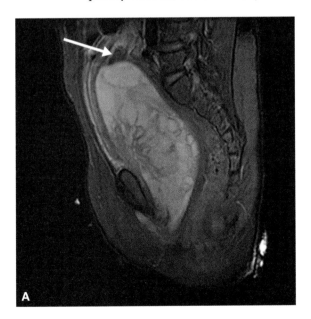 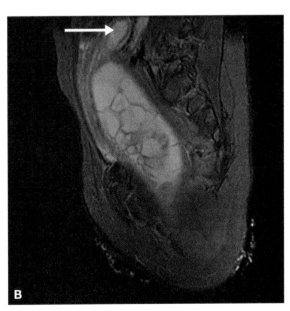

References: Agrons GA, Wagner BJ, Lonergan GJ, et al. From the archives of the AFIP. Genitourinary rhabdomyosarcoma in children: radiologic-pathologic correlation. *Radiographics.* 1997;17(4):919-937.

Kobi M, Khatri G, Edelman M, et al. Sarcoma botryoides: MRI findings in two patients. *J Magn Reson Imaging.* 2009;29(3):708-712.

36   **Answer C.** Clear cell renal sarcoma is a rare tumor and constitutes 4% of primary pediatric malignant renal tumors. It is known as an aggressive tumor with a poor prognosis. Clinically and radiographically, it resembles Wilms tumor. Clear cell sarcoma is seen mainly in young children with a peak incidence between 2 and 3 years of age with a male predominance. The most common site of metastasis at the time of presentation in patients with this tumor is the ipsilateral renal hilar lymph nodes. Treatment consists of nephrectomy and chemotherapy with current long-term survival rate of 60% to 70%. One important distinguishing feature of this tumor is its 40% to 60% incidence of bone metastasis, which is much higher than the 2% incidence of bone metastasis found in Wilms patients. The bone metastasis can be both lytic and sclerotic. Bone is the most common site of distant metastases followed by the lung, retroperitoneum, brain, and liver.

Mesoblastic nephroma can be both benign and aggressive as detailed in the explanations for Questions 24 and 25. Rarely, this lesion may recur locally if incompletely resected or metastasize to the lungs, brain, or bones.

Rhabdoid tumor is a rare highly aggressive renal neoplasm seen exclusively in the pediatric population. Peak incidence of rhabdoid tumor occurs at 11 months of age with a slight male predominance. On imaging, a rhabdoid tumor may present as an enhancing soft tissue renal mass with a similar imaging appearance to a Wilms tumor. As a result, a rhabdoid tumor often cannot be differentiated from a Wilms tumor. More specific imaging characteristics include subcapsular fluid collections with a mildly enhancing intrarenal tumor. Because brain malignancy, often midline and in the posterior fossa, may present concurrently, an MR examination of the head is recommended at the time of diagnosis to assess for concomitant malignancy in this region. Rhabdoid tumor is the renal neoplasm with the worst prognosis, with metastatic disease most commonly involving the lungs. Surgical resection followed by chemotherapy is the current standard of care in pediatric patients with rhabdoid tumor. The survival rate is <15%.

References: Franco A, Dao TV, Lewis KN, et al. A case of clear cell sarcoma of the kidney. *J Radiol Case Rep.* 2011;5(2):8-12.

Lowe LH, Isuani BH, Heller RM, et al. Pediatric renal masses: Wilms tumor and beyond. *Radiographics.* 2000;20(6):1585-1603.

Son J, Lee EY, Restrepo R, et al. Focal renal lesions in pediatric patients. *AJR Am J Roentgenol.* 2012;199(6):W668-W682.

37   **Answer A.** Nephroblastomatosis refers to diffuse or multifocal areas of nephrogenic rests. Although nephrogenic rests can be classified histologically as dormant, sclerosing, hyperplastic, or neoplastic, these types cannot be differentiated by imaging. Anatomically, nephroblastomatosis can be separated into perilobar and intralobar types. Perilobar nephroblastomatosis presents as soft tissue nodules with mild contrast enhancement located at the peripheral portion of the kidney. Most cases of nephroblastomatosis occur sporadically. However, perilobar nephroblastomatosis is associated with Beckwith-Wiedemann syndrome, hemihypertrophy, and Perlman syndrome. Intralobar nephroblastomatosis usually occurs as a single poorly marginated mass that can be found anywhere in the kidney. It is associated with Drash syndrome, sporadic aniridia, and WAGR (Wilms tumor, aniridia, GU anomalies, and mental retardation) syndrome.

Most children with nephroblastomatosis do not develop Wilms tumor. However, 30% to 40% of Wilms tumors are thought to arise from nephrogenic rests. With bilateral Wilms tumors, nephrogenic rests are thought to be involved in as many as 99% of patients. Treatment of nephroblastomatosis is currently controversial, with some advocating chemotherapy, whereas others recommend close surveillance, preferably with MRI, which is more sensitive than US for detecting residual or recurrent nephroblastomatosis.

Reference: Son J, Lee EY, Restrepo R, et al. Focal renal lesions in pediatric patients. *AJR Am J Roentgenol.* 2012;199(6):W668-W682.

38 **Answer C.** The definition of a UTI is the presence of bacteria in the urine, but the term typically refers to infections of the lower urinary tract. Acute pyelonephritis is defined as UTI that involves the kidney. Young children with pyelonephritis often present with nonspecific symptoms such as fever, irritability, and vague abdominal pain. In older children, the findings may be more specific and include fever and associated flank pain. In patients in whom the diagnosis is straightforward, no imaging is needed in the acute phase, but patients are imaged later as part of the standard workup for a UTI to look for renal scarring. In patients in whom there is clinical difficulty in distinguishing an upper from a lower UTI, cortical scintigraphy with Tc-99m DMSA has been advocated as the most sensitive test. In cases of pyelonephritis, this study demonstrates single or multiple areas of lack of renal uptake of the radiotracer. These areas tend to be triangular and peripheral.

US with color Doppler flow is probably now the most common way that pyelonephritis is imaged and can show lack of color Doppler flow in the peripheral affected portions of the kidneys. Pyelonephritis is often not well characterized on routine gray-scale images. Therefore, most patients with clinically suspected acute pyelonephritis have negative US exams. When positive findings of pyelonephritis are found on gray-scale images, they can include congenital anomalies and a variety of changes in the renal parenchyma such as hydronephrosis, renal enlargement, loss of renal sinus fat because of edema, changes in echogenicity due to both edema (hypoechoic) and hemorrhage (hyperechoic), loss of corticomedullary differentiation, and abscess formation. Occasionally, areas of abnormal echogenicity can have a mass-like appearance.

Unenhanced CT is excellent for identifying urinary tract gas, calculi, hemorrhage, renal enlargement, inflammatory masses, and obstruction. Involved regions occasionally appear with lower attenuation related to edema; less frequently, they have pockets of higher attenuation that are thought to represent hemorrhage. The abovementioned findings are frequently absent, however, and unenhanced CT images may appear normal. It is only after contrast material is administered that the diagnostic features of acute bacterial nephritis are revealed. These features are better described in the explanation for Question 28.

Abdominal plain films may provide evidence of gas in the renal area in emphysematous pyelonephritis or abscess and the typical mass-like calcification in end-stage renal tuberculosis (putty kidney). However, there are pitfalls in diagnosing pyelonephritis on plain films such as differentiation of abdominal bowel gas from urinary tract gas and nonvisualization of small urinary tract calcifications overlying normally ossified structures such as the transverse processes of vertebral bodies.

References: Craig WD, Wagner BJ, Travis MD. Pyelonephritis: radiologic-pathologic review. *Radiographics.* 2008;28(1):255-277.

Navarro OM. Genitourinary. In: Donnelly LF, ed. *Fundamentals of Pediatric Imaging.* 3rd ed. Elsevier; 2022:139-174.

39 **Answer A.** The images shown were obtained using a pinhole collimator during a Tc-99m DMSA scan. There is a triangular-shaped photopenic defect in the cortex of the mid- to upper pole of the left kidney (long arrows). Given the clinical history of the patient, these findings are consistent with acute pyelonephritis although similar findings could be seen with chronic renal scarring. There is also some irregularity of the cortex of the lower pole of the left kidney (short arrow). The right kidney is normal.

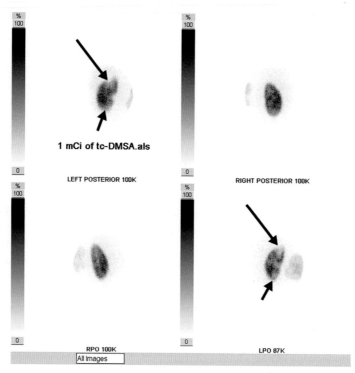

Reference: Navarro OM. Genitourinary. In: Donnelly LF, ed. *Fundamentals of Pediatric Imaging*. 3rd ed. Elsevier; 2022:139-174.

40 **Answer B.** US sensitivities for the diagnosis of adnexal torsion range from 46% to 74%. Investigators have evaluated the value of CT in the diagnosis of ovarian torsion because of its accessibility in emergent situations. However, exposure to pelvic irradiation makes this a less favorable imaging method in young women. MR has been found to be accurate in the diagnosis of adnexal torsion in the context of acute pelvic pain that presents rapidly over <4 hours with accuracies higher than 80%. A repeat US in 4 hours would not be indicated because this would cause a potential delay in the diagnosis of ovarian torsion, which is a surgical emergency. An abdominal radiograph would not be helpful in the diagnosis of ovarian torsion and would expose the patient to needless radiation.

Reference: Béranger-Gibert S, Sakly H, Ballester M, et al. Diagnostic value of MR imaging in the diagnosis of adnexal torsion. *Radiology*. 2016;279(2):461-470.

41 **Answer C.** Figure A is an axial T2-weighted image and Figure B is an axial T1 fat-saturated image obtained after the administration of IV contrast. The right ovary is asymmetrically enlarged when compared to the left ovary on both images. There is a lack of internal T2-weighted signal within the right ovary on the T2-weighted image and lack of internal contrast enhancement on the second image. The follicles within the right ovary are in a peripheral distribution. These features can be compared with the normal size, internal T2 signal, uniform follicle distribution, and internal contrast enhancement of the normal left ovary. The most common but fairly nonspecific finding of a torsed ovary is an enlarged ovary (>4.0 cm in maximal dimension), which is reliably seen both on CT and MRI. An enlarged ovary with a central afollicular stroma (resulting from hemorrhage and edema) and peripherally displaced follicles is a more specific feature of ovarian torsion and can sometimes be identified on contrast-enhanced CT or on fast spin-echo T2-weighted MRI. The torsed ovary is characterized by disrupted blood flow, which is seen as abnormal enhancement after IV contrast agent administration. Heterogeneous minimal or absent enhancement indicates the evolution of ovarian torsion from ischemia to infarction. However, the presence of enhancement does not exclude torsion because a twisted ovary, with its redundant blood supply, can appear to enhance normally, presumably because the torsion is intermittent or of recent onset.

Reference: Duigenan S, Oliva E, Lee SI. Ovarian torsion: diagnostic features on CT and MRI with pathologic correlation. *AJR Am J Roentgenol.* 2012;198(2):W122-W131.

42 **Answer B.** Twisting of the adnexal pedicle as occurs in ovarian torsion obstructs the lymphatic drainage, causing enlargement of the ovary. This is followed by obstruction of the venous drainage resulting in hemorrhagic infarction. Finally, the arterial supply is obstructed resulting in necrosis. This order of vascular compromise explains why vascular flow, especially arterial flow, may be present and detected by pelvic Doppler US examinations in torsed ovaries if the torsion is intermittent or early or partial torsion.

Reference: Reid JR, Paladin A, Davros W, et al. *Rotations in Radiology Pediatric Radiology.* Oxford University Press; 2013.

43 **Answer C.** The US images of the kidneys demonstrate diffusely increased echogenicity of the medullary pyramids bilaterally consistent with medullary nephrocalcinosis. The most common metabolic abnormality responsible for histologic changes in the pyramids that may be depicted as increased echogenicity at sonography is nephrocalcinosis. Nephrocalcinosis primarily affects the renal pyramids, but it can occasionally be appreciated in the cortex as well. Although nephrocalcinosis may eventually progress to involve most of the pyramid, acoustic shadowing is rarely seen. The lack of shadowing may reflect the way in which the calcium is laid down within the pyramid. Acoustic shadowing may be appreciated only in rare cases of extreme involvement of the pyramids or if there is development of associated calculi in the adjacent calices.

There are numerous causes for medullary nephrocalcinosis in children. Most of these conditions are associated with hypercalciuria and include distal renal tubular acidosis and prolonged immobilization.

Reference: Daneman A, Navarro OM, Somers GR, et al. Renal pyramids: focused sonography of normal and pathologic processes. *Radiographics.* 2010;30(5):1287-1307.

44 **Answer C.** In children, the left and right kidney should generally measure within 1 cm of each other. If there is a discrepancy of more than 1 cm, an underlying abnormality should be suspected. Such discrepancies may result from a disorder that causes one of the kidneys to be too small, such as global scarring, or from a process that causes one of the kidneys to be too large, such as renal duplication or acute pyelonephritis. In every case, it is important to compare the patient's renal length with tables that plot normal renal length against age.

Reference: Navarro OM. Genitourinary. In: Donnelly LF, ed. *Fundamentals of Pediatric Imaging.* 3rd ed. Elsevier; 2022:139-174.

45 **Answer C.** The transverse US image shown demonstrates a normal echotexture of both testes, but there is a lack of color Doppler flow in the right testis. These findings are consistent with acute right-sided testicular torsion, and the patient will require prompt diagnosis and treatment as preservation of the affected testis is usually only possible within 6 to 10 hours after onset.

In the early phases of torsion (1-3 hours), testicular echogenicity appears normal. With progression, enlargement of the affected testis and increased or heterogeneous echogenicity are common findings. Testicular viability can be suggested from gray-scale and color Doppler findings. Normal echogenicity with mild testicular enlargement is a good sign of viability, whereas marked enlargement, heterogeneous echotexture, and scrotal wall hypervascularity are signs of testicular infarction and necrosis. In addition, the whirlpool sign, which is an abrupt spiral twist in the course of the spermatic cord at the external ring or in the scrotum, can be seen on testicular US exams. This finding is considered a direct sign of testicular torsion. Note that blood flow can be present in an incompletely torsed testis, although it is usually decreased when compared with a contralateral normal testicle.

Demonstration of blood flow within a normal testis is more difficult in children <2 years of age. Gray-scale US may demonstrate asymmetric enlargement and slightly decreased echogenicity of a torsed testis in this age group. Advanced findings in young children that occur with progressive ischemia and infarction are like those for older patients. These include hemorrhage and necrosis, which may cause increasing asymmetric heterogeneity of the affected testis.

References: Aso C, Enríquez G, Fité M, et al. Gray-scale and color Doppler sonography of scrotal disorders in children: an update. *Radiographics*. 2005;25(5):1197-1214.

Navarro OM. Genitourinary. In: Donnelly LF, ed. *Fundamentals of Pediatric Imaging*. 3rd ed. Elsevier; 2022:139-174.

46 **Answer C.** The US image demonstrates an anechoic fluid tract extending from the anterosuperior aspect of the urinary bladder on the right of the image to the umbilicus, which is on the left of the image (arrow). This is consistent with a urachal remnant. The urachus, or median umbilical ligament, is a midline tubular structure that extends upward from the anterior dome of the bladder toward the umbilicus. It is a vestigial remnant of at least two embryonic structures: the cloaca, which is the cephalic extension of the urogenital sinus (a precursor of the fetal bladder), and the allantois, which is a derivative of the yolk sac. The tubular urachus normally involutes before birth, remaining as a fibrous band with no known function. However, persistence of an embryonic urachal remnant can give rise to various clinical problems, not only in infants and children but also in adults.

Congenital urachal anomalies are twice as common in men as in women. There are four types of congenital urachal anomalies: patent urachus, umbilical-urachal sinus, vesicourachal diverticulum, and urachal cyst. A patent urachus is purely congenital and accounts for about 50% of all cases of congenital anomalies. An umbilical-urachal sinus (15% of cases), vesicourachal diverticulum (3% to 5% of cases), or urachal cyst (about 30% of cases) may close normally after birth but then reopen in association with pathologic conditions that are often categorized as acquired diseases.

Most patients with urachal abnormalities (except those with a patent urachus) are asymptomatic. However, they may become symptomatic if these abnormalities are associated with infection. If a persistent communication exists between the bladder lumen and the umbilicus, urine leakage is usually noted during the neonatal period. Although the normal urachus is most commonly lined by transitional epithelium, urachal carcinoma predominantly manifests as adenocarcinoma (90% of cases), probably because of the metaplasia of the urachal mucosa into columnar epithelium followed by malignant transformation; conversely, 34% of bladder adenocarcinomas are of urachal origin. These tumors are mostly seen in patients 40 to 70 years of age, two-thirds of whom are men.

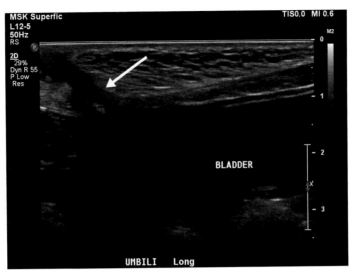

Reference: Yu JS, Kim KW, Lee HJ, et al. Urachal remnant diseases: spectrum of CT and US findings. *Radiographics*. 2001;21(2):451-461.

47 **Answer C.** The images shown demonstrate a horseshoe kidney (HSK). Fusion between the lower poles of each kidney is known to be the most common (>90%) fusion type in HSK. Fusion of the upper poles of each kidney (inverted U shape) is extremely rare.

Wilms tumor has been reported to be the most common type of renal tumor in children with HSK. The incidence of renal tumors arising from HSK has been studied in adult populations and RCC has been found to be the most common. The incidence of RCC in patients with HSK is equal to that in the healthy population; however, the incidence of Wilms tumor in patients with HSK is two times higher than that in the general population.

Patients with HSK are susceptible to associated renal complications. This is due to the abnormal ureteral course secondary to abnormal renal rotation and the relatively high position of the UPJs. The abnormal ureteral course can result in ureteral obstruction or slow drainage of urine (or both), which can lead to hydronephrosis, infections, and stones.

In addition to renal complications, patients with HSK are also prone to extrarenal complications. In one study of patients with HSK, various extrarenal diseases and syndromes were noted to occur in half of the patients studied. These included spinal and pelvic diseases such as vertebral anomalies, anorectal malformations, GU disease, cloacal anomalies, and VATER-VACTERL (Vertebral, Anorectal, Cardiac, TracheoEsophageal, Renal, and Limb anomalies) association. In another study, HSK was known to occur in patients with Turner syndrome, Down syndrome, and Edward syndrome. In other studies, HSK cases were associated with a vertebral anomaly, congenital disease, and Turner syndrome.

Reference: Je BK, Kim HK, Horn PS. Incidence and spectrum of renal complications and extrarenal diseases and syndromes in 380 children and young adults with horseshoe kidney. *AJR Am J Roentgenol*. 2015;205(6):1306-1314.

48 **Answer A.** HSK is a congenital anomaly occurring during the embryonic period of fetal development. Starting at the fourth week of gestation, two embryologic kidneys, known as metanephrons, are located in close proximity in the pelvis. During the seventh and eighth weeks of gestation, the normal kidneys start to ascend from the pelvis and rotate to face medially. However, when an HSK ascends, the inferior mesenteric artery (IMA) inhibits superior migration and rotation of the HSK by blocking the isthmus. On the MR image, a flow void from the IMA (arrow) is seen which drapes over the isthmus of the HSK. Ultimately, the isthmus becomes trapped below the IMA, resulting in a position of the HSK at the level of L3 or lower in the pelvis. In this circumstance, the renal pelvis faces anteriorly instead of medially. Theoretically, HSKs can be found at any location along the path of normal renal ascent from the pelvis to the midabdomen. However, in one study, 98.9% of the HSKs were located at or around the origin of IMA from the aorta, and 1.1% remained in the pelvis.

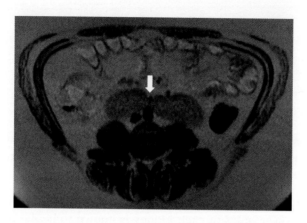

Reference: Je BK, Kim HK, Horn PS. Incidence and spectrum of renal complications and extrarenal diseases and syndromes in 380 children and young adults with horseshoe kidney. *AJR Am J Roentgenol.* 2015;205(6):1306-1314.

49 **Answer D.** An autoamputated wandering calcified ovary (AWCO) is an extremely rare cause of abdominal calcification in the pediatric population. Torsion of an ovary or an ovarian lesion and the adnexa can lead to infarction and necrosis and subsequent amputation of the ovary. An amputated ovary becomes calcified (dystrophic calcification) and may freely float in the peritoneal cavity, which explains why the calcification is noted in the left side of the pelvis (white arrow) on the plain film and in the right side of the pelvis on the CT scan (black arrow). In most cases, a blunt-ending fallopian tube is noted on the involved side as is seen in the left adnexa on the MR image (white arrow). Note that the right ovary is visualized and intact and demonstrates a normal appearance (black arrow). In premenopausal women, the ovaries are usually easily recognized at MRI as ovoid structures with intermediate T2 signal intensity and with high T2 signal intensity follicles. There is no evidence of fat surrounding the calcified ovary on the CT scan as would be found in an ovarian dermoid.

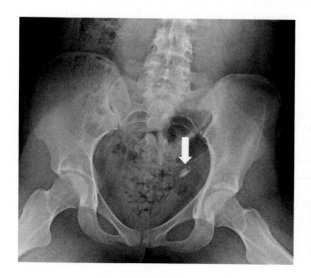

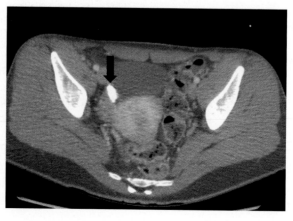

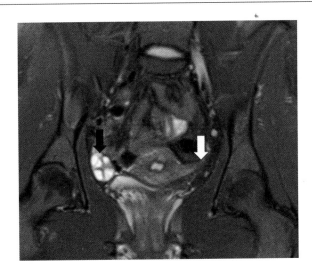

References: Mahajan PS, Ahamad N, Hussain SA. First report of MRI findings in a case of an autoamputated wandering calcified ovary. *Int Med Case Rep J*. 2014;7:49-52.

Nougaret S, Nikolovski I, Paroder V, et al. MRI of tumors and tumor mimics in female pelvis: anatomic pelvic space-based approach. *Radiographics*. 2019;39(4):1205-1229.

Outwater EK, Siegelman ES, Hunt JL. Ovarian teratomas: tumor types and imaging characteristics. *Radiographics*. 2001;21(2):475-490.

50 **Answer D.** The images shown were obtained after contrast administration during a ceVUS exam, which is a well-established, sensitive, and safe US method for detecting and grading VUR and urethral imaging in children. This method does not utilize ionizing radiation in contrast to fluoroscopy and nuclear medicine scintigraphy, which are other modalities used in evaluating for VUR. In 2016, the U.S. Food and Drug Administration (FDA) approved the UCA Lumason (Bracco Diagnostics, Monroe Township, NJ) for pediatric intravesical applications, which is the contrast agent typically administered for these examinations. The images of the kidneys below show a gray-scale image of each kidney with nondilated collecting systems and an adjacent image obtained after administration of contrast agent showing dilated collecting systems consistent with VUR. The bladder is filled with contrast material on the image shown below.

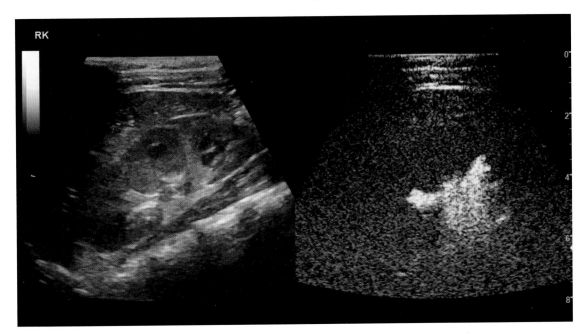

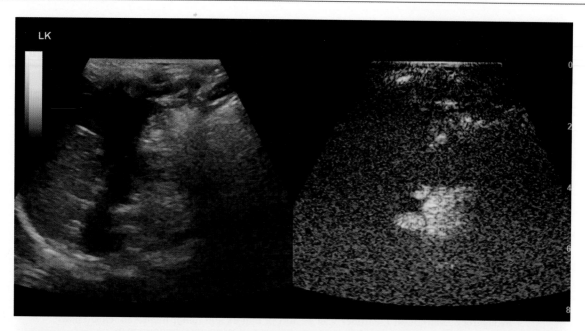

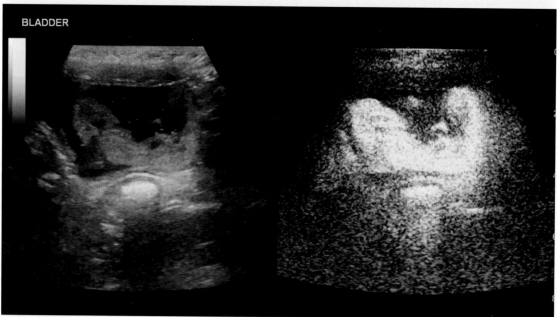

Reference: Toulia A, Aguirre Pascual E, Back SJ, et al. Contrast-enhanced voiding urosonography, part 1: vesicoureteral reflux evaluation. *Pediatr Radiol.* 2021;51(12):2351-2367.

51 **Answer B.** In 2014, a multidisciplinary consensus on the classification of pre- and postnatal urinary tract dilatation (UTD) was developed. Its goal was to provide a standardized system for evaluating and reporting UTD both in the prenatal and postnatal periods with the purpose of determining which children have obstructive uropathy. Other than normal, there are two antenatal categories (UTD A1 and A2-3) and three postnatal categories (UTD P1, P2, and P3). The six common urinary tract descriptors regardless of age are: the anterior-posterior renal pelvic diameter (APRPD), presence or absence of central or central and peripheral calyceal dilatation, renal parenchymal thickness (normal or abnormal), renal parenchymal echogenicity (normal or abnormal), ureteral dilatation (present or absent), and bladder abnormality (present or absent). In this classification system, an APRPD less than 10 mm is normal.

References: Nguyen HT, Benson CB, Bromley B, et al. Multidisciplinary consensus on the classification of prenatal and postnatal urinary tract dilation (UTD classification system). *J Pediatr Urol.* 2014;10(6):982-998.

Nguyen HT, Phelps A, Coley B, et al. 2021 update on the urinary tract dilation (UTD) classification system: clarifications, review of the literature, and practical suggestions. *Pediatr Radiol.* 2022;52:740-751.

52 **Answer B.** The US images demonstrate a heterogeneous, primarily hypoechoic, and ill-defined lesion with calcification and internal vascular flow. Given the clinical history and imaging findings, this lesion is most consistent with a testicular tumor. A painless scrotal mass is the most frequent clinical presentation. US is the best imaging modality to study testicular tumors. A benign tumor is suggested when US shows a mainly cystic component, well-defined borders, echogenic rim, or normal to increased echogenicity lesion when compared to the healthy testicular parenchyma. A malignant tumor is suspected when US shows an inhomogeneous, hypoechoic, poorly circumscribed, and/or diffusely infiltrative lesion. However, these US findings may overlap.

Most intratesticular neoplasms in children (>90%) are germ cell tumors with a stratification according to age. In the first decade of life, yolk sac tumors and teratomas are the most common types, whereas in the second decade, choriocarcinoma is the most common intratesticular neoplasm. Malignant germ cell tumors spread first via the lymphatic system usually through the inguinal ring and spermatic cord to the retroperitoneum. Therefore, an MR or CT examination of the abdomen and pelvis should be performed to evaluate for metastatic disease after diagnosis. Choriocarcinoma has an early hematogenous spread and chest CT is necessary to evaluate for pulmonary metastatic disease when this tumor is diagnosed. There are no specific US findings that suggest a specific histologic diagnosis. Less than 10% of testicular tumors in children are metastatic disease from leukemia or lymphoma. Most extratesticular and not intratesticular scrotal neoplasms in children are due to embryonal rhabdomyosarcomas.

References: Navarro OM. Genitourinary. In: Donnelly LF, ed. *Fundamentals of Pediatric Imaging.* 3rd ed. Elsevier; 2022:139-174.

Sangüesa C, Veiga D, Llavador M, Serrano A. Testicular tumours in children: an approach to diagnosis and management with pathologic correlation. *Insights Imaging.* 2020;11(1):74.

QUESTIONS

1 An 8-year-old male with a history of hip pain presents with a frontal radiograph of the pelvis.

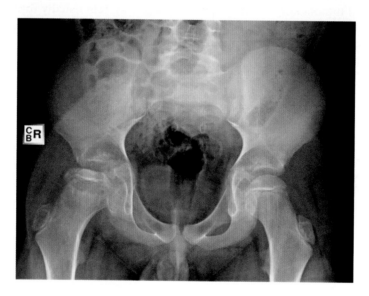

What is the most likely diagnosis?

A. Developmental dysplasia of the hip
B. Slipped capital femoral epiphysis
C. Legg-Calvé-Perthes disease
D. Osteomyelitis

2 What is the stage of the disease in Question 1?

A. Stage 1
B. Stage 2
C. Stage 3
D. Stage 4

3 A 7-year-old male with knee pain presents with an AP radiograph and a coronal image from an MRI of the same knee.

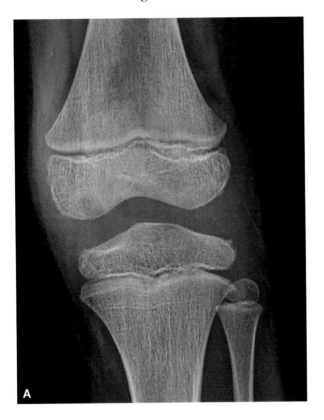

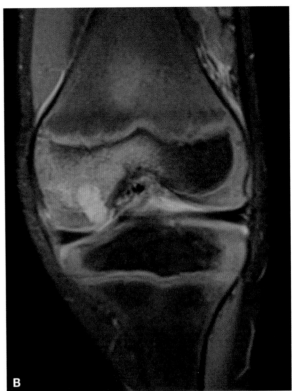

What is the most likely diagnosis?

A. Chondroblastoma
B. Osteomyelitis
C. Osteoid osteoma
D. OCD

4 In what location does osteomyelitis occur most often in children?

A. Metaphysis
B. Diaphysis
C. Epiphysis
D. Intra-articular

5 Osteoarticular osteomyelitis in young children (<4 years of age) involving the epiphyseal cartilage is suggestive of which causative organism?

A. *Staphylococcus aureus*
B. *Streptococcus*
C. *Kingella kingae*
D. *Pseudomonas*

6   A child presents with a radiograph of the elbow following trauma.

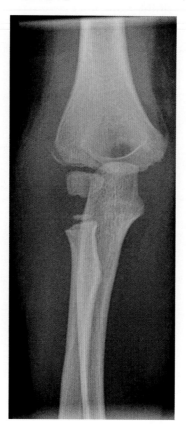

What is the diagnosis?

A. Lateral condylar fracture
B. Supracondylar fracture
C. Medial condylar fracture
D. Lateral epicondylar fracture
E. Medical epicondylar fracture

7   What is the most common age at which the fracture seen in Question 6 occurs?

A. 0 to 3 years
B. 3 to 6 years
C. 5 to 10 years
D. 10 to 15 years

8   The fracture in Question 6 most commonly represents which Salter-Harris fracture type?

A. Salter-Harris II
B. Salter-Harris III
C. Salter-Harris IV
D. Salter-Harris V

9 A 2-year-old with a history of abnormal knee alignment presents with the following radiograph of the knee.

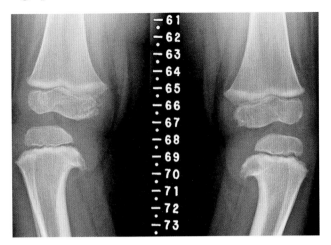

What is the diagnosis?

A. Genu varum
B. Blount disease
C. Rickets
D. Epiphyseal dysplasia

10 Which of the following is an imaging characteristic of the disorder in Question 9?

A. Fracture of the distal femoral metaphysis
B. Absence of the cruciate ligaments
C. Tibial hemimelia
D. Hypertrophy of the medial meniscus

11 A 13-year-old boy with subacute hip pain and joint stiffness presents with an MRI of the pelvis and hip.

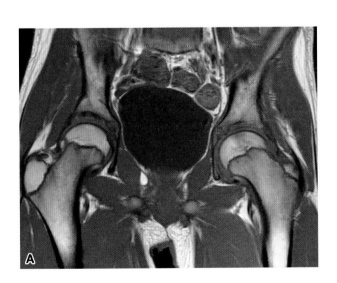
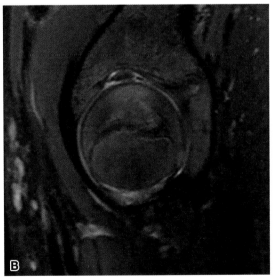

What is the diagnosis?

A. Avascular necrosis
B. Osteomyelitis
C. Idiopathic chondrolysis
D. Bone contusion

12 A 12-year-old male with knee pain presents for a whole-body MRI.

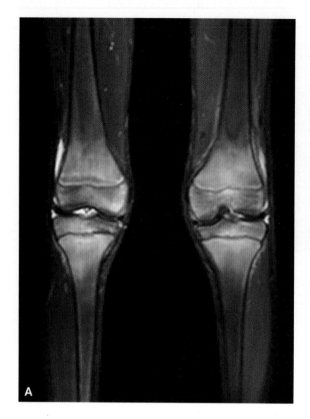 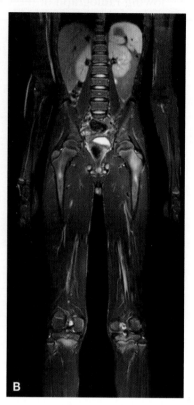

What is the most likely diagnosis?

A. Leukemia
B. Rickets
C. Metastasis
D. Chronic recurrent multifocal osteomyelitis

13 What is the most common location of the bone in the disorder in Question 12?

A. Epiphysis
B. Metaphysis
C. Diaphysis

14 Which of the following conditions is associated with the disorder in Question 12?

A. Autosomal recessive polycystic kidney disease (ARPKD)
B. Wegener granulomatosis
C. Truncus arteriosus
D. Chondroblastoma

15 A child with a history of a congenital foot abnormality presents with the following radiograph.

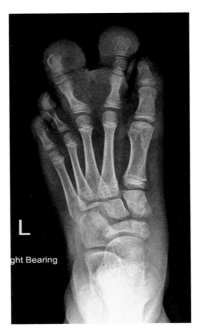

What is the diagnosis?

A. Proteus syndrome
B. Macrodystrophia lipomatosa
C. Neurofibromatosis
D. Hemihypertrophy

16 The following babygram was performed on a stillborn neonate.

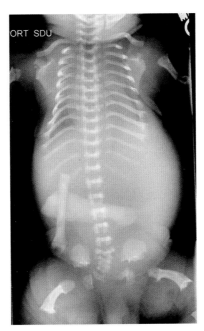

What is the diagnosis?

A. Achondroplasia
B. Jeune syndrome
C. Thanatophoric dysplasia
D. Osteogenesis imperfecta

17 A central nervous system abnormality associated with the disorder in Question 16 is which of the following?

A. Tethered cord
B. Ocular nerve enlargement
C. Megalencephaly
D. Basal ganglia calcification

18 An adolescent with elbow pain presents with a frontal radiograph of the elbow and sagittal MR image from a fluid-sensitive sequence of the elbow.

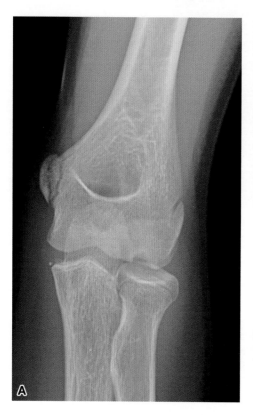 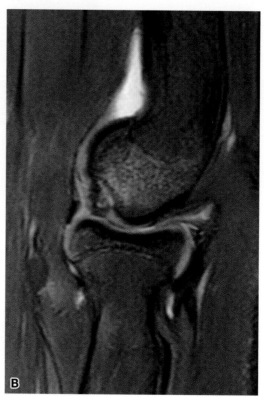

What is the diagnosis?

A. Osteomyelitis
B. Avascular necrosis
C. Osteoid osteoma
D. Osteochondritis dissecans

19 The disorder in Question 18 has a high prevalence of which of the following?

A. Radial head subluxation
B. Supracondylar fracture
C. Olecranon bursitis
D. Lateral epicondylitis

20 In the diagnosis in Question 18, which of the following is a criterion on MRI to diagnose an unstable lesion?

A. Focal defect of 5 mm or more in the meniscus adjacent to the lesion
B. Thin line of hyperintensity within the metaphysis of the bone
C. Small cystic focus of 5 mm or greater in the articular surface of the lesion
D. Low signal extending through the articular cartilage

21 An 8-year-old presents with left hip pain. The following radiograph of the pelvis was performed.

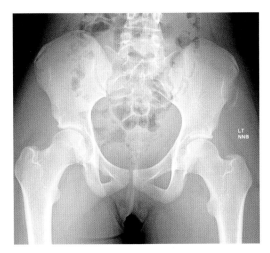

What is the diagnosis?

A. Avulsion of the anterior inferior iliac spine
B. Avulsion of the anterior superior iliac spine
C. Nondisplaced fracture of the femoral neck
D. Fracture of the anterior column of the acetabulum
E. Fracture of the posterior column of the acetabulum

22 Which of the following is *true*?

A. Avulsion from the anterior superior iliac spine is related to the adductor muscles.
B. Avulsion of the anterior inferior iliac spine is related to the hamstrings.
C. Avulsion of the greater trochanter is related to the rectus femoris.
D. Avulsion of the lesser trochanter is related to the iliopsoas muscle.

23 Frontal and lateral radiographs of the tibia/fibula were performed in an infant who presents with skull fracture.

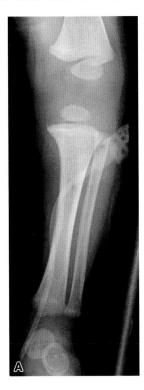
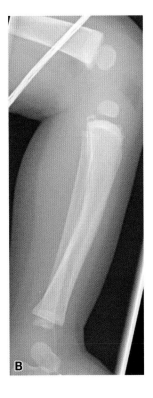

What is the diagnosis?

A. Toddler's fracture
B. Metaphyseal corner fracture
C. Buckle fracture
D. Triplane fracture

24 The mechanism of the fracture in Question 23 is which of the following?

A. Direct trauma to the bone
B. Shearing injury
C. Insufficiency fracture
D. Bending injury

25 Which of the following imaging findings is commonly associated with nonaccidental injury (child abuse)?

A. Buckle fracture of the distal radius
B. Toddler's fracture of the tibia
C. Medial epicondyle avulsion fracture
D. Posterior rib fractures

26 The preferred initial imaging evaluation of infants with suspected nonaccidental injury (child abuse) is:

A. Radiographical skeletal survey
B. Radiographs at site of suspected injury only
C. Whole-body MRI examination
D. Sonographic skeletal survey

27 The following radiograph of the forearm was performed in a patient with a history of an arm deformity.

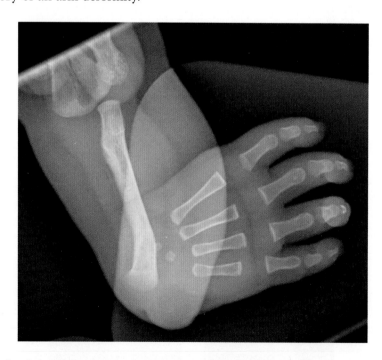

Which of the following is *true* concerning radial dysplasia?

A. It is associated with hypoplasia of the thumb.
B. On physical examination, there is ulnar and palmar deviation of the hand.
C. Development of the radius occurs between the 10th and 12th week of gestation.
D. Bilateral radial dysplasia occurs in <10% of affected children.

28 Which of the following syndromes is associated with radial dysplasia?

A. Holt-Oram syndrome
B. Trisomy 21
C. Achondroplasia
D. Ehlers-Danlos syndrome

29 A teenager presents with right shoulder pain. The following radiograph was obtained.

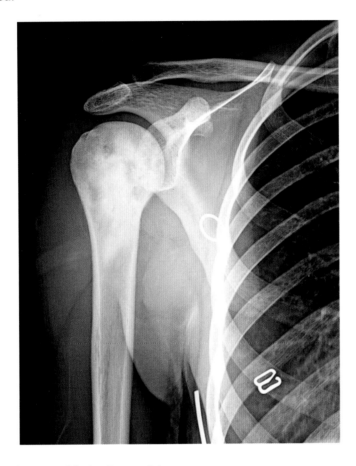

What is the most likely diagnosis?

A. Chondroblastoma
B. Osteoid osteoma
C. Fibrous dysplasia
D. Rhabdomyosarcoma
E. Osteosarcoma

30 When imaging the lesion in Question 29, it is important to image the complete long bone from the proximal joint to the distal joint because:

A. A malignant joint effusion is common and should be evaluated.
B. Skip metastases can be seen in this lesion and should be evaluated.
C. Articular dislocations are common and should be evaluated.
D. Invasion of the ligaments of the joint is common and should be evaluated.

31 Where is the most common site of relapse of the lesion in Question 29?

A. Locally within the bone
B. Lung parenchyma
C. Liver
D. Lymph nodes

32 An 8-week-old infant presents with an abnormal hip click on physical examination. What imaging examination is recommended for further evaluation of this infant?

A. Radiograph of the hips
B. MRI of the hips
C. Ultrasound of the hips
D. CT of the hips

33 The following sonographic image of the hip was obtained in an infant.

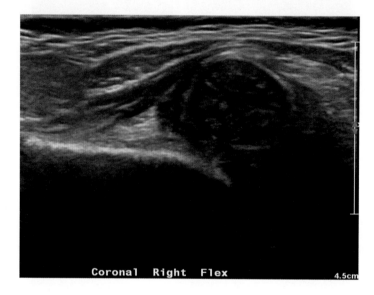

What is the diagnosis?

A. Avascular necrosis
B. Developmental hip dysplasia
C. Traumatic dislocation
D. Transient synovitis

34 Which of the following is a risk factor for developing the condition in Question 33?

A. Congenital heart disease
B. Surfactant deficiency disorder
C. Posterior urethral valves
D. Foot deformity

35 The following frontal radiograph of the thoracolumbar spine was obtained.

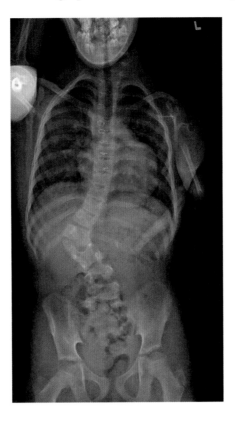

What is the diagnosis?

A. Levoscoliosis of the thoracolumbar spine *without* a vertebral anomaly
B. Levoscoliosis of the thoracolumbar spine *with* a vertebral anomaly
C. Dextroscoliosis of the thoracolumbar spine *without* a vertebral anomaly
D. Dextroscoliosis of the thoracolumbar spine *with* a vertebral anomaly

36 Which of the following concerning structural and nonstructural scoliotic curves is *true*?

A. A structural curve is correctable with ipsilateral bending.
B. A structural curve has vertebral morphologic changes such as wedging and rotation.
C. A nonstructural curve never progresses to a structural curve.
D. A Cobb angle of 15 degrees or more on ipsilateral side-bending views differentiates a structural curve from a nonstructural curve.

37 At what Cobb angle is bracing recommended for treatment of adolescent scoliosis?

A. 10 to 35 degrees
B. 20 to 45 degrees
C. 30 to 55 degrees
D. 40 to 65 degrees

38 A 3-year-old child presents with a limp. The following frontal and lateral radiographs were performed.

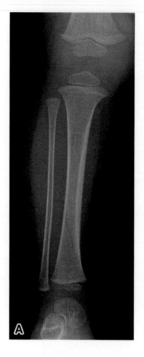 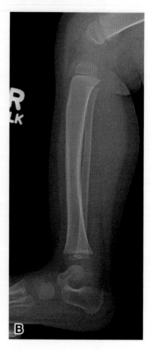

What is the diagnosis?

A. Toddler's fracture of the tibia
B. Buckle fracture of the proximal tibia
C. Buckle fracture of the distal tibia
D. Avulsion fracture of the medial malleolus of the distal tibia

39 A child presents with a short leg. The following radiograph was performed.

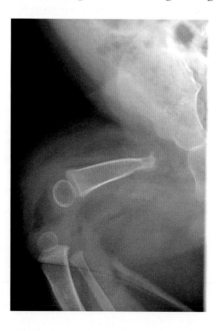

What is the diagnosis?

A. Achondroplasia
B. Osteonecrosis
C. Rhabdomyosarcoma
D. Proximal focal femoral deficiency disorder

40 Which of the following is associated with the disorder in Question 39?

A. Congenital syringomyelia
B. Neuroblastoma
C. Coxa valga deformity
D. Absent cruciate ligaments

41 Frontal and oblique radiographs of the left foot were obtained in a teenager with chronic foot pain.

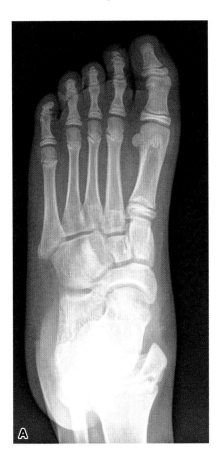 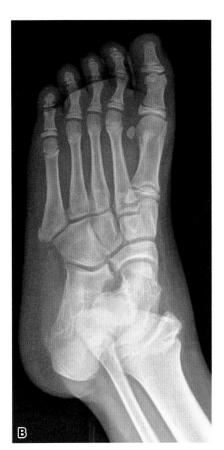

What is the diagnosis?

A. Cuboid fracture
B. Tarsal coalition
C. Equinovarus foot
D. Plantar fasciitis
E. Septic arthritis

42 The condition in Question 41 is bilateral in approximately what percentage of affected individuals?

A. 20%
B. 50%
C. 70%
D. 90%

43 A child with a history of multiple fractures presents with the following radiograph.

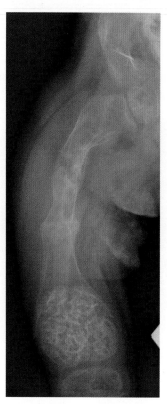

What is the most likely diagnosis?

A. Rickets
B. Scurvy
C. Chronic recurrent multifocal osteomyelitis
D. Osteogenesis imperfecta

44 Which of the following in regard to the diagnosis in Question 43 is the lethal form of the disease due to respiratory insufficiency?

A. Type I
B. Type II
C. Type III
D. Type IV
E. Type V

45 Following treatment, this patient developed dense metaphyseal lines (arrow) within the long bones and a "bone within a bone pattern" within the spine and flat bones. What treatment did this patient receive?

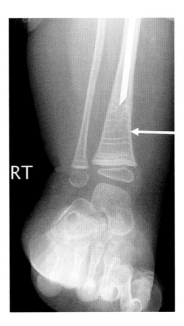

A. NSAID therapy
B. Metronidazole therapy
C. Calcium therapy
D. Bisphosphonate therapy

46 What is the most likely diagnosis?

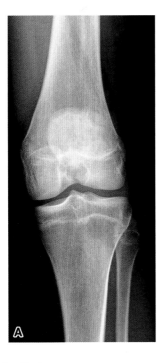 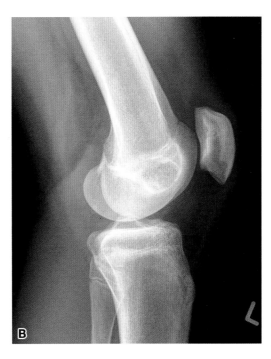

A. Ewing sarcoma
B. Osteosarcoma
C. Fibrous dysplasia
D. Chondroblastoma

47 What is the treatment of the lesion seen in Question 46?

A. Chemotherapy followed by above-the-knee amputation (AKA)

B. Chemotherapy followed by local resection

C. Curettage and bone grafting

D. Chemotherapy only

48 The following sonographic examination was performed of both the right and left hip in an 8-year-old child with hip pain.

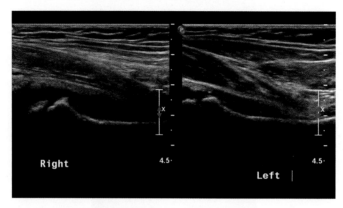

What is the most likely diagnosis?

A. Transient synovitis

B. Fracture of the radial neck

C. Slipped capital femoral epiphysis

D. Osteoid osteoma

49 A child presents with chronic pain in the left knee. Frontal and lateral radiographs of the left knee were performed.

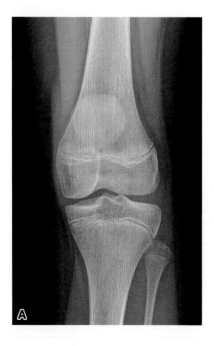 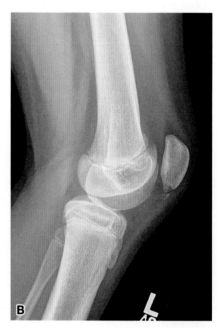

What is the most likely diagnosis?

A. Sinding-Larsen-Johansson syndrome

B. Osgood-Schlatter disease

C. Patellar sleeve avulsion fracture

D. Bipartite patella

50 Which of the following is *true* regarding the diagnosis in Question 49?

    A. It is an osteochondrosis due to traction of the quadriceps tendon.

    B. It most commonly occurs between the ages of 14 and 18 years.

    C. On MRI evaluation, bone marrow edema may be seen in the anterior tibial tubercle.

    D. Initial treatment is rest and NSAIDs.

51 A neonate presents with the following radiographs of the right and left forearm.

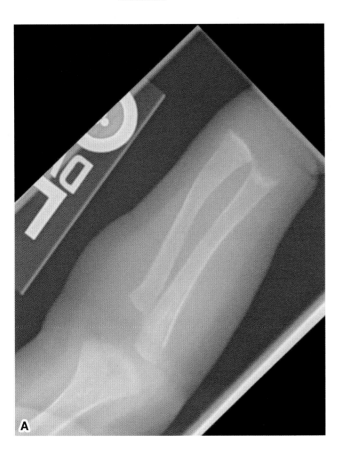
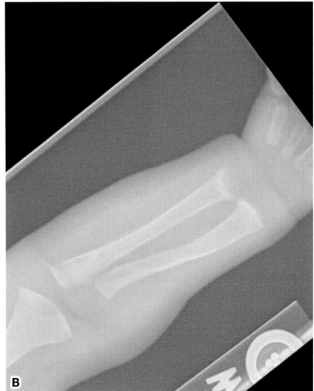

What is the most likely diagnosis?

    A. Legg-Calvé-Perthes disease

    B. Rickets

    C. Scurvy

    D. Osteomyelitis

    E. Osteopetrosis

52 The pathophysiology of the diagnosis in Question 51 is the following:

    A. Vitamin A deficiency

    B. Vitamin C deficiency

    C. Vitamin D deficiency

    D. Vitamin E deficiency

53 A child presents with deformity of the left scapula.

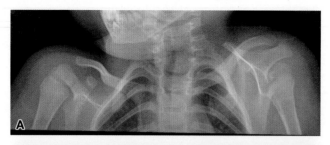

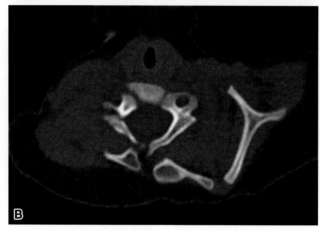

There is a high position of the left scapula. What is this deformity referred to?

A. Osteogenesis imperfecta
B. Osteochondromatosis
C. Paget deformity
D. Sprengel deformity

54 The images in Question 53 also demonstrate this additional finding.

A. Omovertebral bone
B. Butterfly vertebral body
C. Spina bifida
D. Hemivertebrae

55 What syndrome is this imaging finding in Question 53 associated with?

A. Jeune syndrome
B. Ellis-van Creveld syndrome
C. Klippel-Feil syndrome
D. Li-Fraumeni syndrome

56 A neonate presents for evaluation of a suspected skeletal dysplasia. Selected images from a skeletal survey are shown below.

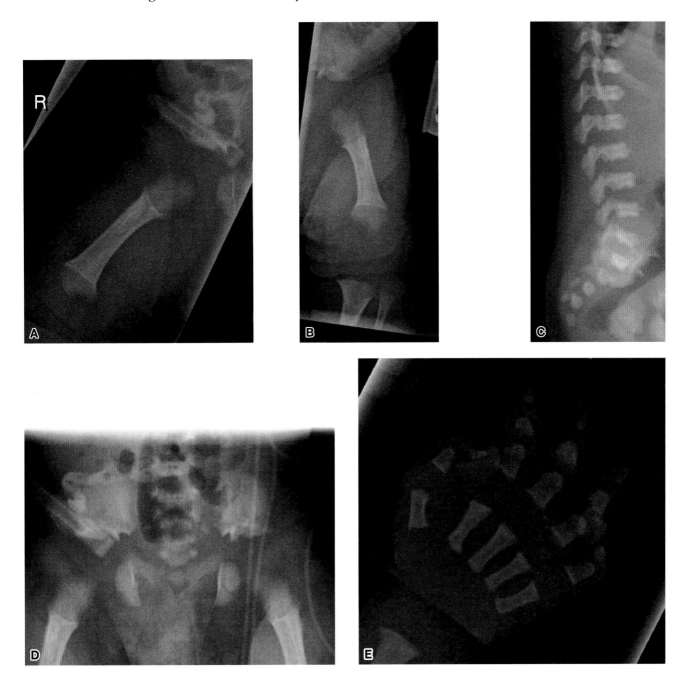

What is the most likely diagnosis?

A. Thanatophoric dysplasia

B. Osteogenesis imperfecta

C. Achondroplasia

D. Ellis-van Creveld syndrome

ANSWERS AND EXPLANATIONS

1 **Answer C.** Legg-Calvé-Perthes (LCP) disease is the result of idiopathic, avascular necrosis of the developing proximal femoral epiphysis that often presents between 4 and 8 years of age. There are four stages of pathogenesis with radiographic correlation: avascularity, revascularization, healing, and residual deformity.

The radiographic pattern of a dense, flattened femoral epiphysis (arrow) with normal acetabular morphology is the imaging hallmark of LCP, thus excluding hip dysplasia as a diagnosis. Slipped capital femoral epiphysis typically occurs in older children (mean age of 13 years), and radiographs reveal an irregularity of the physis that is more pronounced on frog-leg lateral projections. Osteomyelitis of the hip may result in a dense irregular epiphysis. However, there is typically an aggressive, osteolytic appearance to the proximal femur with involvement of the entire hip joint and rapid destruction if not treated urgently.

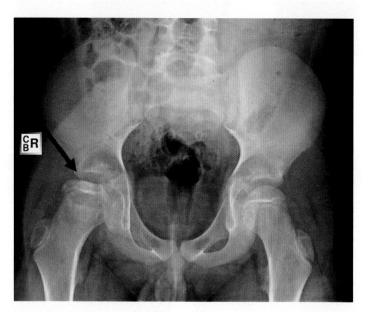

References: Dillman JR, Hernandez RJ. MRI of Legg-Calvé-Perthes disease. *AJR Am J Roentgenol.* 2009;193(5):1394-1407.

Resnick D. *Osteochondroses in Diagnosis of Bone and Joint Disorders.* 4th ed. WB Saunders and Company; 2002:3686-3741.

Salter RB. *Textbook of Disorders and Injuries of the Musculoskeletal System.* 3rd ed. Williams & Wilkins; 1999:339-350.

2 **Answer C.** This case represents a late healing stage of legg-calve-perthes (LCP) disease with dense bone replacing trabecular bone at the middle pillar of the epiphysis. The initial stage 1 of avascularity is radiographically occult. A symptomatic child with normal radiographs may be further evaluated by MRI with a high sensitivity for detecting osteonecrosis, marrow edema, and hip effusion. The figure below represents the different stages of LCP disease. The earliest radiographic finding of a relatively dense epiphysis represents stage 2, revascularization. At this time, children are often asymptomatic. The "crescent sign" that is sometimes seen at stage 2 results from a pathologic, subchondral fracture of the anterosuperior epiphysis (see arrow in **A**). Stage 4 reveals a chronic, residual deformity of the femoral head, often with collapse, fragmentation, and lateral subluxation. Additional findings during disease progression may include a cystic lucency of the subphyseal femoral neck (see arrow in **B**) and coxa magna with a short and widened femoral metaphysis.

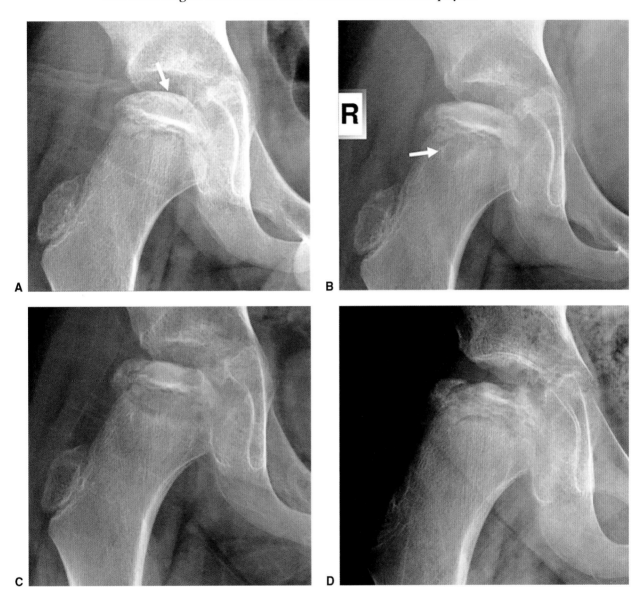

Stages of LCP disease on radiograph. **A:** 2 months; **B:** 4 months; **C:** 7 months; **D:** 10 months.

References: Dillman JR, Hernandez RJ. MRI of Legg-Calvé-Perthes disease. *AJR Am J Roentgenol.* 2009;193(5):1394-1407.

Resnick D. *Osteochondroses in Diagnosis of Bone and Joint Disorders.* 4th ed. WB Saunders and Company; 2002:3686-3741.

Salter RB. *Textbook of Disorders and Injuries of the Musculoskeletal System.* 3rd ed. Williams & Wilkins; 1999:339-350.

3 **Answer B.** The radiograph reveals a geographic, lytic lesion without sclerotic margins (arrows in Figure A and B) involving the epiphysis of the knee, the differential diagnosis of which includes both chondroblastoma and osteomyelitis. However, most chondroblastomas demonstrate a thin sclerotic margin radiographically.

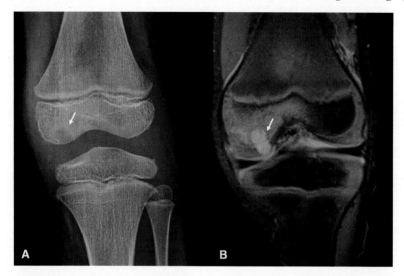

Osteoid osteomas classically appear as a central, lucent lesion or nidus that is often cortically based but can occur in subchondral, intra-articular locations. Nonetheless, absent any surrounding cortical hyperostosis, an osteoid osteoma is unlikely. An osteochondral defect (OCD) should have an irregular fracture lucency, often with sclerotic margins abutting a fragment of subchondral bone, all of which are not present in this case.

The MRI appearance of a fluid signal, solitary lytic lesion centered at the distal epiphysis and cartilage (arrow) with surrounding reactive marrow signal is highly suggestive of osteomyelitis. Rim enhancement of the lytic lesion (not shown) would then suggest an associated abscess. Chondroblastomas also have surrounding T2 hyperintense marrow signal. However, the lesion itself is characteristically lobular with internal matrix that is T2 isointense/hypointense, not present in this case.

Understanding the imaging findings of osteomyelitis is important as the classic clinical history of fever, elevated white blood cell count, and inflammatory markers is not always present.

References: Guillerman RP. Osteomyelitis and beyond. *Pediatr Radiol.* 2013;43(1):S193-S203.

Lyer RS, Chapman T, Chew FS. Pediatric bone imaging: diagnostic imaging of osteoid osteoma. *AJR Am J Roentgenol.* 2012;198:1039-1052.

Weatherall PT, Maale GE, Mendelsohn DB, et al. Chondroblastoma: classic and confusing appearance at MR imaging. *Radiology.* 1994;190:467-474.

4 **Answer A.** The metaphyses of long bones are the most common sites of hematogenous osteomyelitis in children owing to the unique changes in metaphyseal and epiphyseal vascularity with age. In neonates, the epiphysis is at an increased risk of infection as nutrient vessels cross the physis. However, transphyseal extension of metaphyseal osteomyelitis may still occur in children older than 2 years despite the theoretic protection of an avascular physis.

References: Gilbertson-Dahdal D, Wright JE, Krupinski E, et al. Transphyseal involvement of pyogenic osteomyelitis is considerably more common than classically taught. *AJR Am J Roentgenol.* 2014;203:190-195.

Guillerman RP. Osteomyelitis and beyond. *Pediatr Radiol.* 2013;43(1):S193-S203.

5 **Answer C.** The gram-positive cocci (GPC), *S. aureus* followed by *Streptococcus*, are considered the most common pathogens for acute hematogenous osteomyelitis. However, the gram-negative bacillus, *K. kingae*, has an increased prevalence in children younger than 4 years.

MRI is highly sensitive for distinguishing *K. kingae* from GPC in young children when there is focal epiphyseal (and equivalent) cartilage involvement. There is also a diminished inflammatory response and bone marrow/soft tissue reaction with *K. kingae* compared to GPC. *Pseudomonas* and *Escherichia coli* are often associated with osteomyelitis from penetrating trauma, typically within the foot, but this is rare in the intra-articular epiphysis.

References: Gilbertson-Dahdal D, Wright JE, Krupinski E, et al. Transphyseal involvement of pyogenic osteomyelitis is considerably more common than classically taught. *AJR Am J Roentgenol.* 2014;203:190-195.

Guillerman RP. Osteomyelitis and beyond. *Pediatr Radiol.* 2013;43(1):S193-S203.

Kanavaki A, Ceroni D, Tchernin D, et al. Can early MRI distinguish between *Kingella kingae* and gram-positive cocci in osteoarticular infections in young children? *Pediatr Radiol.* 2012;42:57-62.

6 **Answer A.** The crescentic fracture fragment (arrow) arising from the lateral condyle is the typical location of a lateral condylar fracture. This often results from a varus injury to an extended supinated forearm. The more common supracondylar fracture is a horizontal fracture located at the distal humeral metaphysis, often involving the coronoid fossa without involvement of the physis.

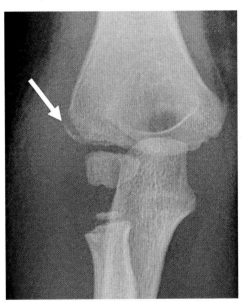

Reference: Green NE. Fractures and dislocations about the elbow. In: Green NE, Swiontkowski MF, eds. *Skeletal Trauma in Children.* 3rd ed. WB Saunders; 2003:257.

7 **Answer C.** Lateral condylar fractures most commonly occur between the ages of 5 and 10 years.

Reference: Green NE. Fractures and dislocations about the elbow. In: Green NE, Swiontkowski MF, eds. *Skeletal Trauma in Children*, 3rd ed. WB Saunders; 2003:257.

8 **Answer C.** Lateral condylar fractures of the elbow are most commonly Salter-Harris IV fractures.

The Milch classification groups lateral condylar fractures into types I and II based on fracture involvement lateral or medial to the capitello-trochlear groove, respectively. A Milch I fracture is lateral to the trochlea and extends through the capitellum. As the capitellum is usually ossified in this age group, it clearly represents a Salter-Harris IV fracture on elbow radiographs. However, the elbow remains stable as the humeroulnar joint is spared.

The Milch II fracture spares the capitellum and extends medial to the capitello-trochlear groove. There has been controversy classifying this fracture type as Salter-Harris IV when the involved trochlear epiphysis is not yet ossified and it appears radiographically as a Salter-Harris II fracture. However, the consensus is that the Milch II fracture pattern is also a Salter-Harris IV fracture as it involves the metaphysis, physis, and unossified trochlear epiphysis. Therefore, nearly all lateral condylar fractures are considered Salter-Harris IV fractures. However, the Milch classification is more important than the Salter-Harris classification for management because Milch II fractures are unstable and require surgical fixation.

This case highlights the more common Milch type II lateral condylar fracture as the metaphyseal fragment (arrow) extends medial to the capitellum. Radiographic evaluation is limited in this age group because of incomplete ossification of the trochlea. As a result, surgical management may rely on the degree of displacement of the metaphyseal fragment (>2 mm).

References: Bache E. Elbow injuries. In: Johnson KJ, Bache E, eds. *Imaging in Pediatric Skeletal Trauma*. Springer; 2008:257-270.

Green NE. Fractures and dislocations about the elbow. In: Green NE, Swiontkowski MF, eds. *Skeletal Trauma in Children*. 3rd ed. WB Saunders; 2003:257.

Letts M, Davidson D. Fractures of the lateral condyle of the humerus in children. *Orthop Knowl Online J*. 2002;1(6). http://orthoportal.aaos.org/oko/article.aspx?article=OKO PED007

9 **Answer B.** Blount disease (tibia vara) is secondary to pathologic stress upon the posteromedial physis of the proximal tibia that results in medial growth suppression and associated tibia vara. As the name tibia vara implies, the lower-extremity bowing (varus) is centered at the proximal tibia. The metaphyseal-diaphyseal angle is >11 degrees (~20 degrees in this case). This angle is drawn from the metaphyseal beak to a line at the physis that is perpendicular to the lateral cortex of the tibial diaphysis (see angle). Although bilateral in this case, Blount disease is often unilateral or asymmetric and has infantile, juvenile, and adolescent presentations. The Langenskiold classification describes six stages of progressive metaphyseal depression, beaking, and fragmentation.

Developmental (physiologic) genu varus (bowing) normally resolves within 6 months of walking or by the age of 2 years. Congenital bowing classically presents as convex posterior and medial bowing of the tibial diaphysis and may be due to intrauterine positioning or skeletal dysplasia. In both cases, there is a normal medial metaphysis of the tibia. As rickets represents deficient mineralization of the growing physis, radiographs should display symmetric widening, cupping, and fraying of the growth plates of the distal femur and proximal and distal tibia (not present in this case).

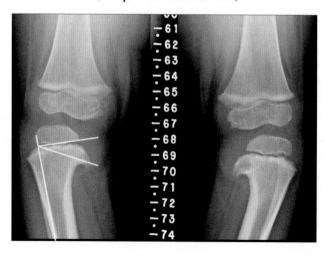

References: Biko DM, Miller AL, Ho-Fung V, et al. MRI of congenital and developmental abnormalities of the knee. *Clin Radiol.* 2012;67:1198-1206.

Cheema FI, Grissom LE, Harcke T. Radiographic characteristics of lower-extremity bowing in children. *Radiographics.* 2003;23:871-880.

10 **Answer D.** Imaging findings of Blount disease include radiographical findings of depression of the medial tibial metaphysis. Additional MRI can better evaluate the growth plate demonstrating bony bridging, delayed ossification of the medial tibial epiphysis, widening of the tibial growth plate, and hypertrophy of the medial meniscus. The hypertrophy of the medial meniscus is likely compensatory due to abnormal forces within the knee.

Reference: Biko DM, Miller AL, Ho-Fung V, et al. MRI of congenital and developmental abnormalities of the knee. *Clin Radiol.* 2012;67:1198-1206.

11 **Answer C.** Idiopathic chondrolysis of the hip (ICH) is a disease of unknown etiology that results in progressive articular cartilage destruction. ICH is often unilateral and presents with spontaneous hip or knee pain with worsening joint stiffness. Neither systemic symptoms nor abnormal inflammatory biomarkers are present. Early radiographs are often normal and performed to exclude more common acute causes of hip pain such as slipped capital femoral epiphysis. Later radiographs 10 to 12 months from symptom onset often reveal degenerative changes of concentric joint space loss, protrusio acetabuli, subchondral cysts, and sclerosis. It is important to distinguish ICH from secondary causes of cartilage loss from juvenile idiopathic arthritis (JIA) or infection. The MRI findings in this case reveal a geographic pattern of T1/T2 signal prolongation confined to the middle third of the subchondral femoral head to the physis (arrows). This pattern is characteristic of early MRI findings of ICH. Synovial enhancement is less commonly reported with ICH compared to JIA. However, this negative finding is not specific. Additional findings of muscle wasting and atrophy are reported with follow-up imaging usually with associated joint contractures. Synovial biopsy is often performed for pathologic confirmation and to exclude infection. The prognosis is variable from spontaneous resolution to significant joint contracture and ankylosis.

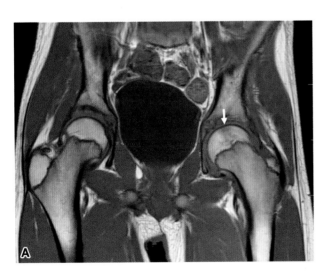
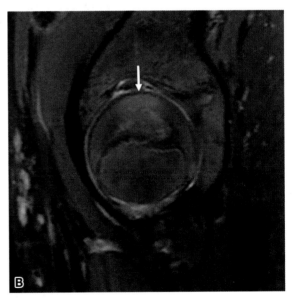

References: Johnson K, Haigh SF, Ehtisham S, et al. Childhood idiopathic chondrolysis of the hip: MRI features. *Pediatr Radiol.* 2003;33:194-199.

Laor T, Crawford AH. Idiopathic chondrolysis of the hip in children: early MRI findings. *AJR Am J Roentgenol.* 2009;192:526-531.

12 **Answer D.** The imaging findings are most suggestive of chronic recurrent multifocal osteomyelitis (CRMO). CRMO is an idiopathic inflammatory disorder most commonly seen in children and adolescents. This disorder is characterized by multiple inflammatory bone lesions that demonstrate a relapsing/remitting pattern. On imaging, these lesions are most often lytic on plain radiographs initially followed by sclerosis in the chronic course. On MRI, the lesions demonstrate bone marrow edema and periostitis. CRMO commonly occurs in the long tubular bone and clavicle but can occur anywhere throughout the skeleton.

Reference: Khanna G, Sato TS, Ferguson P. Imaging of chronic recurrent multifocal osteomyelitis. *Radiographics*. 2009;29:1159-1177.

13 **Answer B.** CRMO most commonly involves the metaphysis and metaphyseal equivalents. This is similar to the distribution of hematogenous spread of osteomyelitis, but CRMO may involve the clavicle.

References: Khanna G, Sato TS, Ferguson P. Imaging of chronic recurrent multifocal osteomyelitis. *Radiographics*. 2009;29:1159-1177.

Mandell GA, Contreras SJ, Conrad K, et al. Bone scintigraphy in the detection of chronic recurrent multifocal osteomyelitis. *J Nucl Med*. 1998;39:1778-1783.

14 **Answer B.** Multiple conditions are associated with CRMO. These include dermatologic conditions such as psoriasis and pyoderma gangrenosum, autoinflammatory disorders such as Takayasu arteritis and Wegener granulomatosis, gastrointestinal syndromes such as inflammatory bowel disease, and genetic syndromes such as Majeed syndrome. CRMO is also associated with SAPHO syndrome (synovitis, acne, pustulosis, hyperostosis, osteitis) and spondyloarthropathies.

Reference: Khanna G, Sato TS, Ferguson P. Imaging of chronic recurrent multifocal osteomyelitis. *Radiographics*. 2009;29:1159-1177.

15 **Answer B.** Lipomatosis of a nerve with macrodactyly is referred to as macrodystrophia lipomatosa. In this disorder, the affected nerve is enlarged by fibrofatty tissue. This can occur without or with macrodactyly (macrodystrophia lipomatosa). Clinically, this disorder is characterized by a slow-growing mass most frequently within the upper extremity. Most cases involve the median nerve in the upper extremity and the medial plantar nerve in the lower extremity. Radiographs of this disorder demonstrate both soft tissue and bony overgrowth in the distribution of a sclerotome (arrows). MRI demonstrates a diffusely enlarged thickened nerve surrounded by adipose tissue.

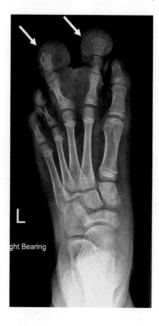

References: Murphey MD, Carroll JF, Flemming DJ, et al. From the archive of the AFIP: benign musculoskeletal lipomatous lesions. *Radiographics*. 2004;24:1433-1466.

Tripathi SK, Nanda SN, Kumar S, et al. Macrodystrophia lipomatosa—a rare congenital anomaly: a case report and review of literature. *Ann Int Med Dent Res*. 2016;2(5):1-3.

16 **Answer C.** Thanatophoric dysplasia is a short-limbed dwarfism caused by a mutation of fibroblast growth factor receptor 3 (*FGFR3*) gene. It is the most common lethal neonatal skeletal dysplasia. In this disorder, the long bones are short and may have a curved "telephone receiver" appearance (arrowheads). The ribs are shortened. Additionally, the vertebral bodies are flattened and may appear H shaped (arrows). This feature can be used to differentiate thanatophoric dysplasia from the short rib polydactyly syndromes such as Jeune syndrome.

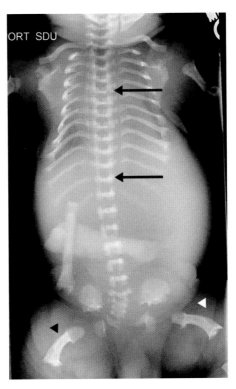

Reference: Miller E, Blaser S, Shannon P, et al. Brain and bone abnormalities of thanatophoric dwarfism. *AJR Am J Roentgenol*. 2009;192:48-51.

17 **Answer C.** The most common central nervous system manifestations of thanatophoric dysplasia are the cloverleaf skull deformity and megalencephaly. Additional central nervous system abnormalities are deep fissures and abnormal sulcation of the temporal lobes, a dysplastic hippocampus, and polymicrogyria.

Reference: Miller E, Blaser S, Shannon P, et al. Brain and bone abnormalities of thanatophoric dwarfism. *AJR Am J Roentgenol*. 2009;192:48-51.

18 **Answer D.** Osteochondritis dissecans (OCD) of the capitellum is a focal injury of the articular cartilage and subchondral bone within the humeral capitellum. It is most commonly seen in this location in throwing athletes and is typically seen in patients between 12 and 17 years old. The suggested etiology of this lesion is repetitive microtrauma. OCD is most commonly seen within the knee.

On plain radiographs, there is most often a subchondral lucent focus (arrow), but there may be fragmentation or sclerosis. MRI best depicts the OCD where the subchondral abnormality is readily visible (arrowhead).

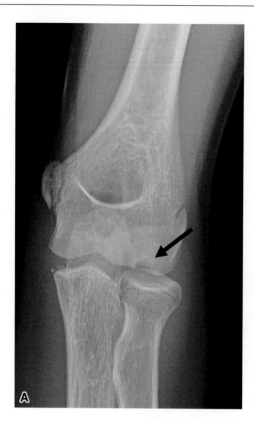

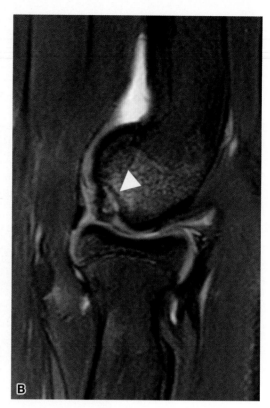

References: Cruz AI, Shea KG, Ganley TJ. Pediatric knee osteochondritis dissecans lesions. *Orthop Clin N Am.* 2016;47:763-775.

Itsubo T, Murakami N, Uemura K, et al. Magnetic resonance imaging staging to evaluate stability of capitella osteochondritis dissecans lesions. *Am J Sports Med.* 2014;42:1972-1977.

Jarret DY, Walters MM, Kleinman PK. Prevalence of capitellar osteochondritis dissecans in children with chronic radial head subluxation and dislocation. *AJR Am J Roentgenol.* 2016;206:1329-1334.

19 **Answer A.** The prevalence of capitellar OCD is increased in children with radial head subluxation. Capitellar OCD is seen in 32% to 33% of children with chronic radial head subluxation likely because of abnormal radiocapitellar mechanics.

Reference: Jarret DY, Walters MM, Kleinman PK. Prevalence of capitellar osteochondritis dissecans in children with chronic radial head subluxation and dislocation. *AJR Am J Roentgenol.* 2016;206:1329-1334.

20 **Answer C.** The criteria for unstable OCD on MRI are the following:

A. Thin line of high signal intensity 5 mm or greater between the OCD and bone
B. Discrete cystic focus 5 mm or greater in diameter beneath the OCD
C. Focal defect with a width of 5 mm or greater in the articular surface of the OCD
D. High-signal-intensity line extending through the articular cartilage and subchondral bone into the OCD

Reference: Cruz AI, Shea KG, Ganley TJ. Pediatric knee osteochondritis dissecans lesions. *Orthop Clin N Am.* 2016;47:763-775.

21 **Answer B.** The image demonstrates a small osseous fragment adjacent to the pelvis consistent with an avulsion fracture of the anterior superior iliac spine (arrow). The anterior superior iliac spine is the attachment point of the sartorius muscle and tensor muscle of the fascia lata. This injury occurs during forceful extension of the hip and is commonly seen in sprinters. Treatment is activity restriction.

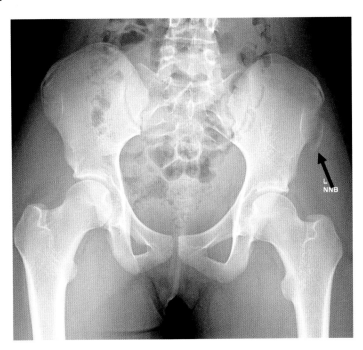

Reference: Stevens MA, El-Khoury GY, Kathol MH, et al. Imaging features of avulsion injuries. *Radiographics*. 1999;19:655-672.

22 **Answer D.** The table below lists the common sites for avulsion injuries of the pelvis and the associated muscular attachments.

Avulsion Fracture	Muscle Attachment
Iliac crest	Abdominal muscles
Anterior superior iliac spine	Sartorius, tensor fasciae latae
Anterior inferior iliac spine	Rectus femoris
Greater trochanter	Hip rotators
Lesser trochanter	Iliopsoas
Ischial tuberosity	Hamstrings
Body/inferior pubic ramus	Adductors, gracilis

Reference: Stevens MA, El-Khoury GY, Kathol MH, et al. Imaging features of avulsion injuries. *Radiographics*. 1999;19:655-672.

23 **Answer B.** The image demonstrates a metaphyseal corner fracture of the proximal tibia (arrow). This is a disk-shaped fracture through the metaphysis where the fracture line is nearly parallel to the physis. The fracture has been described a corner fracture or bucket handle fracture depending on the orientation of the radiographic projection. This fracture has been called a classic metaphyseal lesion (CML) and is common in abused infants particularly <18 months of age. CMLs are considered highly specific for infant child abuse.

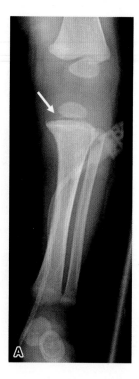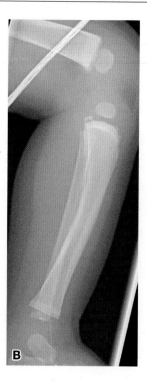

References: Kleinman PK. Diagnostic imaging in infant abuse. *AJR Am J Roentgenol.* 1990;155:703-712.

Lonergan GJ, Baker AM, Morey MK, et al. Child abuse: radiologic-pathologic correlation. *Radiographics.* 2003;23:811-845.

Thackeray JD, Wannemacher J, Adler BH, et al. The classic metaphyseal lesion and traumatic injury. *Pediatr Radiol.* 2016;46:1128-1133.

24 **Answer B.** A metaphyseal corner fracture or CML occurs because of shearing injury, which causes differential horizontal motion across the metaphysis. This shearing force is caused by the to-and-fro movement such as seen in shaking an infant by holding the infant from the feet or hands or shaking an infant while holding the chest and whiplashing their extremities.

References: Lonergan GJ, Baker AM, Morey MK, et al. Child abuse: radiologic-pathologic correlation. *Radiographics.* 2003;23:811-845.

Thackeray JD, Wannemacher J, Adler BH, et al. The classic metaphyseal lesion and traumatic injury. *Pediatr Radiol.* 2016;46:1128-1133.

25 **Answer D.** Although skeletal injuries without an explanation may be concerning for abuse, skeletal imaging findings that are associated with infant nonaccidental injury are metaphyseal corner fractures, rib fractures, sternal fractures, vertebral spinous process fractures, and acromion fractures of the scapula. Metaphyseal corner fractures or CMLs are due to shear injury that can be seen with shaking. Rib fractures in infants are rare injuries given the plasticity of the bones. Given this, rib fractures require substantial force but can be seen with squeezing of the chest. Given the rarity of sternal fractures, vertebral spinous fractures, and acromion fractures of the scapula in infants, these fractures are also concerning for abuse. Skull fracture patterns such as multiple fractures, fractures crossing sutures, and bilateral fractures have also been associated with abusive injury.

References: Kleinman PK. Diagnostic imaging in infant abuse. *AJR Am J Roentgenol.* 1990;155:703-712.

Lonergan GJ, Baker AM, Morey MK, et al. Child abuse: radiologic-pathologic correlation. *Radiographics.* 2003;23:811-845.

26 **Answer A.** All infants with suspected abusive injury should undergo a skeletal survey. Further, a repeat skeletal survey 10 to 14 days following the injury may identify additional injuries that could not be seen on the initial skeletal survey. The recommended views for a skeletal survey of suspected infant abuse are the following:

Axial Skeleton	Appendicular Skeleton
Thorax (anteroposterior [AP], lateral, right and left oblique)	Humerus (AP)
Abdomen (AP to include pelvis)	Forearms (AP)
Lumbosacral spine (lateral)	Hands (posteroanterior [PA])
Skull (frontal and lateral to include cervical spine)	Femur (AP)
	Tibia (AP)
	Feet (AP)

References: Kleinman PK. Diagnostic imaging in infant abuse. *AJR Am J Roentgenol.* 1990;155:703-712.

Lonergan GJ, Baker AM, Morey MK, et al. Child abuse: radiologic-pathologic correlation. *Radiographics.* 2003;23:811-845.

27 **Answer A.** Radial deficiency or dysplasia is also referred to as clubhand due to failure of development of the radius occurring between the fifth and sixth week of gestation. In this disorder, there are varying degrees of dysplasia, but complete absence of the radius is most common. The trapezium, scaphoid, and thumb are usually absent or deformed. The remainder of the carpal bones and the second through fifth ray are most often normal. Radial dysplasia occurs bilaterally in 50% of affected children.

On physical examination, there is commonly radial and ulnar deviation of the hand due to the unopposed flexor carpi ulnaris and brachioradialis.

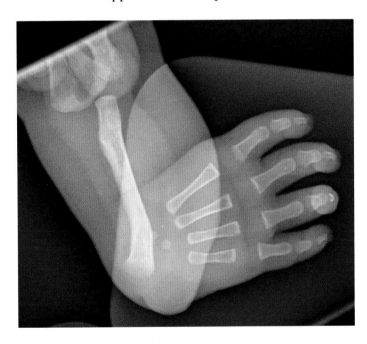

Reference: Laor T. Congenital malformations of bone. In: Slovis TS, ed. *Caffey's Pediatric Diagnostic Imaging.* Elsevier; 2008:2594-2612.

28 **Answer A.** The table below lists syndromes associated with radial dysplasia.

Syndrome	Other Associations
Trisomy 13	Chromosomal abnormalities
Trisomy 18	
Holt-Oram syndrome	Congenital heart disease
Cornelia de Lange syndrome	Mental delay
Seckel syndrome	
Thalidomide embryopathy	Teratogens
Varicella embryopathy	
Fanconi anemia	Blood dyscrasias
Thrombocytopenia absent radius	
VACTERL	

Reference: Laor T. Congenital malformations of bone. In: Slovis TS, ed. *Caffey's Pediatric Diagnostic Imaging*. Elsevier; 2008:2594-2612.

29 **Answer E.** Osteosarcoma is the most common primary malignant bone tumor of childhood. Osteoblastic osteosarcomas are intramedullary and most commonly occur adjacent to the metaphysis of the long bone. Given that there is osteoid, the osteoblastic osteosarcoma is most often sclerotic on plain radiographs (arrow). If the osteosarcoma invades the cortex, it can produce periosteal reaction along with Codman triangles and a "sunburst" appearance of the cortex.

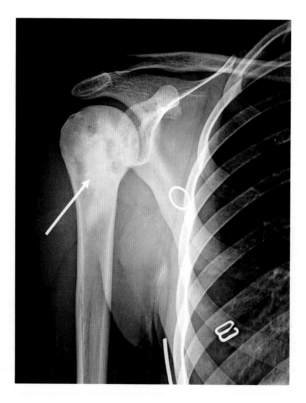

References: Clayer M. Many faces of osteosarcoma on plain radiographs. *ANZ J Surg*. 2015;85:22-26.

Murphey MD, Robbin MR, McRae GA, et al. The many faces of osteosarcoma. *Radiographics*. 1997;17:1205-1231.

30 **Answer B.** In osteosarcoma, skip metastases, which are foci of tumor separate from the primary lesion, can be seen. Because of this, when imaging osteosarcomas, it is important to define the extent of the disease by imaging from the proximal to the distal joint.

Although the physis is sometimes considered a barrier to extension of tumors, 75% to 88% of metaphyseal osteosarcomas extend across the physis to the epiphysis. Joint involvement is seen in nearly 25% of osteosarcomas, but the synovium is not often infiltrated. Malignant joint effusions do occur when the joint is invaded, but this is not the reason that both the proximal and distal joints need to be imaged.

Reference: Murphey MD, Robbin MR, McRae GA, et al. The many faces of osteosarcoma. *Radiographics*. 1997;17:1205-1231.

31 **Answer B.** Approximately 30% to 40% of patients with localized osteosarcoma will develop recurrence. The most common location for recurrence is within the lung (90%), usually occurring within the first 2 to 3 years. After 5 years, relapse of osteosarcoma is rare, occurring in about 2%. Lung metastases may be calcified.

Reference: Luetke A, Meyers PA, Lewis I, et al. Osteosarcoma treatment—where do we stand? A state of the art review. *Cancer Treat Rev*. 2014;40:523-532.

32 **Answer C.** For the evaluation of the hip in patients up to at least 4 months of age, sonographic examination is recommended. After 4 months, an ultrasound may be attempted, but some advocate a radiograph.

Additionally, sonographic evaluation of an infant with risk factor for hip dysplasia should be delayed until 4 to 6 weeks of life to avoid normal instability of the hip present during the first 2 weeks of life.

References: Gerscovich EO. Infant hip in developmental dysplasia: facts to consider for a successful diagnostic ultrasound examination. *Appl Radiol*. 1999;28:18-25.

Harcke HT. Screening newborns for developmental dysplasia of the hip: the role of sonography. *AJR Am J Roentgenol*. 1994;162:395-397.

33 **Answer B.** In this infant, the femoral head (*) is subluxed and the acetabulum is shallow, consistent with developmental dysplasia of the hip. The slope of the acetabulum with respect to the ilium can be evaluated sonographically (lines). The angle (arrow) formed by these two lines is the alpha angle. An alpha angle of >60 degrees is normal. An alpha angle between 50 and 60 degrees may be physiologic during the first 3 months of age and should be followed up. An alpha angle <50 degrees is abnormal.

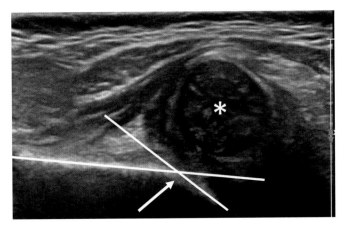

References: Gerscovich EO. Infant hip in developmental dysplasia: facts to consider for a successful diagnostic ultrasound examination. *Appl Radiol*. 1999;28:18-25.

Harcke HT. Screening newborns for developmental dysplasia of the hip: the role of sonography. *AJR Am J Roentgenol*. 1994;162:395-397.

34 **Answer D.** The main risk factors for developmental dysplasia of the hip are breech presentation at birth, family history of hip dysplasia, and postural deformities such as torticollis or a foot deformity. Additionally, physical examination findings of hip instability, limited range of motion, or a hip click may indicate underlying hip dysplasia.

References: Gerscovich EO. Infant hip in developmental dysplasia: facts to consider for a successful diagnostic ultrasound examination. *Appl Radiol.* 1999;28:18-25.

Harcke HT. Screening newborns for developmental dysplasia of the hip: the role of sonography. *AJR Am J Roentgenol.* 1994;162:395-397.

35 **Answer D.** This frontal radiograph of the thoracolumbar spine demonstrates a dextroscoliosis centered at the level of T12-L1. In a dextroscoliosis, there is a rightward curvature of the spine. In a levoscoliosis, there is a leftward curvature of the spine.

Additionally, there is a vertebral segmentation anomaly at L1 (arrow). This bifid vertebral body should be identified with this curve and would be an indication for further imaging with MRI.

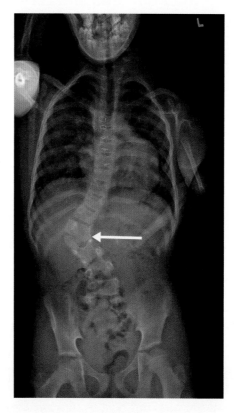

Reference: Kim H, Kim HS, Moon ES, et al. Scoliosis imaging: what radiologists should know. *Radiographics.* 2010;30:1823-1842.

36 **Answer B.** In a structural scoliotic curve, there are vertebral morphologic changes such as wedging and rotation. The structural curve is not correctable with ipsilateral bending. In a nonstructural curve, there are no vertebral morphologic changes. Given this, a nonstructural curve is correctable with ipsilateral bending. Although a nonstructural curve does not usually progress, it can progress to a structural curve because of ligament shortening from decreased growth on the concave side of the curve. Differentiation of a structural from nonstructural scoliotic curvature is a Cobb angle of 25 degrees or more on ipsilateral side-bending.

Reference: Kim H, Kim HS, Moon ES, et al. Scoliosis imaging: what radiologists should know. *Radiographics.* 2010;30:1823-1842.

37 **Answer B.** The Cobb angle is the measurement of the angle between two lines, one of which is at the superior end plate of the superior end vertebral body and the other at the inferior end plate of the inferior end vertebral body. In adolescent idiopathic scoliosis, observation is recommended for a Cobb angle <20 degrees, bracing is recommended when the Cobb angle is between 20 and 45 degrees, and surgery is recommended when the Cobb angle is >45 degrees. The greatest factors suggesting the probability of progression of an adolescent idiopathic scoliosis are spinal growth velocity and the degree of curvature at presentation.

Reference: Kim H, Kim HS, Moon ES, et al. Scoliosis imaging: what radiologists should know. *Radiographics*. 2010;30:1823-1842.

38 **Answer A.** The radiograph demonstrates a lucency extending through the tibial diaphysis (arrow) consistent with a toddler's fracture. This is a nondisplaced fracture of the tibia, which can be radiographically occult. The fracture typical occurs between 9 months and 3 years of age. The most common presenting symptom is refusal to walk or refusal to bear weight on the affected leg. These fractures most often heal without treatment.

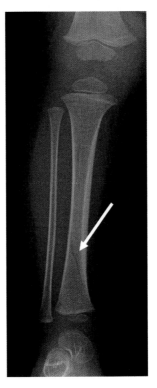

Reference: Donnelly L. Toddler's fracture of the fibula. *AJR Am J Roentgenol*. 2000;175:922.

39 **Answer D.** In the provided image, there is shortening of the femur with tapering of the proximal femur (arrow) and absence of the femoral head. There is also associated dysplasia of the acetabulum. These findings are consistent with the diagnosis of proximal focal femoral deficiency (PFFD) disorder.

PFFD is a rare disorder, which is characterized by failure of development of the proximal femur. In this disorder, there is deficiency of the iliofemoral articulation, limb malrotation, and a leg length discrepancy.

The Aitken classification (table) is the most common classification scheme for this disorder.

Class	Femoral Head	Femoral Segment	Acetabulum
A	Present	Short	Normal
B	Present	Short, usually proximal bony tuft	Developed or moderately dysplastic
C	Absent or very small	Short, usually proximally tapered	Severely dysplastic
D	Absent	Short, deformed	Absent

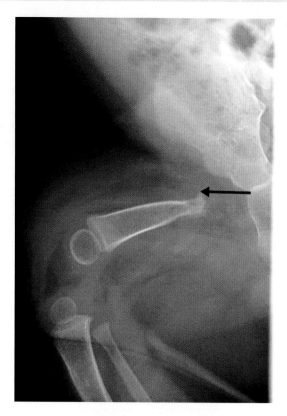

Reference: Biko DM, Davidson R, Pena A, Jaramillo D. Proximal focal femoral deficiency: evaluation by MR imaging. *Pediatr Radiol*. 2012;42:50-56.

40 **Answer D.** In PFFD disorder, there is maldevelopment of the proximal femur. The femoral head may be present or absent. A coxa vara deformity is often present. The acetabulum may be normal, dysplastic, or absent. In the knee, there may be flattening of the distal femoral epiphysis, underdevelopment of the intercondylar notch, and absent cruciates.

References: Biko DM, Davidson R, Pena A, Jaramillo D. Proximal focal femoral deficiency: evaluation by MR imaging. *Pediatr Radiol*. 2012;42:50-56.

Biko DM, Mill AL, Ho-Fung V, et al. MRI of congenital and developmental abnormalities of the knee. *Clin Radiol*. 2012;67:1198-1206.

41 **Answer B.** A tarsal coalition is an abnormality of the foot where two or more tarsal bones are joined by bone, cartilage, or fibrous tissue. In this case, there is irregular sclerosis at the calcaneonavicular joint with decrease in the calcaneonavicular gap (arrow) consistent with a calcaneonavicular tarsal coalition. In approximately 10% of cases, there is an osseous bridge between the calcaneus and the navicular. Additional findings of this disorder are an elongated lateral navicular as it approaches the anterior calcaneus on the lateral view and hypoplasia of the lateral talar head.

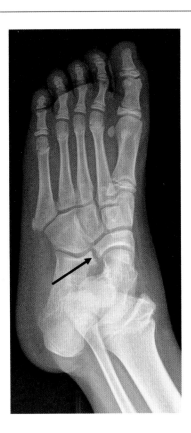

References: Newman JS, Newberg AH. Congenital tarsal coalition: multimodality evaluation with emphasis on CT and MR imaging. *Radiographics.* 2000;20:321-332.

Zaw H, Calder JDF. Tarsal coalitions. *Foot Ankle Clin N Am.* 2010;15:349-364.

42 **Answer B.** Tarsal coalitions are bilateral in approximately 50% of affected individuals. Tarsal coalitions are prevalent in approximately 1% to 2% of the population. Ninety percent of tarsal coalitions involve the talocalcaneal or calcaneonavicular joints.

Reference: Newman JS, Newberg AH. Congenital tarsal coalition: multimodality evaluation with emphasis on CT and MR imaging. *Radiographics.* 2000;20:321-332.

43 **Answer D.** Osteogenesis imperfecta (OI) is a genetic disorder commonly referred to as brittle bone disease. In this autosomal dominant inherited disorder, there are abnormalities in type 1 collagen, which leads to fragile and osteopenic bones.

The severity of this disorder is variable depending on the classification (see answer to Question 44). The disorder is suspected clinically in children who present with repeated or unexplained fractures or fractures with minor trauma.

On imaging, patients with OI demonstrate osteopenia, fractures, and bone deformities. The bone deformities occur because of the plasticity of the bones. Other findings include hyperplastic callus formation, ossification of the interosseous membrane, and "popcorn" calcifications. "Popcorn" calcifications (arrow) usually occur in the metaphysis and epiphysis of the bone and are believed to result from microtrauma leading to disordered maturation of the growth plate.

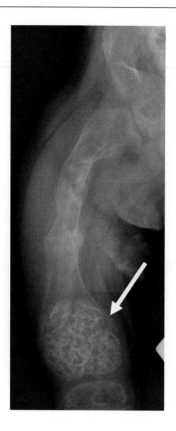

References: Forlino A, Marini JC. Osteogenesis imperfect. *Lancet*. 2016;387:1657-1671.

Renaud A, Aucourt J, Weill J. Radiographic features of osteogenesis imperfecta. *Insights Imaging*. 2013;4:417-429.

Trejo P, Rauch F. Osteogenesis imperfecta in children and adolescents—new developments in diagnosis and treatment. *Osteoporos Int*. 2016;27:3427-3437.

44 **Answer B.** The table describes the four main types of OI.

Type of OI	Features
Type 1	*Mild*
	Fractures, minor deformities
	Normal stature
	Blue sclerae
	Dentinogenesis imperfecta may be present.
Type 2	*Lethal*
	Fractures in utero
	Death due to respiratory insufficiency
Type 3	*Severe*
	Fractures, major deformities
	Very short stature
	Dentinogenesis imperfecta is frequent.
Type 4	*Moderate*
	Fractures
	Short stature
	Variable sclerae
	Dentinogenesis imperfecta may be present.

Reference: Renaud A, Aucourt J, Weill J. Radiographic features of osteogenesis imperfecta. *Insights Imaging*. 2013;4:417-429.

45 **Answer D.** Bisphosphonate therapy is the most common medical treatment for children with OI. Bisphosphonate therapy consists of cyclic intravenous infusion. The result of this therapy on imaging is dense metaphyseal lines in the long bones, which are parallel to the growth plate (arrow). Each line will correspond to the administration of the intravenous bisphosphonate. In the spine and long bones, bisphosphonate therapy results in a "bone within a bone" appearance.

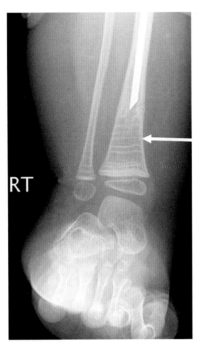

References: Renaud A, Aucourt J, Weill J. Radiographic features of osteogenesis imperfecta. *Insights Imaging.* 2013;4:417-429.

Trejo P, Rauch F. Osteogenesis imperfecta in children and adolescents—new developments in diagnosis and treatment. *Osteoporos Int.* 2016;27:3427-3437.

46 **Answer D.** The image demonstrates a well-circumscribed epiphyseal tumor within the distal femur (arrows in Figure A and B). Given the age of the patient and the epiphyseal location, the diagnosis is most likely a chondroblastoma.

A chondroblastoma is an uncommon benign cartilaginous tumor most often occurring in the epiphysis or apophysis of long bones. It is most commonly seen in the femur. On plain film evaluation, the tumor is a well-defined oval or round lytic lesion located within the epiphysis or apophysis. On MRI, the tumor is lobulated and heterogeneous with associated bone marrow edema. It may have a characteristic thin hypointense rim corresponding to siderosis within the tumor.

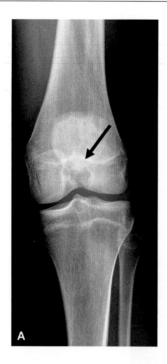
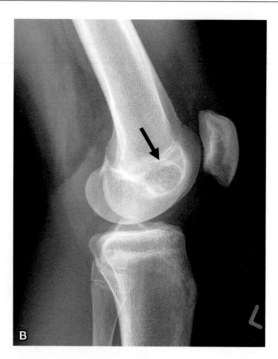

References: DeMattos CBR, Angsanunstsukh C, Akrader A, et al. Chondroblastoma and chondromyxoid fibroma. *J Am Acad Orthop Surg.* 2013;21:225-233.

Wooten-Gorges SL. MR imaging of primary bone tumors and tumor-like conditions in children. *Magn Reson Clin N Am.* 2009;17:469-487.

47 **Answer C.** Curettage and bone grafting is the recommended treatment for a chondroblastoma. Tumors sometimes may be widely excised when in bones such as the ribs or fibula. Recurrence rates of chondroblastoma are variable within the literature, ranging from 5% to 40%.

Reference: DeMattos CBR, Angsanunstsukh C, Akrader A, et al. Chondroblastoma and chondromyxoid fibroma. *J Am Acad Orthop Surg.* 2013;21:225-233.

48 **Answer A.** The image demonstrates an effusion of the right hip (arrow). In a patient of this age with hip pain and a hip effusion, the most likely diagnosis is transient synovitis. Transient synovitis of the hip is an acute but transient inflammation of the synovium of the hip. It typically occurs in patients 3 to 8 years old who present with hip pain, poor joint mobility, and a limp.

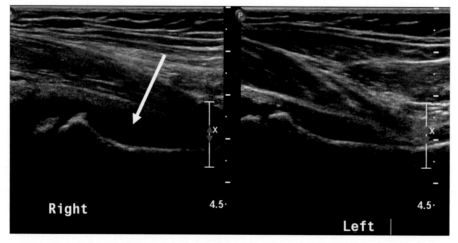

Reference: Paruso S, DiMartino A, Tarantino CC, et al. Transient synovitis of the hip: ultrasound appearance. *J Ultrasound.* 2011;14:92-94.

49 **Answer A.** Sinding-Larsen-Johansson syndrome is an osteochondrosis of the inferior pole of the patella commonly seen between the ages of 10 and 14 years. It is similar to Osgood-Schlatter disease given that it is a result of repetitive microtrauma due to stress at the insertion of the patellar tendon on the lower pole of the patella. Imaging findings include fragmentation of the inferior pole of the patella (arrow) along with inflammation in Hoffa fat pad (arrowhead). It can be distinguished from patellar sleeve avulsion given the clinical history of chronic knee pain.

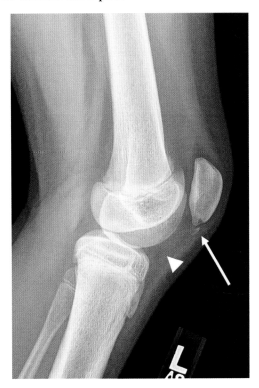

References: Dupuis CS, Westra SJ, Makris J, et al. Injuries and conditions of the extensor mechanism of the pediatric knee. *Radiographics.* 2009;29:877-886.

Kuehnast M, Mahomed N, Mistry B. Sinding-Larsen-Johansson syndrome. *SAJCH.* 2012;6:90-92.

50 **Answer D.** As noted in Answer 49, Sinding-Larsen-Johansson syndrome is an osteochondrosis of the inferior pole of the patella due to traction of the patellar ligament resulting in microtrauma. It is most commonly seen between the ages of 10 and 14 years. On MRI, there is edema of the inferior pole of the patella and proximal patellar tendon. Initial treatment is rest and anti-inflammatory medication such as nonsteroidal anti-inflammatory drugs (NSAIDs).

References: Dupuis CS, Westra SJ, Makris J, et al. Injuries and conditions of the extensor mechanism of the pediatric knee. *Radiographics.* 2009;29:877-886.

Kuehnast M, Mahomed N, Mistry B. Sinding-Larsen-Johansson syndrome. *SAJCH.* 2012;6:90-92.

51   **Answer B.** The images demonstrate flaring and fraying of the metaphysis (arrow) consistent with rickets.

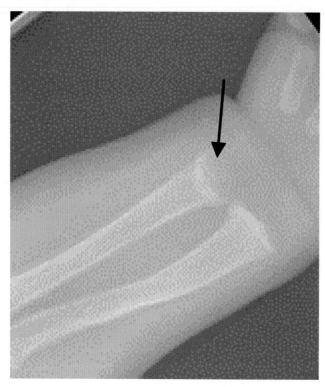

Findings in scurvy are a dense zone of provisional calcification, a ring epiphysis, spurring of the metaphysis, and subperiosteal hemorrhage.

52   **Answer C.** The most common cause of rickets is vitamin D deficiency. A major source of vitamin D is cutaneous photosynthesis due to sunlight exposure. Although vitamin D fortification in the United States includes milk and milk products, vitamin D supplied by these sources is not adequate. Inadequate sunlight exposure leading to a deficiency in vitamin D is therefore a common cause of rickets.

Vitamin C deficiency is the cause of scurvy.

References: Chang CY, Rosenthal DI, Mitchell DM, Handa A, Kattapuram SV, Huang AJ. Imaging findings of metabolic bone disease. *Radiographics*. 2016;36(6):1871-1887.

Shore RM, Chesney RW. Rickets: part I. *Pediatr Radiol*. 2013;43:140-151.

Shore RM, Chesney RW. Rickets: part II. *Pediatr Radiol*. 2013;43:152-172.

53   **Answer D.** A Sprengel deformity is a congenital malformation of the scapula related to a developmental arrest of the intrauterine normal scapular descent, which normally descends to the thorax by the end of the third month of intrauterine life. This gives rise to a high position of the scapula (arrow), leading to significant shoulder asymmetry and limited abduction.

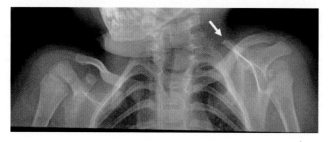

54 **Answer A.** The CT image demonstrates an omovertebral bone (arrow). An omovertebral bone is associated with a Sprengel deformity in one-third of children. It is a bone that extends from the medial border of the scapula to the spinous process, lamina, or transverse process of C5 to C7. A Sprengel deformity is also associated with vertebral body fusions.

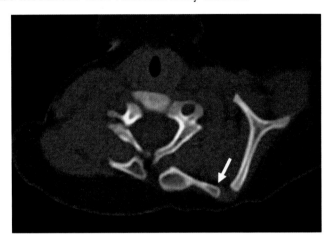

55 **Answer C.** A Sprengel deformity may be sporadic but is most commonly associated with Klippel-Feil syndrome. Klippel-Feil syndrome classically consists of a short neck, limitation of the movement of the head and neck, and a low posterior hairline. There are fusion anomalies of cervical vertebral bodies. The syndrome is also associated with congenital heart defects, deafness, learning disabilities, and renal anomalies.

Jeune syndrome and Ellis-van Creveld syndrome are short rib skeletal dysplasias.

Li-Fraumeni syndrome is an autosomal dominant disorder caused by a mutation of the *TP53* gene associated with pediatric malignancies such as osteosarcoma, brain tumors, adrenocortical carcinoma, and leukemia.

References: Azouz EM. CT demonstration of omovertebral bone. *Pediatr Radiol.* 2007;37(4):404.

Kamal YA. Sprengel deformity: an update on the surgical management. *Pulsus J Surg Res.* 2018;2(2):64-68.

Tiwari R, Singh AK, Somwaru AS, Menias CO, Prasad SR, Katabathina VS. Radiologist's primer on imaging of common hereditary cancer syndromes. *Radiographics.* 2019;39(3):759-778.

56 **Answer C.** The images demonstrate findings consistent with achondroplasia. Achondroplasia is the most common nonlethal dysplasia. It is characterized by shortening of the long bones, with proximal portions being more affected (rhizomelia), flaring of metaphyses (arrow), and short fingers with widely separated second and third digits (trident hand). Additionally, the pelvic cavity is short and broad (champagne glass appearance) with squaring of iliac wings (elephant ear–shaped iliac wings). The acetabular roofs are flat and horizontal. The spine demonstrates progressive decrease in the interpedicular distance craniocaudally in the lumbar spine (lines) with posterior vertebral body scalloping and an anterior bullet-shaped configuration (arrowhead).

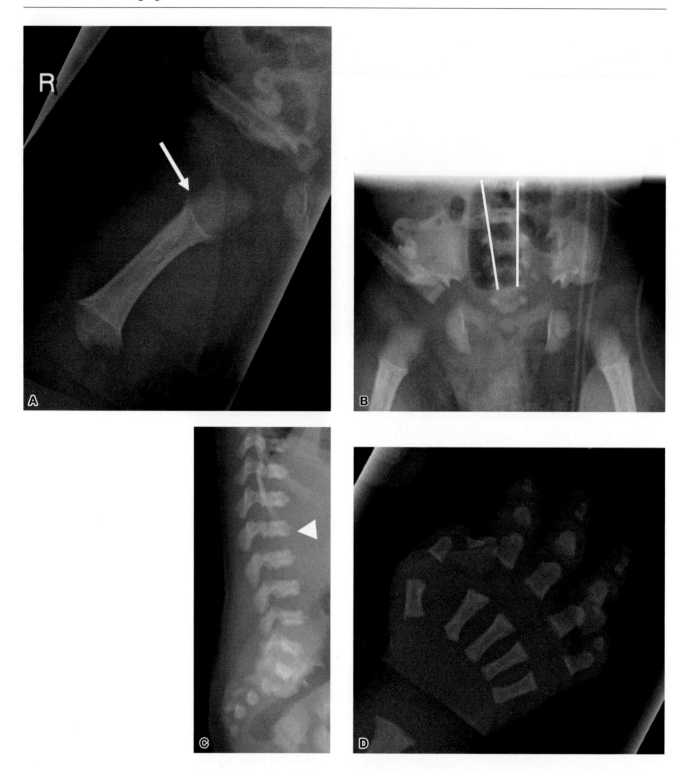

Reference: Panda A, Gamanagatti S, Jana M, Gupta AK. Skeletal dysplasias: a radio-graphic approach and review of common non-lethal skeletal dysplasias. *World J Radiol*. 2014;6(10):808.

1   A full-term newborn presents with respiratory distress shortly after birth. Physical examination reveals decreased breath sounds on the left side of the chest, and the abdomen appears scaphoid. The following chest X-ray is performed. What is the most common type of diaphragmatic hernia in this setting?

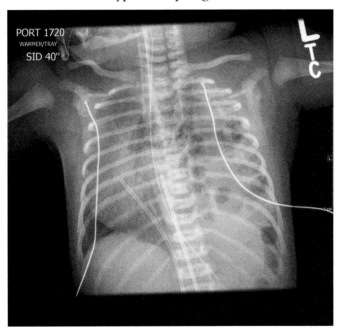

A. Eventration
B. Morgagni
C. Bochdalek
D. Central

2 What is the most likely diagnosis for this infant with respiratory distress?

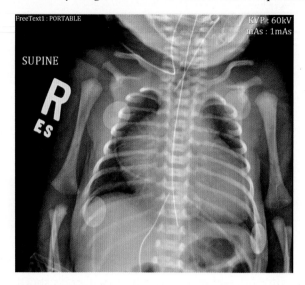

A. Hypoplastic left heart syndrome
B. Tetralogy of Fallot
C. Transposition of the great arteries
D. Ebstein anomaly

3 A 3-month-old female presents with recurrent episodes of pneumonia in the left lower lobe. A contrast-enhanced CT scan of the chest is performed. What is the most likely diagnosis?

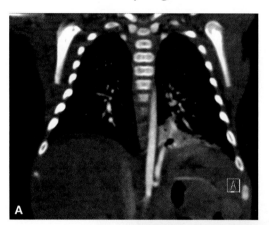
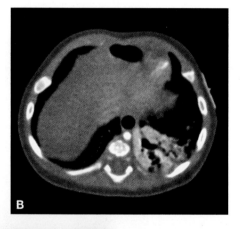
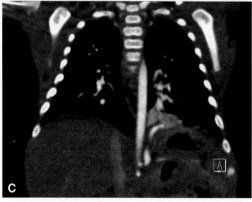

A. Bronchopulmonary sequestration
B. Congenital lobar overinflation
C. Swyer-James syndrome
D. Scimitar syndrome

4 The fetal MRI performed at 30 weeks gestational age and the chest radiograph performed shortly after delivery demonstrate a lesion in the left lung. What is the most likely diagnosis?

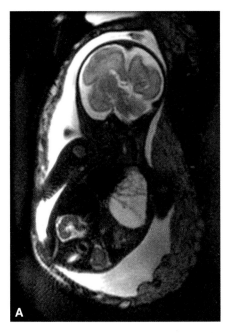

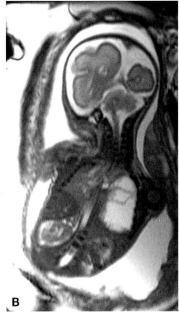

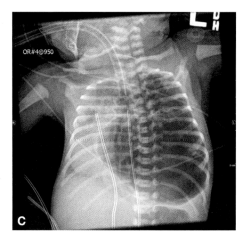

A. Congenital lobar overinflation
B. Congenital diaphragmatic hernia
C. Congenital pulmonary airway malformation
D. Posttraumatic pneumatocele

5 A fetal MRI is performed on a 30-week gestational age fetus. What is the most likely diagnosis?

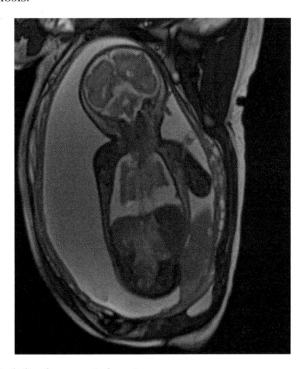

A. Congenital diaphragmatic hernia
B. Pulmonary sequestration
C. Bronchopulmonary foregut malformation
D. Fetal pleural effusion

6 A 2-month-old male presents with progressive respiratory distress and a history of recurrent lung infections. What is the most likely diagnosis?

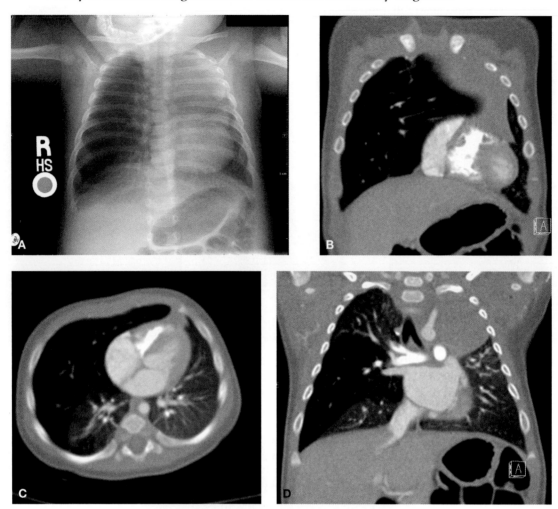

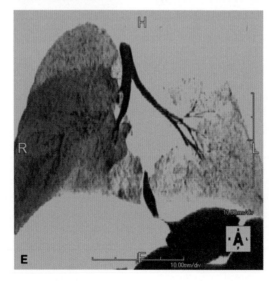

A. Congenital lobar overinflation
B. Congenital diaphragmatic hernia
C. Congenital pulmonary airway malformation
D. Posttraumatic pneumatocele

7 A 6-year-old boy presents with dysphagia and recurrent respiratory infections. What is the most likely diagnosis?

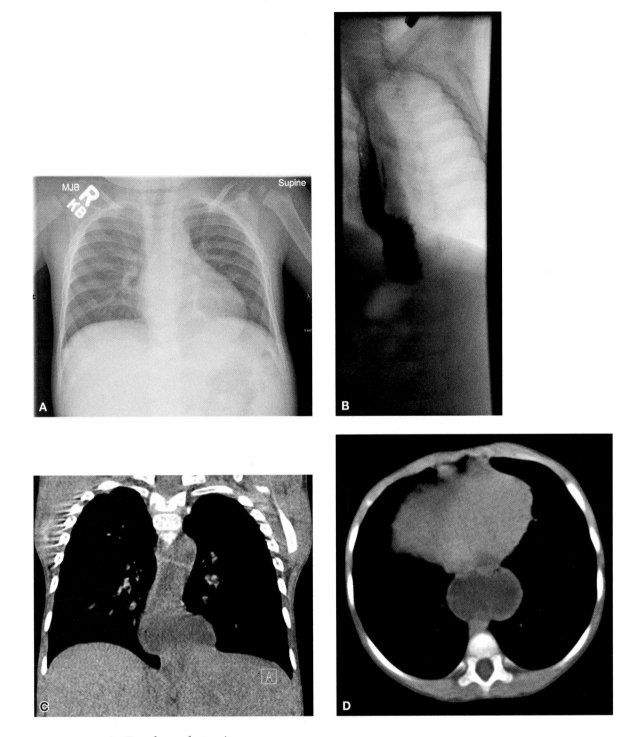

A. Esophageal atresia
B. Esophageal diverticulum
C. Esophageal duplication cyst
D. Esophageal stricture

8 Which of the following thoracic lesions is classically located in the posterior mediastinum?

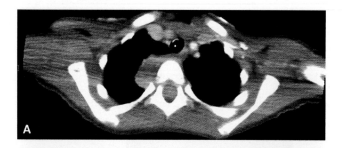

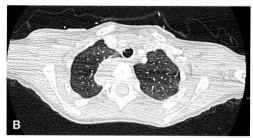

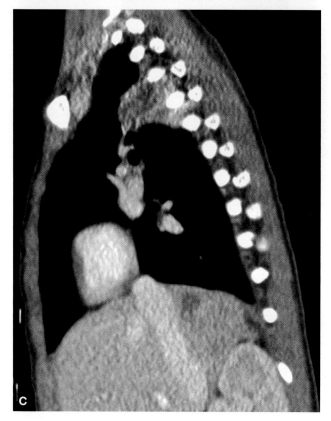

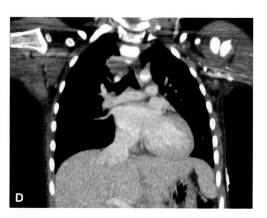

A. Mature teratoma
B. Neuroblastoma
C. Foregut duplication cyst
D. Lymphoma

9 What is the most common infective agent in the setting of round pneumonia?

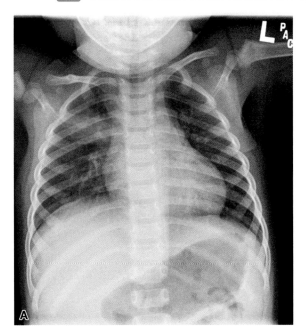
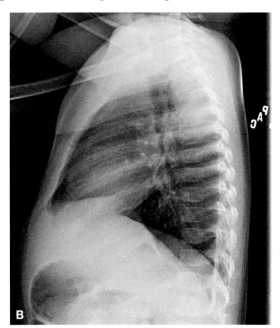

A. *Staphylococcus aureus*
B. *Streptococcus pneumoniae*
C. *Klebsiella pneumoniae*
D. *Mycoplasma pneumoniae*

10 A 6-month-old female presents with intermittent stridor and increased work of breathing. In the setting of suspected foreign body aspiration, what is the next best step?

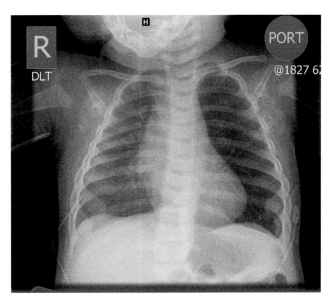

A. Administer broad-spectrum IV antibiotics
B. Perform bronchoscopy
C. Perform lateral decubitus chest radiographs
D. Perform chest CT

11 A 10-year-old female presents with recurrent lung infection. What is the most likely diagnosis?

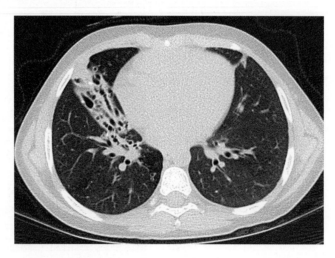

    A. Pulmonary tuberculosis
    B. Metastatic Wilms tumor
    C. Cystic fibrosis
    D. Cavitary pneumonia

12 A 19-month-old male presents with a history of cystic nephroma and DICER1 mutation. What is the most likely primary lung malignancy demonstrated?

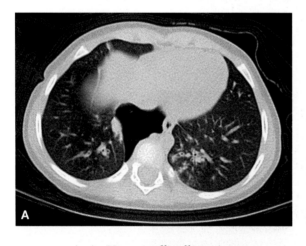
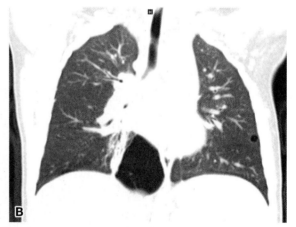

    A. Non–small cell carcinoma
    B. Mesothelioma
    C. Pleuropulmonary blastoma
    D. Ewing sarcoma

13 What anatomic structure is depicted by the yellow arrow in a neonate with situs inversus? The ultrasound correlation of the anatomic structure is provided.

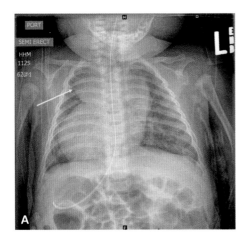 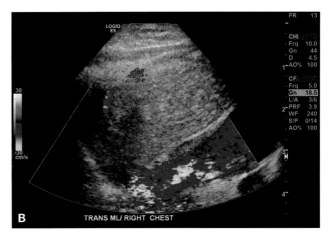

A. Ascending aorta
B. Right pulmonary outflow tract
C. Thymus
D. Esophagus

14 What are the top differential diagnoses for an anterior mediastinal mass?

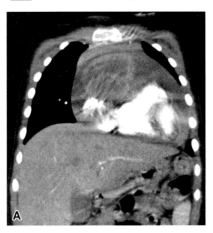 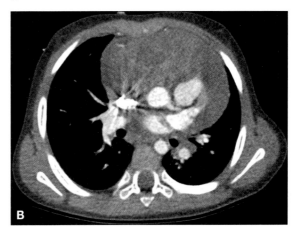

A. Teratoma, foregut duplication cyst, lymphoma
B. Teratoma, thymoma, lymphoma
C. Aortic aneurysm, neuroblastoma, thyroid carcinoma
D. Bronchogenic cyst, paraganglioma, thymoma

15 A 17-year-old female presents with an abnormal chest radiograph. What is the most likely diagnosis?

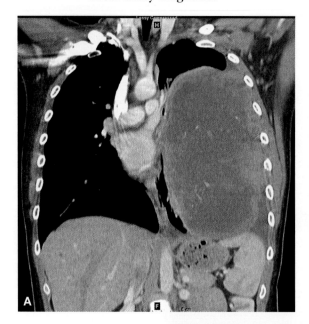

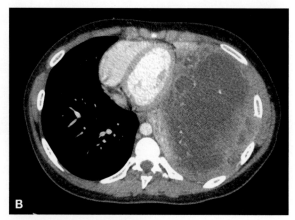

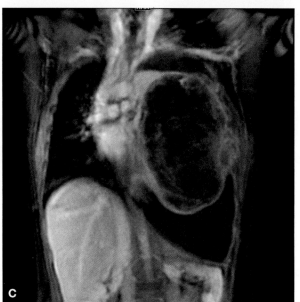

A. Small cell lung carcinoma
B. Mesothelioma
C. Ewing sarcoma
D. Neurofibroma

16 A 4-year-old female presents after liver transplant and airspace disease on chest imaging. What is the most likely infectious etiology based on the following imaging findings?

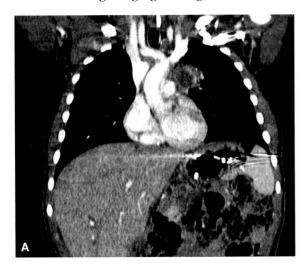 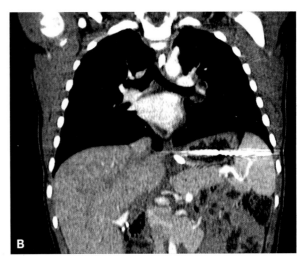

A. *Haemophilus influenzae*
B. *Streptococcus pneumoniae*
C. *Mycobacterium tuberculosis*
D. *Neisseria gonorrhoeae*

17 A 3-year-old female presents with abdominal mass felt by the patient's grandmother. What is the most likely malignancy present?

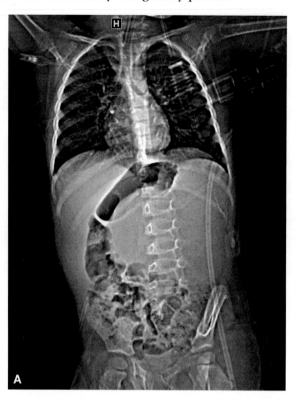

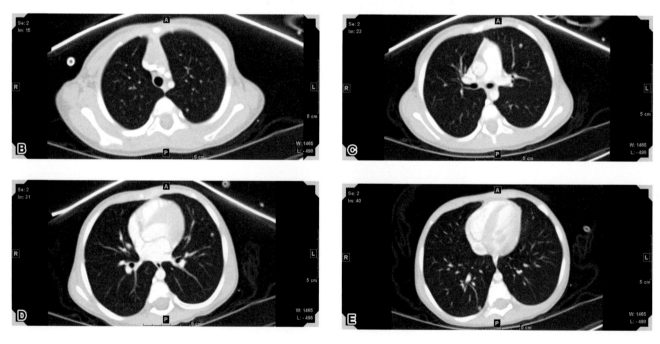

A. Lymphoma
B. Mature retroperitoneal teratoma
C. Colon carcinoma
D. Wilms tumor

18 A 14-year-old male presents with a chest wall deformity. What measurement is commonly calculated to determine if the patient qualifies for surgical intervention?

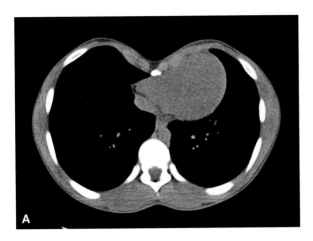 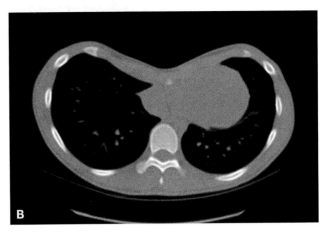

A. Haller index
B. Quantitative lung index
C. Lung heart ratio
D. Congenital pulmonary airway malformation volume ratio

19 What surgical procedure was performed on this patient?

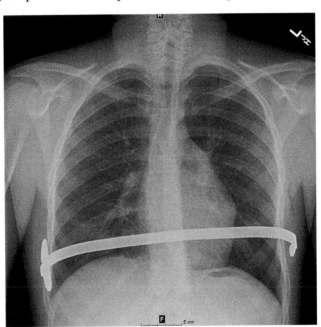

A. Video-assisted thoracoscopic surgery
B. Nuss procedure
C. Ravitch procedure
D. Pleurodesis

20   A 5-day-old presents with decreased respiratory effort and increased oxygen requirements. What is the most likely diagnosis?

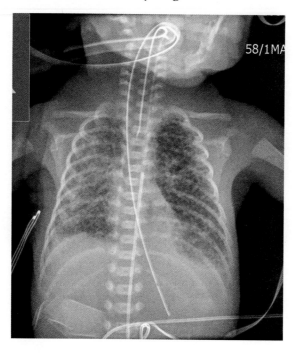

A. Meconium aspiration
B. Transient tachypnea of the newborn
C. Pulmonary interstitial emphysema
D. Pneumatocele

21   A 14-year-old male is imaged after placement of a central venous catheter. What congenital vascular variant is present?

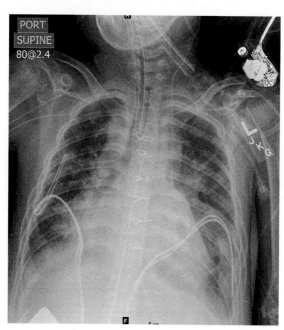

A. Vertical vein
B. Scimitar vein
C. Persistent left-sided superior vena cava
D. Pulmonary sling

22 A newborn presents with increased work of breathing. Within what thoracic compartment is air abnormally located?

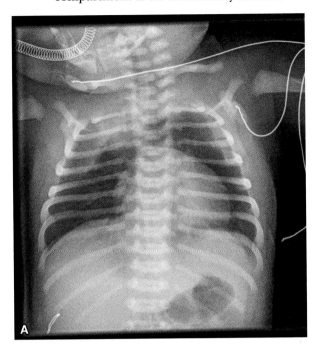

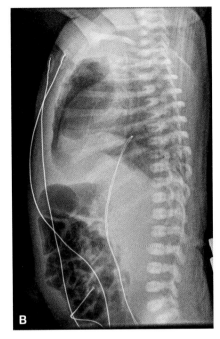

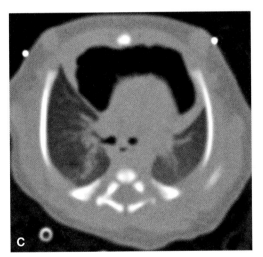

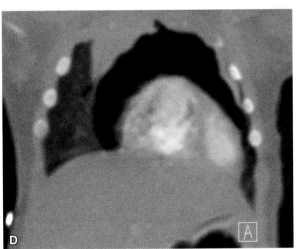

A. Mediastinum
B. Pericardium
C. Pleura
D. Peritoneum

23 A 17-year-old male presents with sepsis. What is the most likely diagnosis?

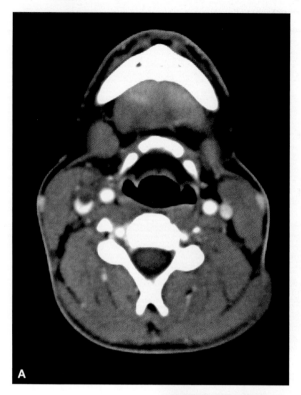

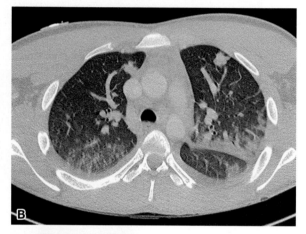

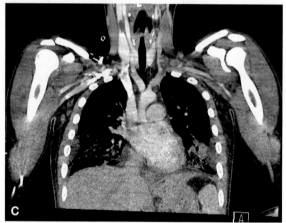

A. Pulmonary artery embolism
B. Lemierre syndrome
C. Aspergillosis
D. Legionnaires disease

24 A newborn male is diagnosed with multiple anomalies prenatally. After delivery, a nasogastric tube is inserted and a chest radiograph is obtained. What is the diagnosis?

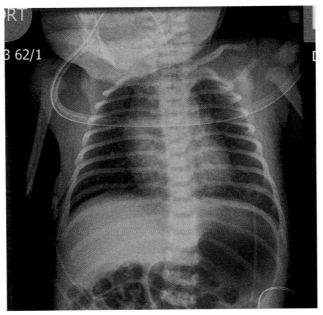

A. Malposition of the nasogastric tube into the tracheal airway
B. Esophageal atresia and tracheoesophageal fistula
C. Choanal atresia
D. Pyriform aperture stenosis

25 What is the most common subtype of esophageal atresia and tracheoesophageal fistula?

A. Proximal fistula, distal atresia
B. Isolated fistula, H-type
C. Isolated esophageal atresia
D. Distal fistula, proximal atresia

26 A newborn presents with history of meconium-stained amniotic fluid. What complication in this setting leads to higher morbidity and mortality?

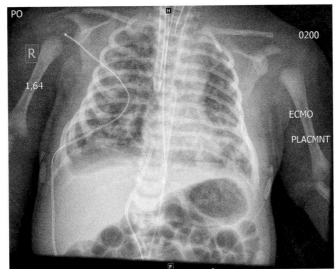

A. Reactive airway disease
B. Air leak
C. Pulmonary interstitial emphysema
D. Pulmonary hypertension

27 A 12-year-old male presents with recurrent lung disease. What is the most likely diagnosis?

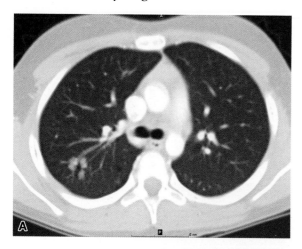 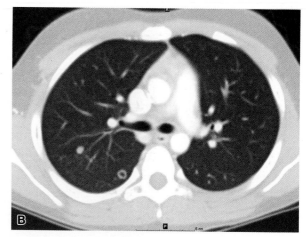

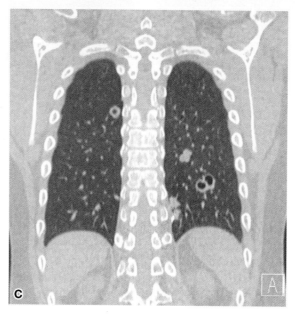

A. Posttransplant lymphoproliferative disorder
B. Tuberculosis
C. Aspergillosis
D. Papillomatosis

28 A 3-month-old male presents with a left humerus fracture. In addition to posterior rib fractures, what other fractured bone is considered highly specific for nonaccidental trauma or child abuse?

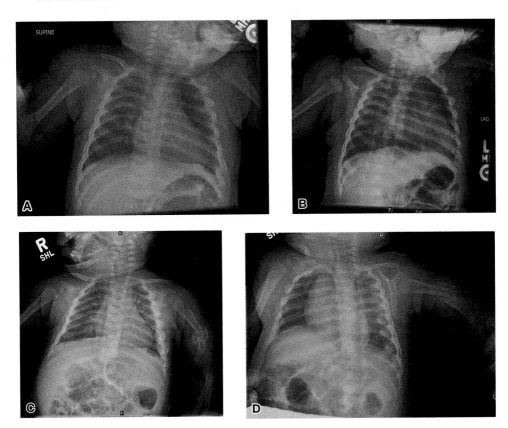

A. Long bone
B. Scapula
C. Pelvis
D. Clavicle

29 A 16-year-old male presents from outside the hospital after a motor vehicle collision (car hit tree). What is the most appropriate next step?

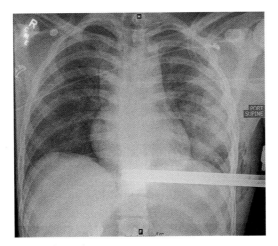

A. Chest ultrasound
B. Abdominal ultrasound
C. CT angiography of the chest
D. Surgical consultation

30 What is the diagnosis?

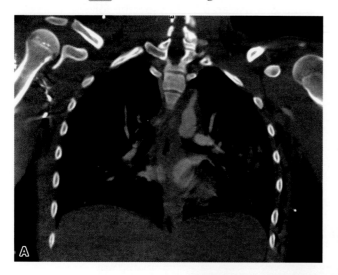

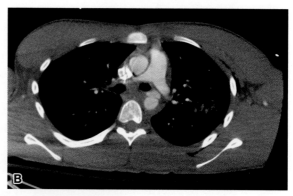

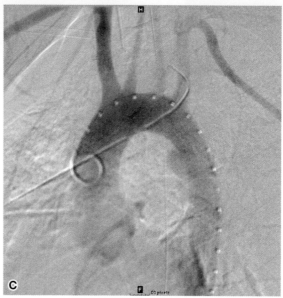

A. Aortic dissection
B. Aortic pseudoaneurysm
C. Tracheal rupture
D. Tension pneumothorax

ANSWERS AND EXPLANATIONS

1 **Answer C.** The clinical presentation and radiographic findings are consistent with a diaphragmatic hernia in a newborn. The chest X-ray images demonstrate a large lucency in the left hemithorax, mediastinal shift to the right, and bowel loops within the thoracic cavity. Diaphragmatic hernias are typically classified as either congenital or acquired. Congenital diaphragmatic hernias (CDHs) are often diagnosed antenatally or in the immediate postnatal period. The most common type of CDH is a Bochdalek hernia, which occurs due to a defect in the posterolateral aspect of the diaphragm. On chest X-ray, CDH typically presents as a large lucency in the affected hemithorax, usually the left side, representing herniated abdominal contents (e.g., bowel loops) within the thoracic cavity. The mediastinum may be shifted to the contralateral side due to the herniated contents. Bowel gas patterns can often be visualized within the thorax. Prompt recognition and management are crucial, as CDH is associated with significant morbidity and mortality due to pulmonary hypoplasia and pulmonary hypertension. Surgical correction is the mainstay of treatment in most cases.

References: Deprest J, Brady P, Nicolaides K, et al. Prenatal management of the fetus with isolated congenital diaphragmatic hernia in the era of the TOTAL trial. *Semin Fetal Neonatal Med.* 2014;19(6):338-348.

Mullassery D, Ba'ath ME, Jesudason EC, Losty PD. Value of liver herniation in prediction of outcome in fetal congenital diaphragmatic hernia: a systematic review and meta-analysis. *Ultrasound Obstet Gynecol.* 2010;35(5):609-614.

2 **Answer D.** Ebstein anomaly is a rare congenital heart defect that affects the tricuspid valve, which separates the right atrium and right ventricle of the heart. The following are the chest X-ray findings in Ebstein anomaly:

1. Cardiomegaly: Ebstein anomaly often presents with a marked enlargement of the right atrium and ventricle, leading to cardiomegaly on chest X-ray.
2. Right atrial enlargement: The right atrium is often significantly enlarged and can be seen as an increased convexity of the right cardiac border on chest X-ray.
3. Right ventricular enlargement: The right ventricle may also be enlarged, causing a bulging of the lower right heart border on chest X-ray.
4. Pulmonary artery enlargement: Due to increased blood flow and pressure in the right ventricle, the pulmonary artery may be enlarged and its branches may be more prominent on chest X-ray.
5. "Snowman" appearance: In severe cases of Ebstein anomaly, there may be a characteristic "snowman" appearance on chest X-ray, where the enlarged right atrium and ventricle form a rounded shape resembling a snowman.

It's important to note that chest X-ray findings alone are not enough to diagnose Ebstein anomaly definitively, and further testing such as echocardiography and cardiac catheterization may be required for diagnosis.

Reference: Ferguson EC, Krishnamurthy R, Oldham SA. Classic imaging signs of congenital cardiovascular abnormalities. *Radiographics.* 2007;27(5):1323-1334.

3 **Answer A.** The CT images reveal a well-defined noncommunicating mass in the left lower lung with systemic arterial supply arising from the descending thoracic aorta. No bronchial communication is identified. This represents a bronchopulmonary sequestration (BPS). BPS is a rare congenital malformation characterized by a nonfunctioning mass of lung tissue that lacks normal communication with the tracheobronchial tree and receives its blood supply from a systemic artery, typically arising from the descending thoracic aorta. On contrast-enhanced CT scan, BPS typically appears as a well-defined noncommunicating mass within the lung parenchyma, often located in the lower lobes. The mass may be solid or cystic and may contain air or fluid. Systemic arterial supply can often be identified within the lesion. Differentiating BPS from other lung lesions, such as pulmonary hamartoma, pulmonary artery aneurysm, or bronchogenic cyst, is important for appropriate management. Surgical resection is the treatment of choice for symptomatic cases of BPS to prevent recurrent infections and complications.

References: Berrocal T, Madrid C, Novo S, et al. Congenital anomalies of the tracheobronchial tree, lung, and mediastinum: embryology, radiology, and pathology. *Radiographics*. 2004;24(1):e17.

Franco J, Aliaga R, Domingo ML, et al. Diagnosis of pulmonary sequestration by spiral CT angiography. *Thorax*. 1998;53(12):1089-1092.

4 **Answer C.** The imaging findings described are consistent with congenital pulmonary airway malformation (CPAM), also known as congenital cystic adenomatoid malformation (CCAM). CPAM is a developmental anomaly of the lung characterized by multicystic, nonfunctioning lung tissue with various degrees of airway and vascular involvement. On chest X-ray, CPAM typically presents as a multicystic lesion with well-defined borders and variable cyst sizes distributed throughout the affected lung segment. The rest of the lung fields typically appear normal. CPAM is usually diagnosed in infancy or early childhood and may present with respiratory distress, infection, or as an incidental finding. Surgical resection is the standard treatment for symptomatic cases to prevent complications such as infection, cystic enlargement, or malignant transformation. Differentiating CPAM from other congenital lung lesions, such as pulmonary sequestration, congenital lobar emphysema, or CDH, is important for appropriate management.

5 **Answer D.** Fetal pleural effusion refers to the accumulation of fluid within the pleural space of the fetus. It can occur due to various causes, such as lymphatic obstruction, infection, or chromosomal abnormalities. On prenatal ultrasound, fetal pleural effusion appears as a fluid-filled lesion within the thorax, adjacent to the heart. The fluid collection is often seen shifting with fetal movements. On MRI, the effusion demonstrates high-T2 signal.

CDH is characterized by an abnormal opening in the diaphragm, allowing abdominal organs to herniate into the thoracic cavity. CDH typically appears as a solid mass or a cystic lesion within the thorax, and it is associated with other abnormalities such as lung hypoplasia.

Pulmonary sequestration refers to an aberrant mass of lung tissue with its own blood supply. It typically presents as a solid lesion within the lung parenchyma and is not associated with pleural fluid accumulation.

Bronchopulmonary foregut malformation is a rare congenital anomaly involving abnormal communication between the bronchial tree and the gastrointestinal tract. It usually presents with complex cystic or solid lesions within the mediastinum or lung parenchyma.

Therefore, based on the given information, the most likely diagnosis is fetal pleural effusion. Further evaluation and management would be required to determine the underlying cause and potential impact on fetal well-being. Fetal intervention such as thoracentesis can be performed to allow for lung development and to evaluate the contents of the pleural effusion.

Reference: Rustico MA, Lanna M, Coviello D, Smoleniec J, Nicolini U. Fetal pleural effusion. *Prenat Diagn*. 2007;27(9):793-799.

6 **Answer A.** There is hyperinflation of the right upper lobe with displacement of the mediastinum to the contralateral side. The left lung appears normal. The clinical history and imaging findings described are consistent with congenital lobar overinflation (CLO). CLO is a rare developmental anomaly characterized by overinflation of one or more lobes of the lung due to partial bronchial obstruction or bronchial cartilage deficiency. On chest X-ray, CLO typically presents as hyperinflation of the affected lobe(s), often with displacement of the mediastinum to the contralateral side. The remaining lungs appear normal. CLO is usually diagnosed in infancy or early childhood and may present with respiratory distress, recurrent lung infections, or failure to thrive. Surgical resection is the treatment of choice to relieve the compression of surrounding structures and prevent complications. Differentiating CLO from other congenital lung lesions, such as pulmonary sequestration, CPAM, or CDH, is important for appropriate management.

References: Berrocal T, Madrid C, Novo S, et al. Congenital anomalies of the tracheobronchial tree, lung, and mediastinum: embryology, radiology, and pathology. *Radiographics.* 2004;24(1):e17.

Stigers KB, Woodring JH, Kanga JF. The clinical and imaging spectrum of findings in patients with congenital lobar emphysema. *Pediatr Pulmonol.* 1992;14(3):160-170.

7 **Answer C.** The images demonstrate a contrast-enhanced CT scan of the chest and reveal a well-defined, fluid-filled cystic lesion adjacent to the esophagus. The cystic lesion is lined by smooth muscle and appears to communicate with the esophageal lumen. The imaging findings described are consistent with an esophageal duplication cyst. Esophageal duplication cysts are rare congenital anomalies that result from the incomplete separation of the foregut during embryonic development. They are usually lined by smooth muscle and are located adjacent to the esophagus. On contrast-enhanced CT scan, an esophageal duplication cyst appears as a well-defined, fluid-filled cystic lesion. Importantly, it may communicate with the esophageal lumen, which helps differentiate it from other cystic lesions in the mediastinum. Esophageal duplication cysts can cause symptoms such as dysphagia, respiratory infections, and chest pain. Surgical resection is usually recommended to alleviate symptoms and prevent complications. Differentiating an esophageal duplication cyst from other esophageal abnormalities, such as esophageal atresia, esophageal diverticulum, or esophageal stricture, is important for appropriate management.

References: Callahan MJ, Taylor GA. CT of the pediatric esophagus. *AJR Am J Roentgenol.* 2003;181(5):1391-1396.

Wiechowska-Kozłowska A, Wunsch E, Majewski M, et al. Esophageal duplication cysts: endosonographic findings in asymptomatic patients. *World J Gastroenterol.* 2012;18(11):1270-1272.

8 **Answer B.** CT demonstrates a heterogeneous right paraspinal mass. There is involvement of the right neural foramina at the levels of T3-T5. Neurogenic tumors represent more than 60% of posterior mediastinal masses. Neuroblastomas and ganglioneuroblastomas are malignant tumors that occur most commonly in children and originate from the sympathetic ganglia. Schwannomas and neurofibromas are benign lesions that arise from the intercostal nerve sheath.

Ganglioneuromas are benign lesions that arise from the sympathetic ganglia and are most common in young adults. Lesions that arise from paraganglionic cells include pheochromocytomas and paragangliomas. A spinal meningocele is a herniation of the meninges through a vertebral column defect or through a foramina. These are most commonly located posteriorly and in the lumbosacral region. Although rare, an anterior spinal meningocele will appear to be a posterior mediastinal mass on imaging. Thoracic teratomas and lymphomas typically occur in the anterior mediastinum. Foregut duplication cysts are typically located in the middle mediastinum.

References: Durand C, Baudain P, Nugues F, Bessaguet S. Mediastinal and thoracic MRI in children. *Pediatr Pulmonol Suppl.* 1999;18:60.

Nakazono T, White CS, Yamasaki F, et al. MRI findings of mediastinal neurogenic tumors. *AJR Am J Roentgenol.* 2011;197(4):W643-W652.

9 **Answer B.** Round pneumonia, also known as focal or lobar pneumonia, is a type of lung infection characterized by a rounded or oval-shaped consolidation of lung tissue. It is most commonly seen in children but can occur in individuals of any age. Round pneumonia is typically caused by bacterial pathogens, with *S. pneumoniae* being the most common culprit.

The infection begins as a localized area of inflammation and consolidation within a specific lung lobe or segment. Unlike typical lobar pneumonia, which affects an entire lobe, round pneumonia is confined to a smaller area. This localized consolidation appears as a rounded opacity on imaging studies such as chest X-ray or CT scan. The affected lung tissue may appear homogeneous and dense, without air bronchograms.

The name "round pneumonia" stems from the characteristic appearance of the infection on imaging. The rounded or oval shape results from the localized inflammation and consolidation, which may lack the typical lobar distribution seen in other types of pneumonia.

Clinical features of round pneumonia may include fever, cough, rapid breathing (tachypnea), and chest pain. These symptoms can vary in severity depending on the extent of the infection and the individual's overall health. In children, round pneumonia is often associated with milder symptoms compared to typical lobar pneumonia.

Treatment for round pneumonia typically involves antibiotic therapy to target the underlying bacterial infection. The choice of antibiotics depends on the suspected or identified pathogen. With appropriate treatment, the infection resolves, and lung function returns to normal.

It is important to differentiate round pneumonia from other causes of round lung opacities, such as lung abscesses, tumors, or other inflammatory conditions. Imaging studies, along with clinical features and the response to antibiotic therapy, help in establishing the diagnosis of round pneumonia.

References: Kim YW, Donnelly LF. Round pneumonia: imaging findings in a large series of children. *Pediatr Radiol.* 2007;37(12):1235-1240.

Wagner AL, Szabunio M, Hazlett KS, et al. Radiologic manifestations of round pneumonia in adults. *AJR Am J Roentgenol.* 1998;170(3):723-726.

10 **Answer C.** When a foreign body is aspirated into the respiratory tract, it can cause significant clinical symptoms and complications. Chest X-ray is often the initial imaging modality used to evaluate foreign body aspiration. The decubitus views of the chest can help identify some key findings of foreign body aspiration including:

Unilateral hyperinflation: If the foreign body obstructs the bronchus of one lung, it can lead to air trapping and hyperinflation of that lung. This results in increased lung volume on the affected side compared to the contralateral lung.

Mediastinal shift: Unilateral hyperinflation caused by foreign body aspiration can cause a shift of the mediastinum toward the contralateral side.

Atelectasis: In some cases, the foreign body can cause complete or partial obstruction of the bronchus, leading to collapse of the affected lung segment or lobe, resulting in atelectasis. Atelectasis may manifest as an area of increased opacity or decreased lung volume on chest X-ray.

Air trapping: In cases where the foreign body is obstructing a smaller airway or bronchiole, it can cause air trapping in the distal lung segments. This can be seen as areas of increased lucency on the chest X-ray, representing overinflated lung segments.

Radiodense foreign body: If the foreign body is radiopaque, such as a metal object, it may be visible directly on the chest X-ray. The foreign body can appear as a discrete opacity within the airway or lung parenchyma.

It is important to note that not all foreign bodies are radiopaque, and some may not be visualized on chest X-ray. In these cases, further imaging with techniques such as bronchoscopy or CT scan may be necessary to confirm the presence and location of the foreign body.

Prompt recognition and appropriate management of foreign body aspiration are crucial to prevent complications such as pneumonia, abscess formation, or respiratory compromise.

References: Capitanio MA, Kirkpatrick JA. The lateral decubitus film. An aid in determining air-trapping in children. *Radiology.* 1972;103(2):460-462.

Passàli D, Lauriello M, Bellussi L, et al. Foreign body inhalation in children: an update. *Acta Otorhinolaryngol Ital.* 2010;30(1):27-32.

11 **Answer C.** Cystic fibrosis (CF) is a genetic disorder that primarily affects the respiratory and gastrointestinal systems. On chest radiography, CF often presents with bronchial wall thickening and dilation, predominantly in the upper lobes of the lungs. This finding is indicative of bronchiectasis, which is a common complication of CF. The lungs may also show increased opacities due to mucus plugging and recurrent lung infections. Additionally, a "tram-track" appearance can be observed, which refers to parallel lines formed by the thickened bronchial walls. These findings are caused by chronic inflammation, recurrent infections, and impaired mucus clearance in CF.

While tuberculosis (TB) can cause lung opacities and occasionally bronchiectasis, the clinical presentation in this case, including chronic symptoms, recurrent infections, and failure to thrive, is more suggestive of CF. Asthma typically presents with reversible airway obstruction and may not demonstrate the same degree of bronchial wall thickening and dilation seen in CF. Therefore, the most likely diagnosis in this case is CF.

References: Helbich TH, Heinz-peer G, Fleischmann D, et al. Evolution of CT findings in patients with cystic fibrosis. *AJR Am J Roentgenol.* 1999;173(1):81-88.

Maffessanti M, Polverosi R, Dalpiaz G, et al. *Diffuse Lung Diseases: Clinical Features, Pathology, HRCT.* Springer Verlag; 2006.

12 **Answer C.** Pleuropulmonary blastoma (PPB) is a rare and aggressive malignant tumor that primarily affects the lungs and pleura (the lining of the chest cavity). It is predominantly seen in children and is associated with genetic alterations, including mutations in the DICER1 gene.

DICER1 is a gene involved in the production of microRNAs, which are small RNA molecules that regulate gene expression. Mutations in the DICER1 gene can disrupt the normal microRNA processing and lead to the development of various tumors, including PPB.

Children with DICER1 mutations have an increased risk of developing PPB, along with other tumors such as ovarian Sertoli-Leydig cell tumors, cystic nephroma, and multinodular goiter. Therefore, the presence of DICER1 mutations is an important consideration in the evaluation and management of pediatric patients with PPB.

PPB is classified into three types: Type I, Type II, and Type III, based on the histological features and clinical behavior. Type I PPB is predominantly cystic, Type II is a mixture of cystic and solid components, and Type III is predominantly solid with minimal cystic areas. Type III PPB is the most aggressive form and carries the highest risk of metastasis.

The treatment of PPB involves a multimodal approach, including surgery, chemotherapy, and sometimes radiation therapy. Early diagnosis and appropriate management are crucial for optimizing outcomes in patients with PPB.

Given the association between PPB and DICER1 mutations, genetic counseling and testing may be recommended for individuals with a personal or family history suggestive of DICER1-related tumors. Identifying DICER1 mutations in affected individuals and their family members can aid in surveillance and early detection of potential tumor development.

Reference: Priest JR, Williams GM, Hill DA, Dehner LP, Jaffe A. Pulmonary cysts in early childhood and the risk of malignancy. *Pediatr Pulmonol.* 2009;44(1):14-30.

13 **Answer C.** The thymus is an organ located in the anterior mediastinum, behind the sternum and in front of the heart. It plays a vital role in immune system development, particularly in the maturation of T cells. The imaging features of the thymus can vary depending on the age of the patient.

In infants and young children, the thymus is relatively large and prominent. Following are the imaging features of the thymus in different age groups:

Neonates and Infants

On chest X-ray, the thymus appears as a soft tissue density in the anterior mediastinum.

It typically has a bilateral triangular shape, with the apex pointing toward the head and the base tapering toward the diaphragm.

The thymus may extend superiorly and be visible behind the manubrium of the sternum.

It can have variable thickness and density, ranging from homogeneous to slightly heterogeneous.

Children and Adolescents

As children grow older, the thymus gradually involutes and becomes less prominent. On imaging, the thymus may appear smaller and less dense compared to the neonatal period. It may have a more rounded or oval shape rather than the triangular shape seen in infants. The thymus is still usually identifiable on imaging, but it becomes less conspicuous.

It is important to note that the appearance of the thymus can be influenced by various factors, such as body habitus, patient position during imaging, and underlying medical conditions. Additionally, abnormalities of the thymus, such as thymic tumors or thymic cysts, can manifest with different imaging features.

Imaging modalities such as chest X-ray, ultrasound, CT scan, or MRI can be used to evaluate the thymus and detect any abnormalities if present. The imaging findings should be interpreted in conjunction with the clinical context to guide appropriate management.

References: Nasseri F, Eftekhari F. Clinical and radiologic review of the normal and abnormal thymus: pearls and pitfalls. *Radiographics.* 2010;30(2):413-428.

Nishino M, Ashiku SK, Kocher ON, et al. The thymus: a comprehensive review. *Radiographics.* 2006;26(2):335-348.

14 **Answer B.** Anterior mediastinal masses in children can arise from various etiologies, including developmental, neoplastic, inflammatory, or infectious causes. Here are some common anterior mediastinal masses seen in children:

Thymic Masses

Thymomas: These are rare tumors arising from the thymus gland. They are usually slow growing and may present with symptoms such as cough, chest pain, or superior vena cava syndrome.

Thymic cysts: These are benign cystic lesions within the thymus and are often asymptomatic. They can be congenital or acquired.

Germ Cell Tumors

Teratomas: These are neoplasms that arise from germ cells and can contain various tissue types. In the anterior mediastinum, they are typically benign in children but can be malignant in adults.

Seminomas: These are malignant germ cell tumors that predominantly affect males and are rare in children.

Yolk sac tumors: These tumors typically occur in young children and may produce alpha-fetoprotein (AFP), which can be elevated in the blood.

Lymphomas

Hodgkin lymphoma: It can present as an anterior mediastinal mass in children, often associated with symptoms such as cough, chest pain, or superior vena cava syndrome.

Non-Hodgkin lymphoma: Certain subtypes, such as lymphoblastic lymphoma or Burkitt lymphoma, can manifest as anterior mediastinal masses in children.

Neurogenic Tumors

Neuroblastoma: Although neuroblastoma typically arises in the adrenal glands or sympathetic ganglia, it can occasionally occur within the anterior mediastinum.

Ganglioneuroma: It is a benign tumor arising from sympathetic ganglion cells and can occur in the mediastinum.

Other Masses

Foregut cysts: These are congenital cystic lesions derived from foregut structures, such as bronchogenic cysts or esophageal duplication cysts.

Castleman disease: It is a rare lymphoproliferative disorder that can present as a mediastinal mass, especially in children with multicentric Castleman disease.

Imaging modalities such as chest X-ray, ultrasound, CT scan, or MRI are typically used to evaluate anterior mediastinal masses. The specific characteristics, location, and associated findings on imaging can provide valuable information for further evaluation, including biopsy or surgical resection if necessary.

Reference: Ranganath SH, Lee EY, Restrepo R, Eisenberg RL. Mediastinal masses in children. *AJR Am J Roentgenol.* 2012;198(3):W197-W216.

15 **Answer C.** Ewing sarcoma is a malignant bone tumor that can occur in the chest, including the ribs, sternum, or other bones in the thoracic cavity. When Ewing sarcoma arises in the chest, it can present as a primary chest wall tumor. Here are some key features of Ewing sarcoma involving the chest:

Imaging Findings

Chest X-ray: Ewing sarcoma may appear as a destructive or lytic lesion in the affected bone. It can cause cortical thinning, cortical destruction, and sometimes periosteal reaction. Soft tissue mass or swelling may be visible as well.

CT scan: CT can provide detailed images of the chest wall, bones, and surrounding structures. It can demonstrate the extent of bone destruction, soft tissue involvement, and potential invasion into nearby structures.

MRI: MRI is useful for evaluating the soft tissue extent of the tumor, assessing the involvement of adjacent structures, and determining the presence of skip lesions. It can also help in preoperative planning and assessing the response to treatment.

Clinical Presentation

Chest pain: Patients may experience localized pain in the chest wall, which can be persistent or worsen with activity.

Swelling or palpable mass: A visible or palpable mass or swelling may be present in the affected area.

Difficulty breathing: Large tumors or involvement of the ribs can cause mechanical compression of the lungs, leading to respiratory symptoms.

Metastatic Evaluation

Ewing sarcoma has a propensity for metastasis, commonly involving the lungs, bones, and bone marrow. Therefore, imaging studies such as chest CT, bone scintigraphy, and bone marrow biopsy are typically performed to evaluate for metastatic spread.

The diagnosis of Ewing sarcoma is confirmed through a combination of clinical, radiological, and histopathological findings. Biopsy of the tumor is required to establish the definitive diagnosis and to differentiate Ewing sarcoma from other chest wall tumors or bone malignancies.

Treatment typically involves a multidisciplinary approach, including chemotherapy, surgery, and radiation therapy, depending on the extent of disease and the patient's individual characteristics. Prognosis can vary depending on various factors such as tumor size, location, metastasis, and response to treatment.

It is important to consult with an oncologist and a specialized sarcoma team for the management and treatment planning of patients with Ewing sarcoma involving the chest.

References: Saenz NC, Hass DJ, Meyers P, et al. Pediatric chest wall Ewing's sarcoma. *J Pediatr Surg.* 2000;35(4):550-555.

Tateishi U, Gladish GW, Kusumoto M, et al. Chest wall tumors: radiologic findings and pathologic correlation: part 2. Malignant tumors. *Radiographics.* 2003;23(6):1491-1508.

16   **Answer C.** Imaging plays a crucial role in the diagnosis and evaluation of pediatric TB. Here are the common imaging findings seen in pediatric patients with TB:

Chest X-ray

Primary complex: In primary TB, which occurs after initial infection, the chest X-ray may show lymphadenopathy, especially hilar or mediastinal lymphadenopathy. It can also show consolidation, which appears as homogeneous opacities usually in the middle or lower lung zones. Ghon focus, a small parenchymal lesion with adjacent lymphadenopathy, may also be seen.

Progressive disease: In progressive or advanced TB, the chest X-ray may show larger areas of consolidation, cavitation (formation of air-filled spaces within the lung), and bronchial wall thickening. These findings are more commonly observed in older children and adolescents.

CT Scan

CT scan is more sensitive and specific than a chest X-ray in detecting the extent of TB infection and associated complications.

It can reveal additional findings such as tree-in-bud opacities, representing small centrilobular nodules connected by thin branching linear opacities, which indicate small airway involvement.

CT can also help identify the presence of cavitary lesions, bronchial wall thickening, pleural effusion, and lymphadenopathy more accurately than a chest X-ray.

Other Imaging Modalities

MRI: MRI is less commonly used for evaluating pediatric TB, but it may be helpful in assessing complications like spinal involvement, spinal cord compression, or central nervous system TB.

Ultrasound: Ultrasound can aid in evaluating peripheral lymph nodes for enlargement or abscess formation.

Nuclear medicine: Techniques like positron emission tomography (PET) scans may be used in selected cases to assess the extent of disease and response to treatment.

References: Jeong YJ, Lee KS. Pulmonary tuberculosis: up-to-date imaging and management. *AJR Am J Roentgenol.* 2008;191(3):834-844.

Leung AN. Pulmonary tuberculosis: the essentials. *Radiology.* 1999;210(2):307-322.

17 **Answer D.** Wilms tumor, also known as nephroblastoma, is a common pediatric kidney tumor. Although it primarily arises in the kidneys, it can metastasize to other organs, including the lungs. Pulmonary involvement of Wilms tumor is referred to as pulmonary Wilms tumor. Here are some key points regarding pulmonary Wilms tumor:

Imaging Findings

Chest X-ray: Pulmonary Wilms tumor typically appears as single or multiple pulmonary nodules or masses on a chest X-ray. These nodules can range in size and may have well-defined or irregular margins.

CT scan: CT imaging provides better characterization of the pulmonary lesions. Pulmonary Wilms tumor can appear as solid or partially cystic masses with enhancement. They may have irregular borders and can be associated with surrounding ground-glass opacities or consolidation.

Clinical Presentation

Pulmonary Wilms tumor is often asymptomatic, especially in the early stages. It is typically identified during routine imaging or surveillance for primary Wilms tumor. If symptoms are present, they may include cough, shortness of breath, chest pain, or hemoptysis.

Diagnostic Evaluation

Imaging: Chest X-ray and CT scan are commonly used to detect and evaluate pulmonary Wilms tumor. These imaging studies help assess the number, size, and characteristics of pulmonary nodules or masses.

Biopsy: A biopsy of the pulmonary lesions is usually required to confirm the diagnosis of pulmonary Wilms tumor. It can be performed using image-guided percutaneous needle biopsy or surgical excision of the lung nodules.

Management

Pulmonary Wilms tumor is managed in conjunction with the primary kidney tumor. Treatment typically involves a multimodal approach, including chemotherapy, surgery, and radiation therapy, tailored to the extent of disease and individual patient factors.

Chemotherapy: Chemotherapy is typically initiated to shrink both the primary kidney tumor and any metastatic pulmonary lesions. It helps facilitate surgical resection and improve outcomes.

Surgery: Surgical resection of the primary Wilms tumor and any accessible pulmonary metastatic lesions is performed whenever feasible.

Radiation therapy: Radiation therapy may be considered for cases with residual disease or when complete surgical resection is not achievable.

References: Guermazi A. *Imaging of Kidney Cancer.* Springer Verlag; 2006.

Lowe LH, Isuani BH, Heller RM, et al. Pediatric renal masses: Wilms tumor and beyond. *Radiographics.* 2000;20(6):1585-1603.

18 **Answer A.** See answer for Question 19.

19 **Answer B.** Pectus excavatum is a congenital chest wall deformity characterized by concave depression of the sternum, resulting in cosmetic and radiographic alterations. The Haller index (maximal transverse diameter/narrowest anteroposterior length of chest) is used to assess the severity of incursion of the sternum into the mediastinum. A normal Haller index is 2.5. Significant pectus excavatum has an index >3.25, representing the standard for determining candidacy for repair.

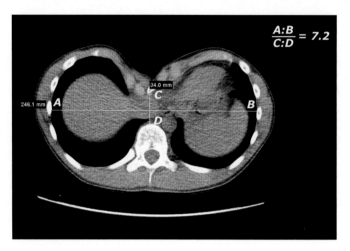

Surgical options include metal bar insertion, rib osteotomies, disconnection of the sternum from costal cartilages, and even reversal of the sternum. The Nuss procedure is a minimally invasive procedure where a concave bar is inserted substernally. It has largely replaced the Ravitch procedure, which was significantly more invasive.

References: Haller AJ, Kramer SS, Lietman SA. Use of CT scans in selection of patients for pectus excavatum surgery: a preliminary report. *J Pediatr Surg*. 1987;22(10):904-906.

Jaroszewski DE, Fonkalsrud EW. Repair of pectus chest deformities in 320 adult patients: 21 year experience. *Ann Thorac Surg*. 2007;84(2):429-433.

20 **Answer C.** Chest radiograph demonstrates left lung hyperinflation and multiple rounded lucencies in the left lung. Pulmonary interstitial emphysema (PIE) refers to the abnormal location of air within the pulmonary interstitium and lymphatics. It typically results from rupture of overdistended alveoli following barotrauma in infants who have hyaline membrane disease. Meconium aspiration is encountered in term infants and presents with high lung volumes, asymmetric patchy lung opacities, and occasionally pneumothorax because of small airway obstruction. Transient tachypnea of the newborn (TTN), also known as retained fetal fluid or wet lung disease, presents in the neonate as tachypnea for the first few hours of life, lasting up to 1 day. The images in TTN typically demonstrate pulmonary edema and small pleural effusions. Pneumatoceles are intrapulmonary air-filled cystic spaces that can have a variety of sizes and appearances. They may contain air-fluid levels and are mainly associated with the etiologic triad of prematurity, respiratory distress syndrome (RDS), and mechanical ventilation therapy.

References: Cleveland RH. A radiologic update on medical diseases of the newborn chest. *Pediatr Radiol*. 1996;25(8):631-637.

Greenough A, Dixon AK, Roberton NR. Pulmonary interstitial emphysema. *Arch Dis Child*. 1984;59(11):1046-1051.

21 **Answer C.** Right upper extremity peripherally inserted central catheter (PICC) line is coiled back upon itself with tip at the level of the right brachial artery. Left internal jugular vein catheter tip terminates in the lower portion of a persistent left-sided superior vena cava (PLSVC). A PLSVC is the most common congenital venous anomaly in the chest and can result in a right-to-left shunt.

The majority of cases are asymptomatic and the presence of the vessel is only identified incidentally during CT scanning of the chest or as a result of line placement as in this example. There are different possible drainage sites:

1. Coronary sinus: functionally insignificant because venous return from the head, neck, and upper limbs is delivered to the right atrium
2. Left atrium: results in a right-to-left shunt, which is usually not large enough to cause cyanosis or symptoms

References: Kellman GM, Alpern MB, Sandler MA, et al. Computed tomography of vena caval anomalies with embryologic correlation. *Radiographics.* 1988;8(3):533-556.

Pretorius PM, Gleeson FV. Case 74: right-sided superior vena cava draining into left atrium in a patient with persistent left-sided superior vena cava. *Radiology.* 2004;232(3):730-734.

22 **Answer A.** There is air in the mediastinum with mass effect and deviation of the thymus to the right. Pneumomediastinum is the presence of extraluminal gas within the mediastinum. Gas may originate from the lungs, trachea, central bronchi, esophagus, and peritoneal cavity and track from the mediastinum to the neck or abdomen. Etiologies include blunt or penetrating chest trauma, surgery, esophageal perforation, tracheobronchial perforation, barotrauma, infection, and idiopathic.

A pneumopericardium can usually be distinguished from pneumomediastinum, because air in the pericardial sac should not rise above the anatomic limits of the pericardial reflection on the proximal great vascular pedicle. Also, on radiographs obtained with the patient in the decubitus position, air in the pericardial sac will shift immediately, whereas air in the mediastinum will not shift in a short interval between films.

Occasionally, it may not be possible to distinguish pneumopericardium from pneumomediastinum on plain film.

References: Bejvan SM, Godwin JD. Pneumomediastinum: old signs and new signs. *AJR Am J Roentgenol.* 1996;166(5):1041-1048.

Karoui M, Bucur PO. Images in clinical medicine. Pneumopericardium. *N Engl J Med.* 2008;359(14):e16.

23 **Answer B.** Lemierre syndrome is a rare and potentially life-threatening condition characterized by a deep neck space infection, typically originating from the oropharynx, and subsequent septic thrombophlebitis of the internal jugular vein. Here are the typical imaging findings seen in Lemierre syndrome:

CT Scan of the Neck

Soft tissue infection: CT can show evidence of a localized oropharyngeal infection, such as tonsillitis or peritonsillar abscess. There may be thickening of the soft tissues of the oropharynx with inflammatory changes and edema.

Internal jugular vein thrombosis: CT can demonstrate thrombus within the internal jugular vein, which may appear as a filling defect or an enlarged, hyperdense vein. The thrombus can extend superiorly to involve the adjacent sigmoid sinus or inferiorly into the brachiocephalic vein.

Lymphadenopathy: Enlarged cervical lymph nodes may be present due to reactive inflammation.

CT or MRI of the Chest:

Pulmonary involvement: Imaging of the chest is often performed to evaluate for septic emboli, which can occur in the lungs. CT or MRI may reveal multiple nodules or consolidations scattered throughout the lung fields. These pulmonary lesions can range in size and may demonstrate peripheral or peribronchial distribution.

Pleural effusion: In some cases, Lemierre syndrome can lead to the development of a pleural effusion, which can be visualized on imaging studies.

Contrast-Enhanced Computed Tomography (CECT) of the Abdomen:
Abdominal involvement: Although less common, Lemierre syndrome can lead to the formation of septic emboli in the liver or other intra-abdominal organs. CECT can help identify these embolic lesions.

Reference: O'Brien WT, Lattin GE, Thompson AK. Lemierre syndrome: an all-but-forgotten disease. *AJR Am J Roentgenol.* 2006;187(3):W324.

24 **Answer B.** Esophageal atresia is a congenital anomaly where the esophagus does not form a continuous tube, resulting in a separation or blockage of the esophageal lumen. It is often associated with a tracheoesophageal fistula (TEF), an abnormal connection between the esophagus and the trachea. Here are some key points regarding the imaging features of esophageal atresia:

Prenatal Ultrasound:
Prenatal ultrasound can sometimes identify esophageal atresia during routine fetal screening. Polyhydramnios (excess amniotic fluid) may be present due to the inability of the fetus to swallow amniotic fluid, which leads to impaired fluid absorption.

Immediate Postnatal Evaluation:
Clinical presentation: Newborns with esophageal atresia may exhibit excessive drooling, choking, or coughing during feeding. The inability to pass a nasogastric tube into the stomach is a strong indicator of esophageal atresia.

Plain Radiographs:
Chest X-ray: The presence of a coiled or coiled-up nasogastric tube in the upper chest is highly suggestive of a TEF. Air may also be seen within the stomach, indicating a patent distal esophagus.

 Abdominal X-ray: Air-filled bowel loops may be seen in the upper abdomen due to the presence of a distal TEF.

Contrast Esophagram (Upper Gastrointestinal Series):
Once the clinical suspicion of esophageal atresia is raised, a contrast esophagram is performed. A radiopaque contrast agent is administered orally, and serial images are obtained. The esophagram can reveal the site of esophageal interruption, the presence and location of the TEF, and any associated anomalies. The contrast agent may not pass beyond the level of the atresia, and there may be a blind-ending upper esophageal pouch.

Additional Imaging:
CT or MRI: In some cases, additional imaging modalities such as CT or MRI may be utilized to further evaluate the anatomy and associated anomalies, especially in complex cases or when surgical planning is necessary. Timely diagnosis and management of esophageal atresia are crucial to prevent complications such as aspiration pneumonia and malnutrition. Surgical repair is the treatment of choice, and the specific surgical approach depends on the type and severity of the atresia as well as the presence of associated anomalies.

25 **Answer D.** There is a feeding tube with its tip at the level of the T3 vertebral body. There is gas in the stomach and bowel loops. Esophageal atresia refers to an absence in contiguity of the esophagus because of an inappropriate division of the primitive foregut into the trachea and esophagus. This is the most common congenital anomaly of the esophagus. It is frequently associated with a TEF. The types of esophageal atresia/TEF can be divided into:

• Proximal atresia with distal fistula: 85%
• Isolated esophageal atresia: 8% to 9%
• Isolated fistula (H-type): 4% to 6%

- Double fistula with intervening atresia: 1% to 2%
- Proximal fistula with distal atresia: 1%

The presence of air in the stomach and bowel in the setting of esophageal atresia implies that there is a distal fistula if feeding tube insertion has been attempted. This may show the tube blind looping and turning back at the upper thoracic part of the esophagus or heading into the trachea and/or bronchial tree.

Esophageal atresias are frequently associated with various other anomalies (50% to 75% of cases). They include:

- Other intestinal atresias
  - Duodenal atresia
  - Jejunoileal atresia
  - Anal atresia
- Annular pancreas
- Pyloric stenosis
- VACTERL association inclusive of congenital cardiac anomalies
- CHARGE syndrome
- Increased incidence of chromosomal anomalies such as
  - Trisomy 21
  - Trisomy 18

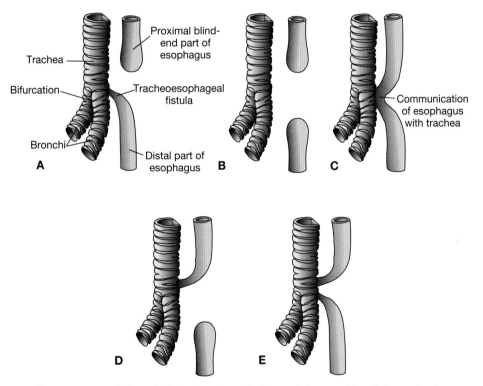

Reference: Berrocal T, Madrid C, Novo S, et al. Congenital anomalies of the tracheobronchial tree, lung, and mediastinum: embryology, radiology, and pathology. *Radiographics.* 2004;24(1):e17.

26 **Answer D.** Bilateral interstitial and airspace opacities are most compatible with meconium aspiration. Extracorporeal membrane oxygenation (ECMO) catheters are in place. Meconium aspiration syndrome (MAS) occurs secondary to intrapartum or intrauterine aspiration of meconium, usually in the setting of fetal distress and usually in term or postterm infants. The mortality rate for MAS resulting from severe parenchymal pulmonary disease and pulmonary hypertension is as high as 20%. Other complications include air leak syndromes (e.g., pneumothorax, pneumomediastinum, pneumopericardium), which occur in 10% to 30% of infants with MAS. The neurologic disabilities of survivors are not due primarily to the aspiration of meconium but rather due to in utero pathophysiology, including chronic hypoxia and acidosis.

Reference: Ghidini A, Spong CY. Severe meconium aspiration syndrome is not caused by aspiration of meconium. *Am J Obstet Gynecol.* 2001;185(4):931-938.

27 **Answer D.** There are well-defined, rounded, pulmonary nodules, many with cavitation, located in both lungs. Tracheobronchial or recurrent respiratory papillomatosis is a disease caused by the human papillomavirus (HPV). Imaging typically demonstrates airway wall (e.g., laryngeal, tracheal) thickening or nodularity and multiple pulmonary nodules and masses. The larger nodules are more likely to cavitate. The posterior, dependent lungs are more likely to be seeded. Most nodules grow slowly; however, rapid growth may represent conversion to squamous cell carcinoma.

References: Jhun BW, Lee K-J, Jeon K, et al. The clinical, radiological, and bronchoscopic findings and outcomes in patients with benign tracheobronchial tumors. *Yonsei Med J.* 2014;55(1):84-91.

Marchiori E, Zanetti G, Mauro Mano C. Tracheobronchial papillomatosis with diffuse cavitary lung lesions. *Pediatr Radiol.* 2010;40(7):1301-1302; author reply 1303.

28 **Answer B.** In addition to the left humerus fracture, there are nondisplaced fractures of the left fifth, sixth, and seventh lateral ribs without associated callus formation. The high-specificity skeletal fractures for nonaccidental trauma (NAT) include:

- Bucket handle or corner fractures
- Ribs (especially posterior)
- Scapula (e.g., acromion)
- Spine (especially spinous processes)
- Sternum

The classical metaphyseal corner or bucket handle fracture is virtually pathognomonic for NAT. Rib fractures are very common and highly specific for NAT in children <2 years old. Fractures of the acromion, sternum, and spinous processes are so rare in other conditions and therefore are considered a high specificity for NAT.

Rib fractures are easily overlooked on radiographs. These fractures are usually not evident on radiographs in the acute stage, as little displacement occurs. They are typically identified in the healing stage as a result of callus formation. It is imperative to routinely include oblique views of the chest while performing the skeletal survey to adequately diagnose rib fractures in the setting of NAT.

References: Kleinman PL, Kleinman PK, Savageau JA. Suspected infant abuse: radiographic skeletal survey practices in pediatric health care facilities. *Radiology.* 2004;233(2):477-485.

Lonergan GJ, Baker AM, Morey MK, et al. From the archives of the AFIP. Child abuse: radiologic-pathologic correlation. *Radiographics.* 2003;23(4):811-845.

29 **Answer C.** CT angiography (CTA) of the chest. Approximately 25% of deaths from blunt trauma arise from chest injuries, although up to 50% of deaths are at least partially related to thoracic injuries. It is essential to diagnose and treat emergent thoracic injuries quickly, and imaging plays an essential role in diagnosing these injuries. The imaging manifestations of thoracic trauma are diverse and include musculoskeletal, pleural, pulmonary, and mediastinal findings. The most devastating injury to the thorax from blunt trauma is acute aortic injury or transection, and the most common thoracic injury is a rib fracture. ACR Appropriateness Criteria topic on "Blunt Chest Trauma—Suspected Aortic Injury" supports the use of chest CTA in combination with chest radiography without reservation. The authors reported evidence that CTA is highly sensitive (with a high negative predictive value) in evaluating suspected traumatic aortic injury when there are no signs of direct aortic injury. CTA is also highly specific for aortic injury, such that most centers have now abandoned invasive aortography in the initial assessment of patients with suspected aortic injury from trauma.

References: Calhoon JH, Trinkle JK. Pathophysiology of chest trauma. *Chest Surg Clin N Am.* 1997;7(2):199-211.

Ungar TC, Wolf SJ, Haukoos JS, et al. Derivation of a clinical decision rule to exclude thoracic aortic imaging in patients with blunt chest trauma after motor vehicle collisions. *J Trauma.* 2006;61(5):1150-1155.

30 **Answer B.** Chest radiography demonstrates an abnormally widened mediastinum. CTA of the chest and aortic angiography demonstrate pseudoaneurysm formation at the isthmus of the descending thoracic aorta.

Trauma to the aorta may result in:

- Aortic laceration: a tear in the intima, which may extend through the vessel wall; the tear is typically transverse.
- Aortic transection: laceration of all three layers of the vessel wall, also known as aortic rupture
- Aortic pseudoaneurysm: aortic rupture contained by adventitia or periaortic tissue
- Aortic intramural hematoma: hematoma within the wall of the aorta

An aortic dissection is a longitudinal tear in the aortic wall and is rarely a sequela of trauma.

Aortic pseudoaneurysms are contained ruptures of the aorta in which the majority of the aortic wall has been breached, and luminal blood is held in only by a thin rim of the remaining wall or adventitia. They typically occur from focal aortic transection. The pseudoaneurysms typically occur along the undersurface of the aortic isthmus at or near the site of the ductus arteriosus. The isthmus is a portion of the proximal descending thoracic aorta between the left subclavian artery origin and the ligamentum arteriosum. Tethering of the aorta by the ligamentum arteriosum is believed to account for the high frequency of aortic injury in this region. Aortic injury is a surgical emergency. Treatment is with an aortic stent graft or open repair. An aortic stent graft is demonstrated in the following image.

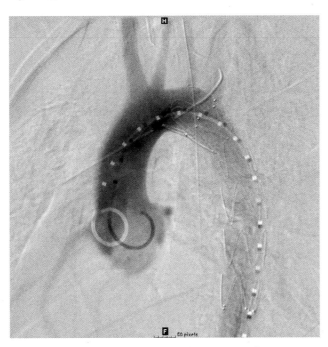

References: Creasy JD, Chiles C, Routh WD, et al. Overview of traumatic injury of the thoracic aorta. *Radiographics.* 1997;17(1):27-45.

Kuhlman JE, Pozniak MA, Collins J, et al. Radiographic and CT findings of blunt chest trauma: aortic injuries and looking beyond them. *Radiographics.* 1998;18(5):1085-1106.

Brain

1   A 1-day-old infant male born at 39 weeks of gestational age presents with a history of abnormal prenatal ultrasound and MRI. What is the correct diagnosis?

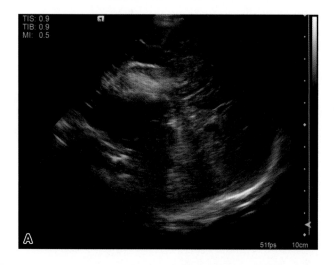 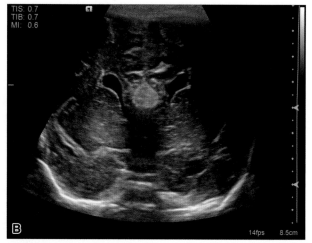

A. Holoprosencephaly
B. Dandy-Walker sequence
C. Agenesis of the corpus callosum
D. Septo-optic dysplasia

2 A 15-year-old female presents with seizure disorder and evaluation for VP shunt malfunction.

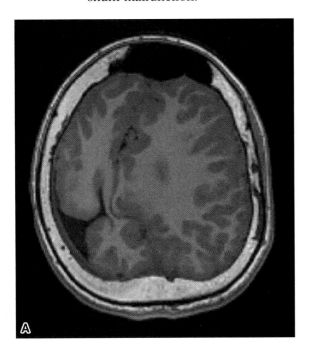
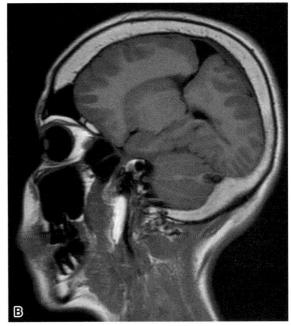

Schizencephaly is commonly associated with which of the following cerebral anomalies?

A. Holoprosencephaly
B. Agenesis of the corpus callosum
C. Lissencephaly
D. Gray matter heterotopia

3 A 2-year-old female presents to the emergency department with increased head circumference and possible VP shunt malfunction.

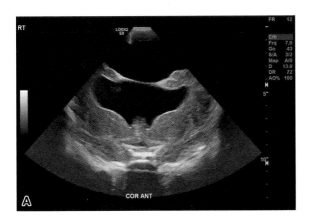
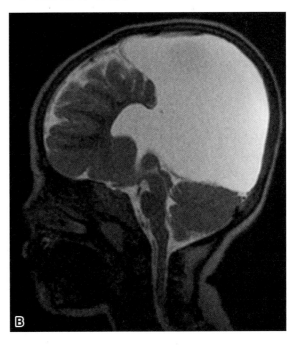

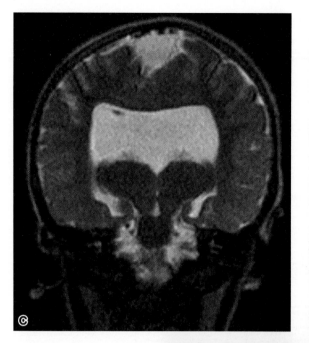

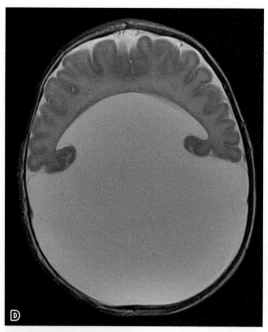

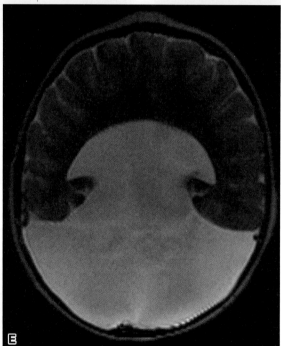

Which subtype of holoprosencephaly is depicted in this case?

A. Alobar

B. Semilobar

C. Lobar

D. Septo-optic dysplasia

4 A 4-year-old female presents with headache.

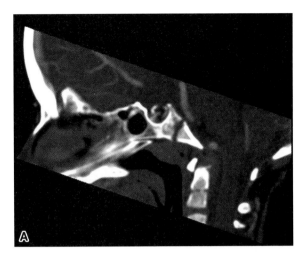

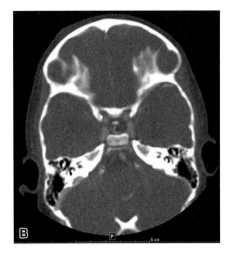

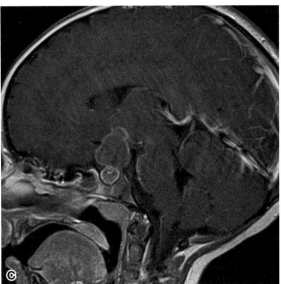

What is the most likely diagnosis?

A. Chordoma

B. Langerhans cell histiocytosis

C. Anterior communicating artery aneurysm

D. Craniopharyngioma

5 A 4-year-old male presents with precocious puberty, early penile growth, and testicular enlargement.

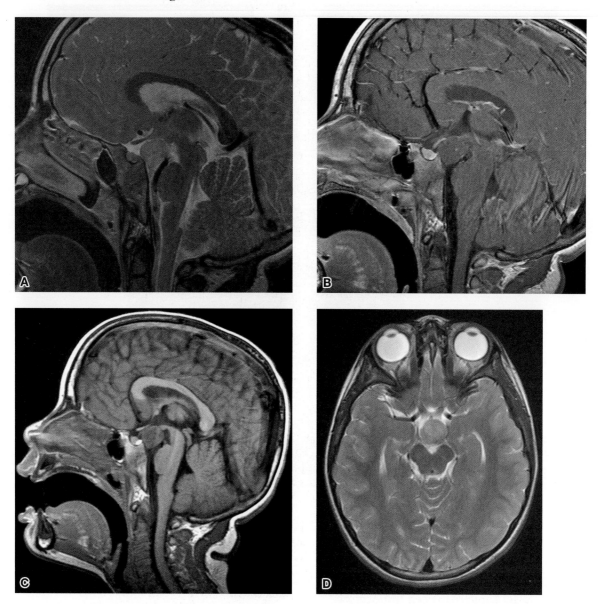

What is the most likely diagnosis?

A. Lipoma

B. Hypothalamic hamartoma

C. Langerhans cell histiocytosis

D. Germinoma

6 A 15-year-old female presents with daily headaches for 1 week and vomiting.

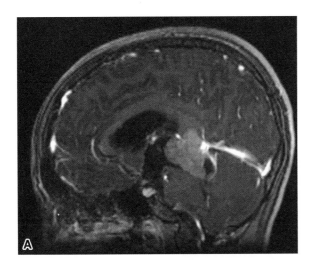
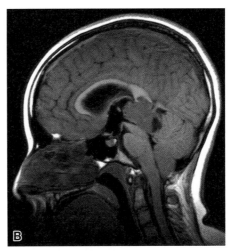
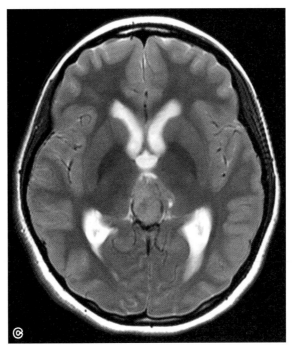

What is the most likely diagnosis?

A. Pineoblastoma

B. Craniopharyngioma

C. Meningioma

D. Ependymoma

7 Pineal region tumors may cause which of the following?

A. Diabetes insipidus

B. Parinaud syndrome

C. Gynecomastia

D. Seborrheic dermatitis

8 An 11-year-old male presents with vomiting, dizziness, headache, and personality changes.

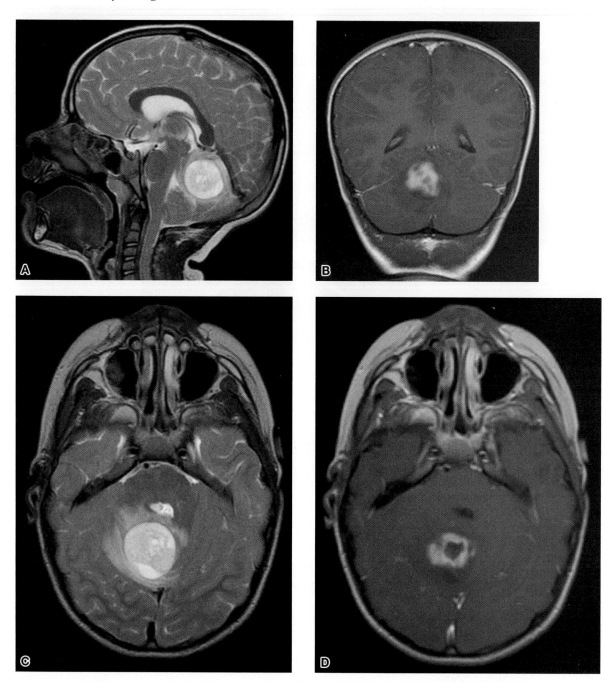

What is the most likely diagnosis?

A. Medulloblastoma
B. Pilocytic astrocytoma
C. Meningioma
D. Dermoid cyst

9 A 12-year-old male presents with progressive ataxia of the past few weeks.

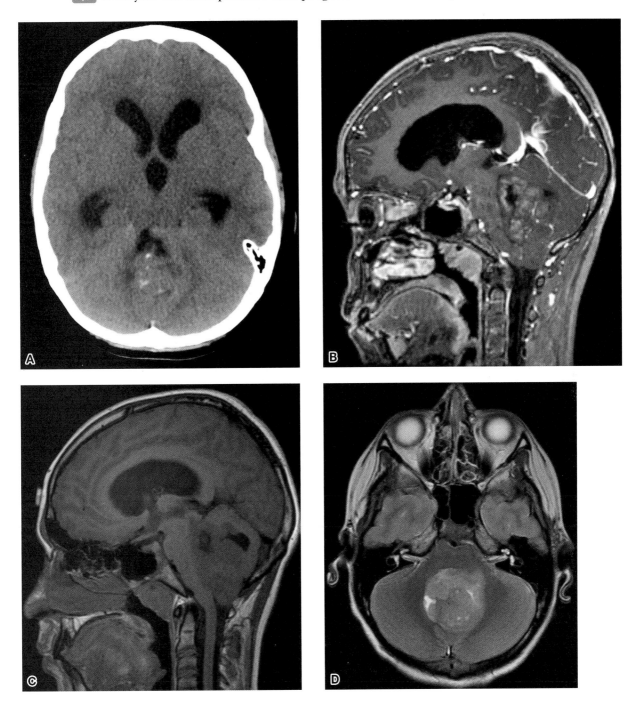

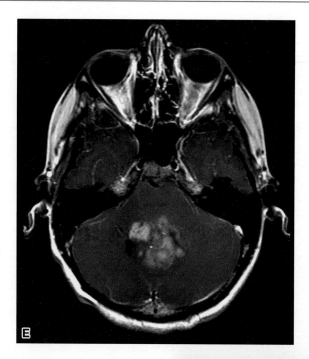

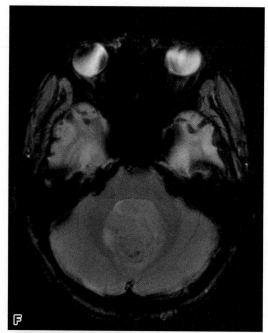

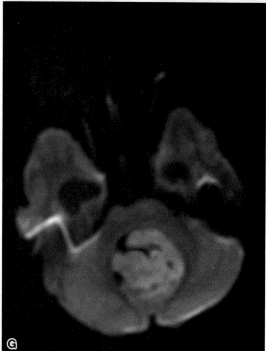

What is the most likely diagnosis?

A. Pineoblastoma
B. Medulloblastoma
C. Pilocytic astrocytoma
D. Hemangioblastoma

10 What is the next best step?

A. Spine imaging to exclude drop metastases
B. Cerebral angiography to delineate feeding vessels
C. Chemotherapy
D. Surgical resection

11 A 2-day-old female presents with abnormal antenatal imaging. Images shown are from fetal MRI performed at 22 weeks of gestational age and sagittal MRI of the brain performed at 2 days of age.

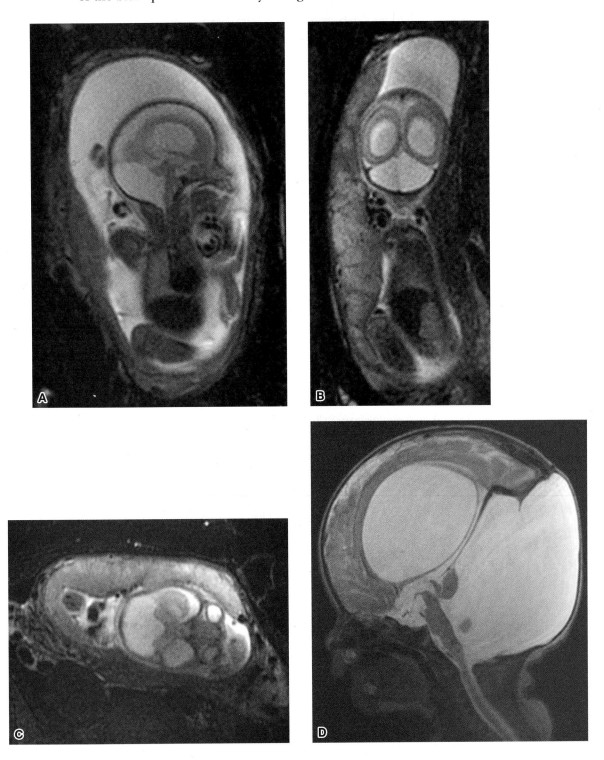

What is the most likely diagnosis?

A. Neurofibromatosis type 1
B. Chiari II malformation
C. Dandy-Walker malformation
D. Subarachnoid cyst

12 A 4-year-old male patient presents with a history of developmental delay. What is the diagnosis?

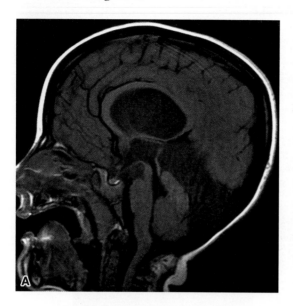 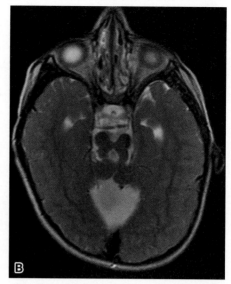

A. Dandy-Walker malformation
B. Posterior fossa arachnoid cyst
C. Mega cisterna magna
D. Joubert syndrome

13 A 5-month-old female presents for the evaluation of congenital fibrosis of extraocular muscles.

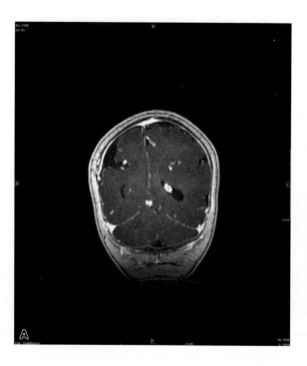 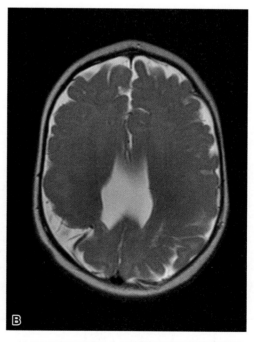

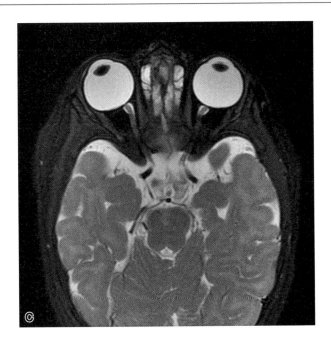
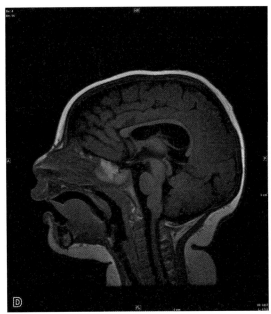

What is the most likely diagnosis?

A. Absence of the corpus callosum
B. Neurofibromatosis type 1
C. Lobar holoprosencephaly
D. Septo-optic dysplasia

14 An 18-year-old male presents with imaging for follow-up of congenital brain abnormality. What syndrome is demonstrated?

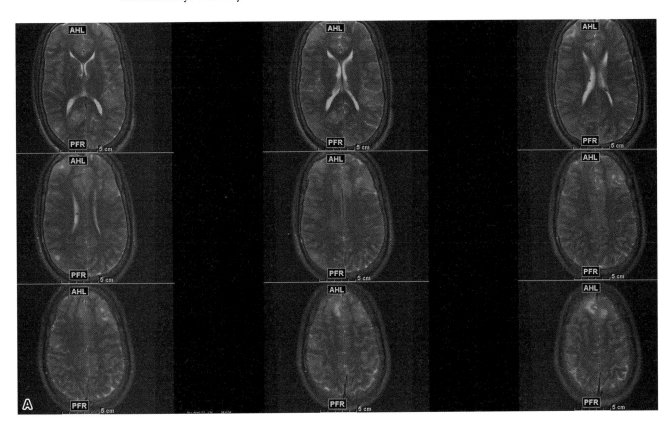

A. Sturge-Weber syndrome
B. Tuberous sclerosis
C. Neurofibromatosis type 2
D. Neurofibromatosis type 1

15 In this syndrome, what is the next most common body system affected?

A. Genitourinary
B. Gastrointestinal
C. Cardiovascular
D. Pulmonary

16 A term infant was born with hydrocephalus, which was originally diagnosed at 20 weeks of gestation on fetal ultrasound.

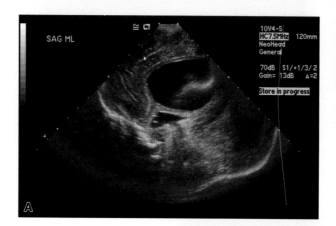
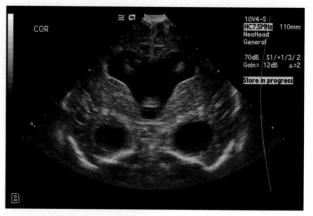
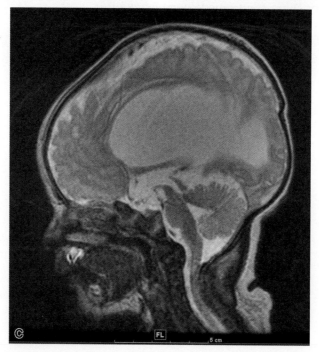

What is the most likely etiology of this congenital hydrocephalus?

A. Chiari I malformation
B. Chiari II malformation
C. Aqueductal stenosis
D. Down syndrome

17 A 6-year-old female presents from outside hospital with a history of newly diagnosed brain mass.

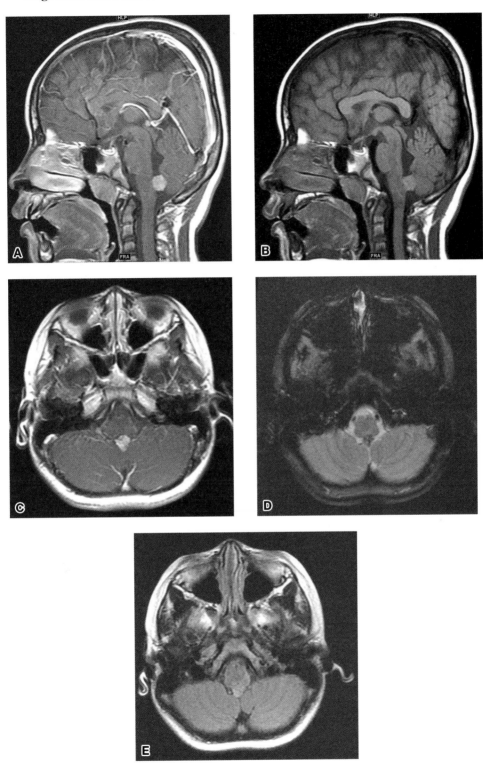

What is the most likely diagnosis?

A. Choroid plexus papilloma
B. Hemangioblastoma
C. Juvenile pilocytic astrocytoma
D. Metastatic neuroblastoma

18 A 24-day-old female presents with macrocephaly.

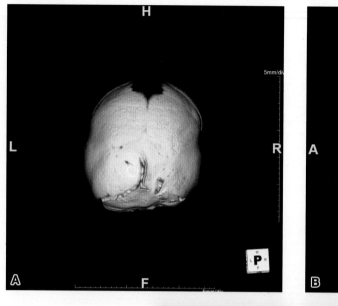

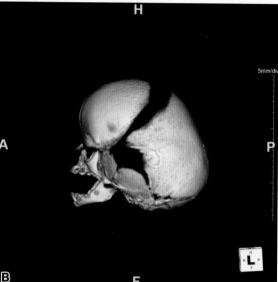

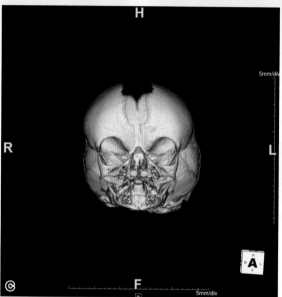

What is the diagnosis?

A. Langerhans cell histiocytosis
B. Multiple myeloma
C. Myelodysplasia
D. Craniosynostosis

19 A 2-week-old male presents with a history of nasal congestion.

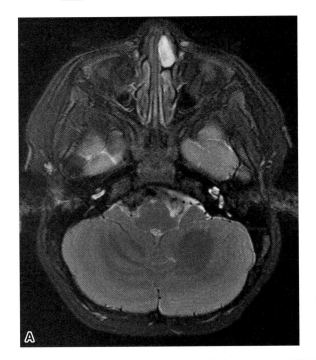

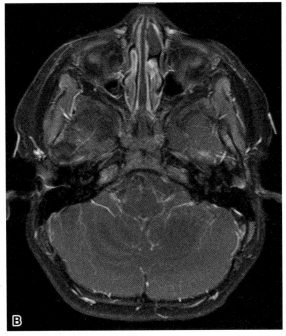

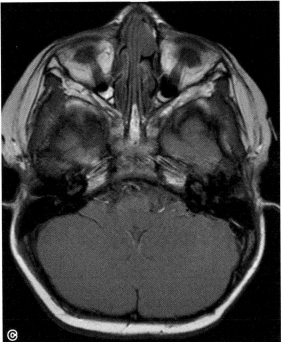

What is the diagnosis?

A. Glioma

B. Encephalocele

C. Fungal infection

D. Angiofibroma

20 A 17-year-old male status post fell from a second-story window. What is the diagnosis?

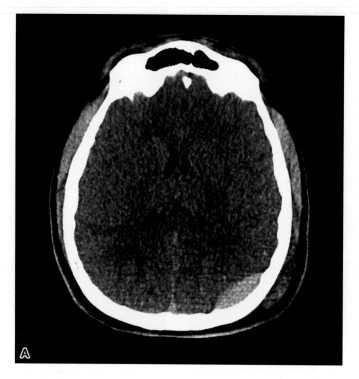

A. Meningocele
B. Epidural hematoma
C. Langerhans cell histiocytosis
D. ADEM

21 A 1-year-old female presents with high-output congestive heart failure and increased head size.

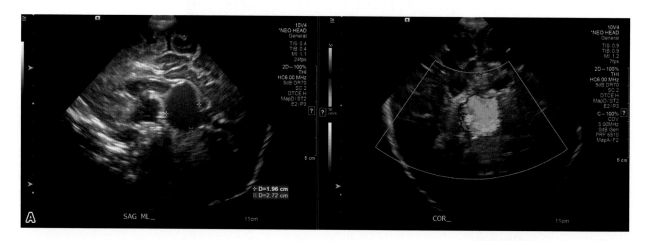

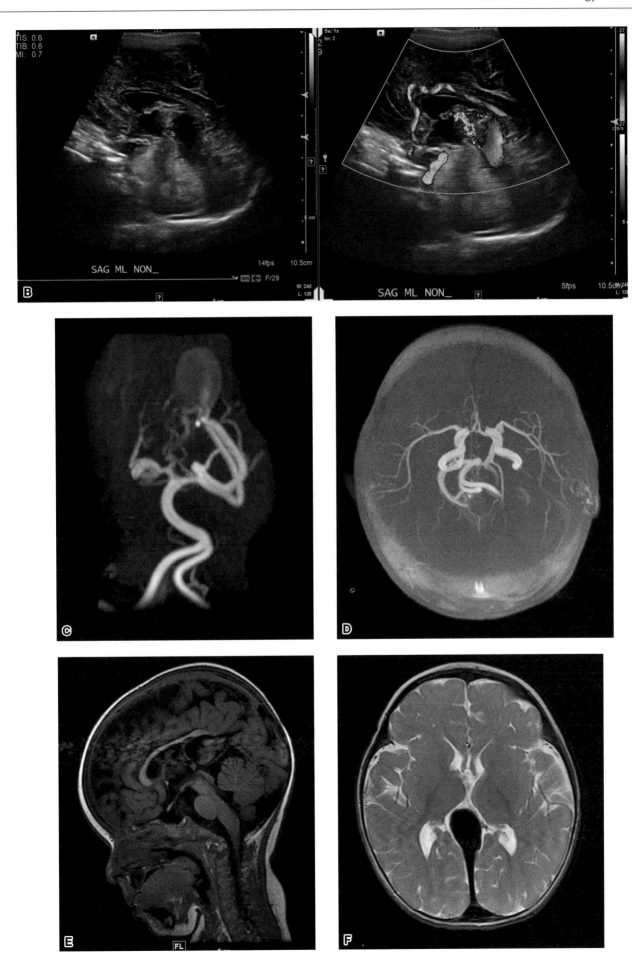

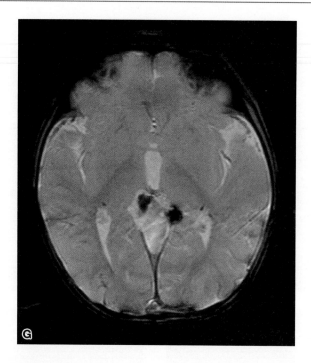

What is the diagnosis?

A. Dural venous thrombosis
B. Pineoblastoma
C. Trilateral retinoblastoma
D. Vein of Galen aneurysmal malformation

22 What is the most appropriate next step for management?

A. Embolization
B. Surgical resection
C. Radiotherapy
D. Thermal ablation

23 A 1-day-old female presents with abnormal antenatal ultrasound and microcephaly.

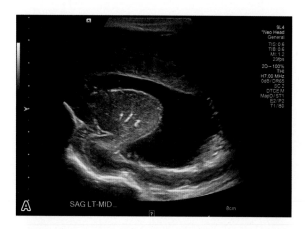

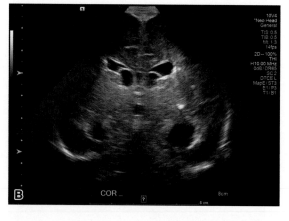

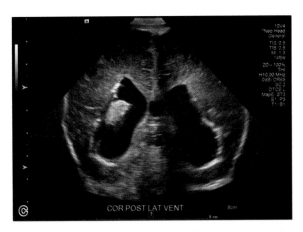

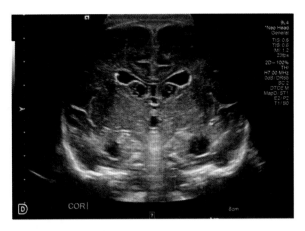

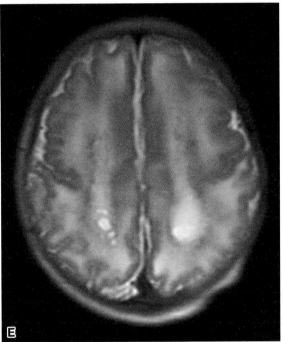

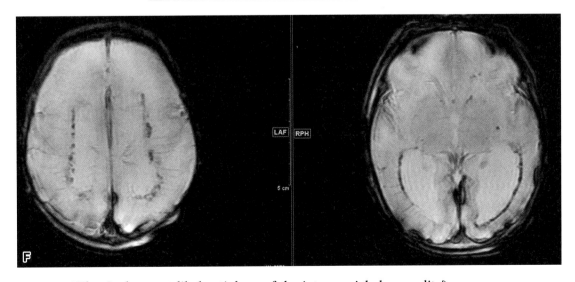

What is the most likely etiology of the intracranial abnormality?

A. Cytomegalovirus (CMV) infection
B. Middle cerebral artery (MCA) infarction
C. Congenital aqueductal stenosis
D. Sturge-Weber syndrome

24   A 3-month-old presents with failure to thrive.

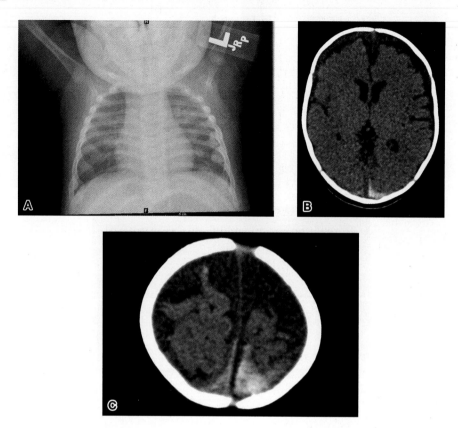

What is the most likely diagnosis?

A. Nonaccidental trauma (child abuse)
B. Osteogenesis imperfecta
C. Congenital syphilis
D. Hemophilia

25 A 7-month-old male presents with palpable nodules on the parietal scalp, as well as on the left maxillary alveola.

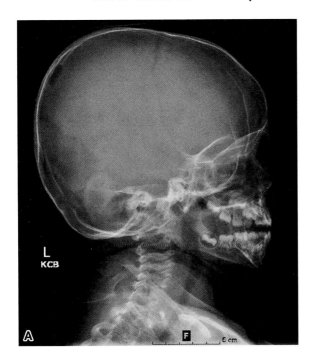

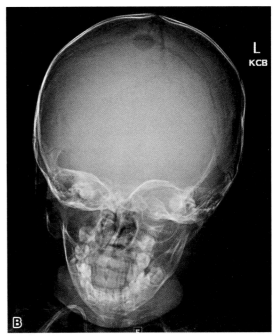

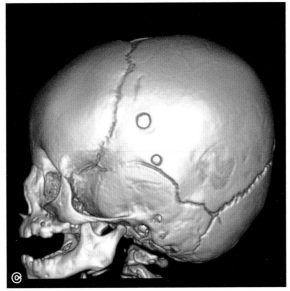

What is the most likely diagnosis?

A. Multiple myeloma
B. Langerhans cell histiocytosis
C. Neuroblastoma metastatic disease
D. Cephalohematoma

26 A 6-year-old male presents with left foot tremor.

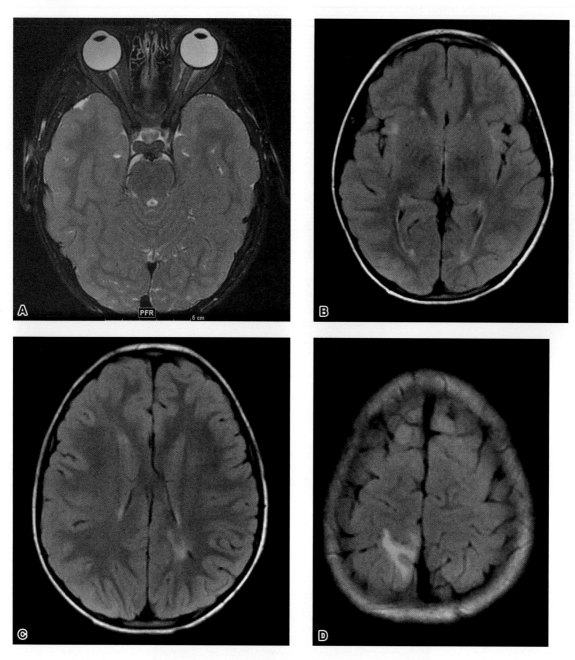

What is the most likely diagnosis?

A. Multiple sclerosis
B. Leukodystrophy
C. Acute disseminated encephalomyelitis
D. TORCH infection

27 An 11-year-old male presents with headache and visual disturbance.

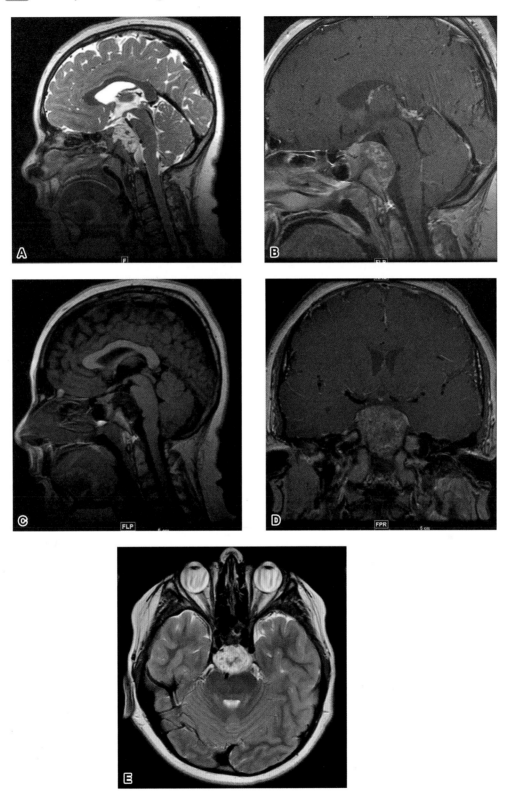

What is the most likely diagnosis?

A. Pineoblastoma

B. Teratoma

C. Chordoma

D. Neuroblastoma

Head and Neck

28 A 4-year-old male transferred from outside hospital with sore throat and stiff neck. After review of the neck radiograph, what is the recommended next step?

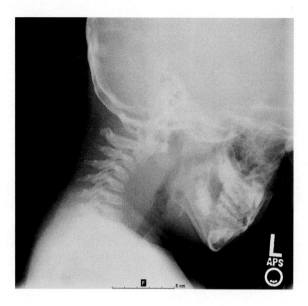

A. Surgery consultation
B. CT neck with contrast
C. IV antibiotics
D. IV steroids

29 What is the diagnosis?

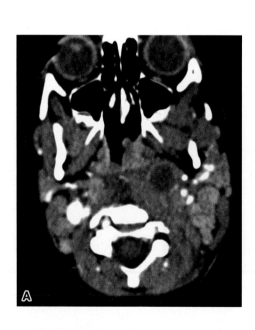
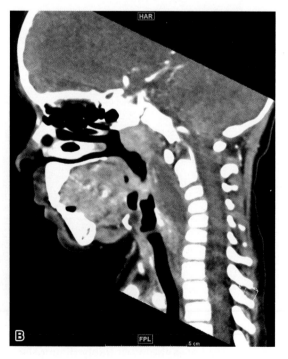

A. Croup
B. Retropharyngeal abscess
C. Retained foreign body
D. Epiglottitis

30 A 4-week-old male presents with a history of trisomy 21 and respiratory distress. What is the most likely diagnosis?

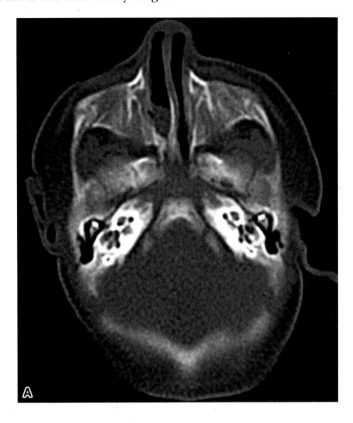

A. Choanal atresia
B. Nasal dermoid
C. Nasolacrimal duct mucocele
D. Nasal encephalocele

31 An otherwise healthy 15-year-old boy presents with symptoms of left nasal congestion. What is the most likely diagnosis?

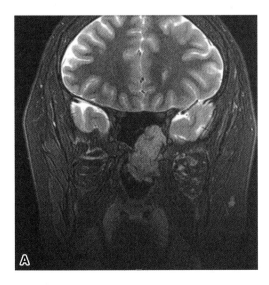
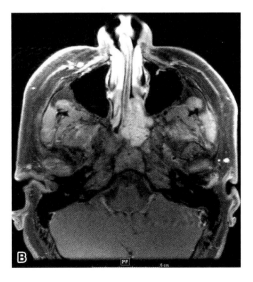

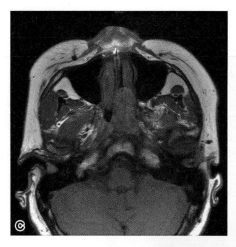

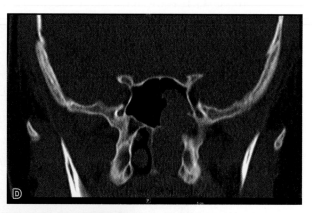

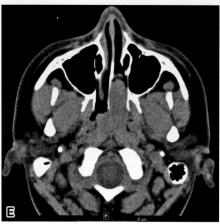

A. Rhabdomyosarcoma

B. Langerhans cell histiocytosis

C. Sinonasal aspergillosis

D. Juvenile nasopharyngeal angiofibroma

32 What is the most common feeding vessel of this mass?

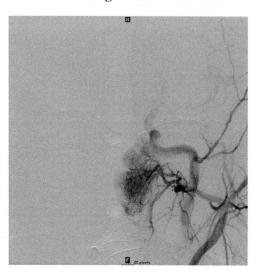

A. Internal maxillary artery

B. Ophthalmic artery

C. Facial artery

D. Vertebral artery

33 A 4-month-old male presents with abnormal ophthalmic examination. What is the most likely diagnosis?

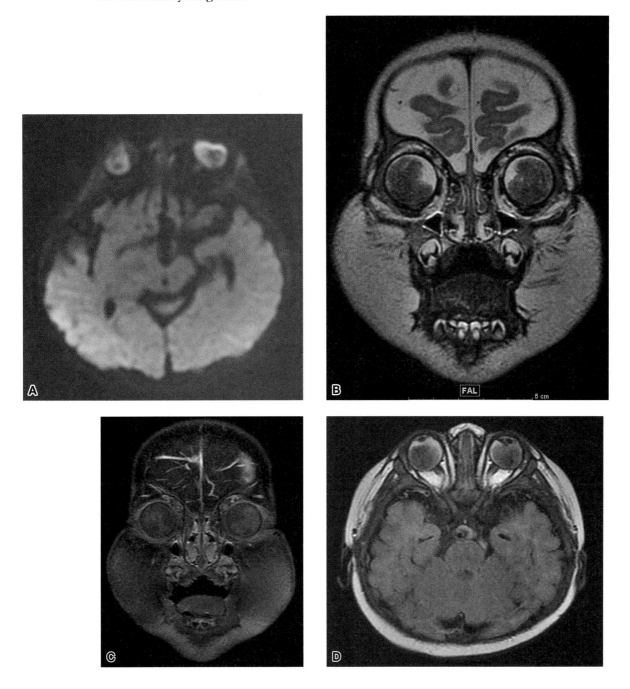

A. Persistent primary hyperplastic vitreous
B. Retinoblastoma
C. Retinopathy of prematurity
D. Orbital toxocariasis

34 A 3-year-old male presents with left neck mass. What is the most likely diagnosis?

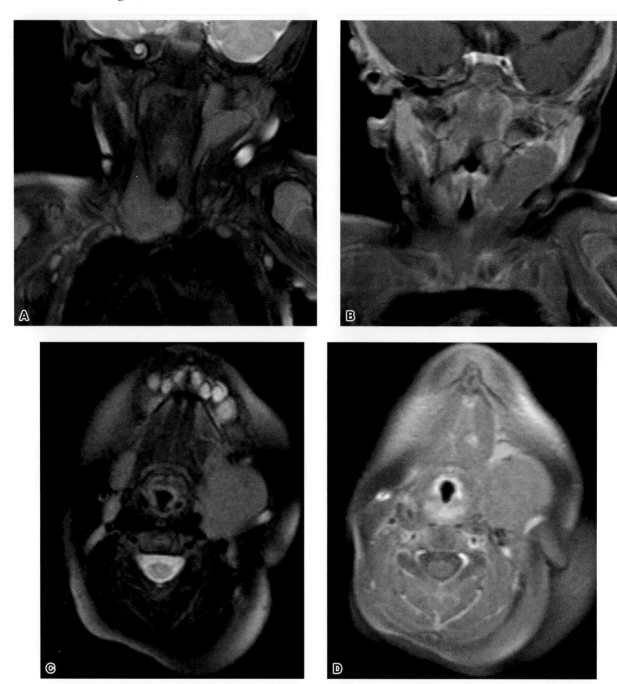

A. Rhabdomyosarcoma
B. Ectopic thymus
C. Papillary thyroid carcinoma
D. Thyroglossal duct cyst

35 A 4-year-old male presents with right facial swelling. Which salivary gland is most likely involved?

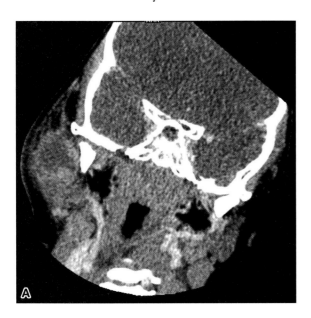
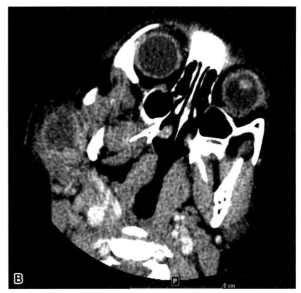

A. Parotid
B. Submandibular
C. Sublingual
D. Minor

36 A 4-year-old female presents with neck mass in the suprasternal notch. What is the most likely diagnosis?

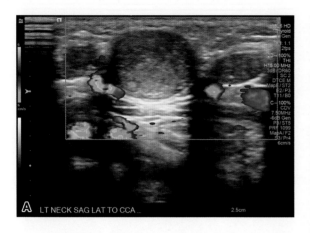

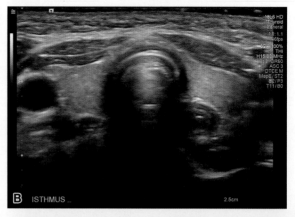

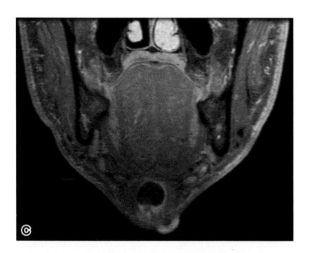

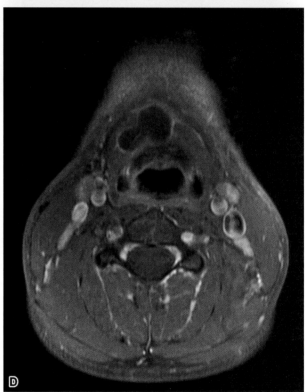

A. Thyroglossal duct cyst
B. Thyroiditis
C. Ectopic thymus
D. Branchial apparatus cyst

37 A 2-month-old presents with antenatally diagnosed neck mass. What is the most likely diagnosis?

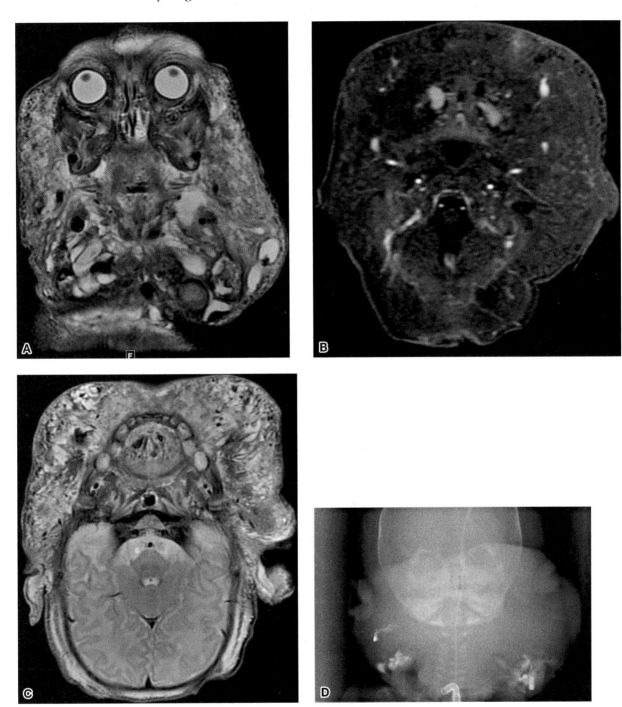

A. Cervical teratoma
B. Venolymphatic malformation
C. Thyroglossal duct cyst
D. Second branchial cleft cyst

38 A 29-day-old female presents with right neck swelling. What is the most likely diagnosis?

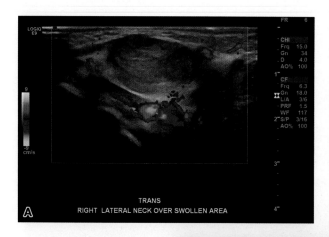

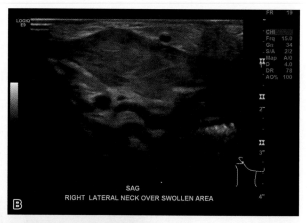

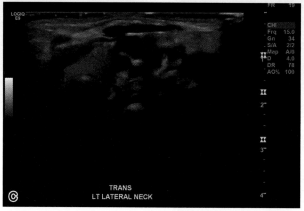

A. Lymphoma

B. Hemangioma

C. Fibromatosis colli

D. Lymphadenitis

Spine

39 A 20-year-old pregnant female is carrying a fetus of 20 weeks gestational age.

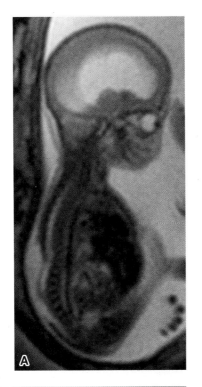

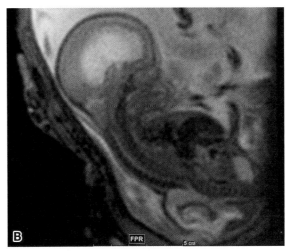

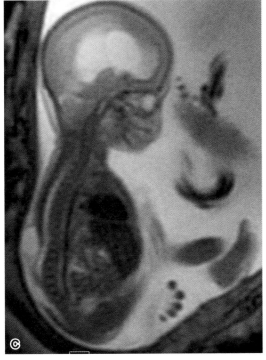

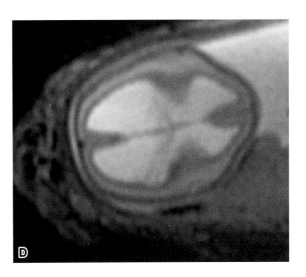

What is the most likely diagnosis?

A. Dandy-Walker malformation
B. Megalencephaly
C. Chiari I malformation
D. Chiari II malformation

40 A 3-year-old female presents with short stature.

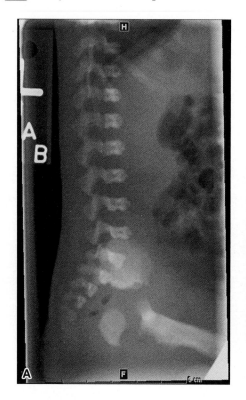

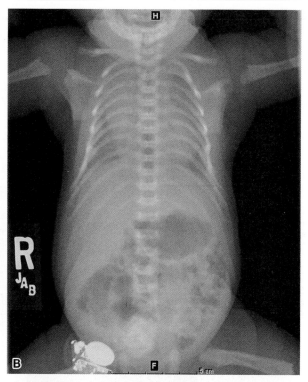

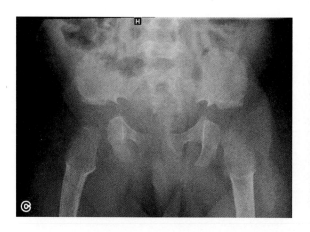

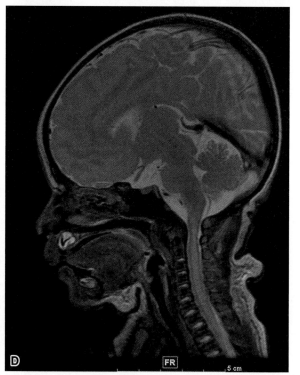

What is the most likely diagnosis?

A. Jeune syndrome

B. Achondroplasia

C. Thanatophoric dwarfism

D. Ollier disease

41 An 18-year-old male presents with a history of chronic osteomyelitis and back pain.

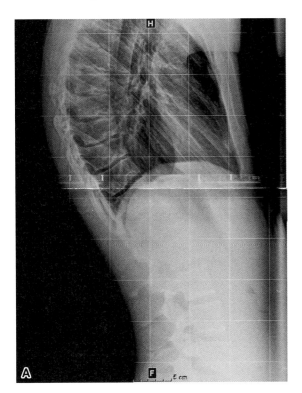

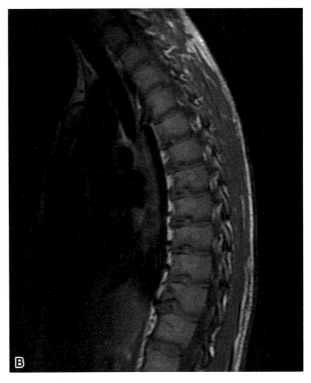

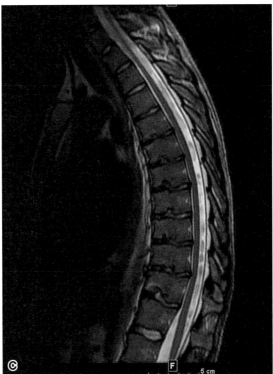

What is the most likely diagnosis?

A. Discitis osteomyelitis
B. Vertebral compression fracture
C. Vertebral hemangioma
D. Scheuermann disease

42 A 9-year-old male presents with multiple anomalies.

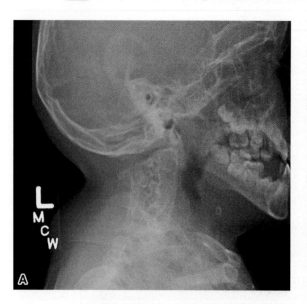 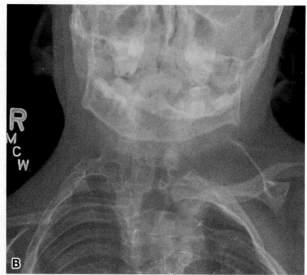

What is the most likely diagnosis?

A. Klippel-Feil syndrome
B. Morquio syndrome
C. Gorham disease
D. Osteogenesis imperfecta

43 A 15-year-old male presents with back pain and progressive lower extremity weakness.

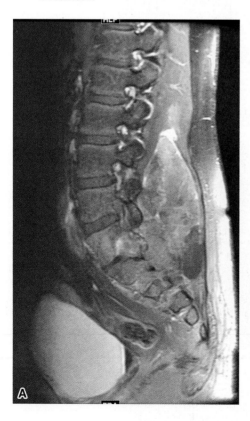 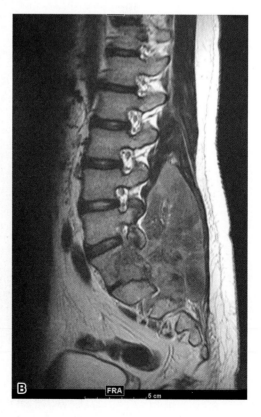

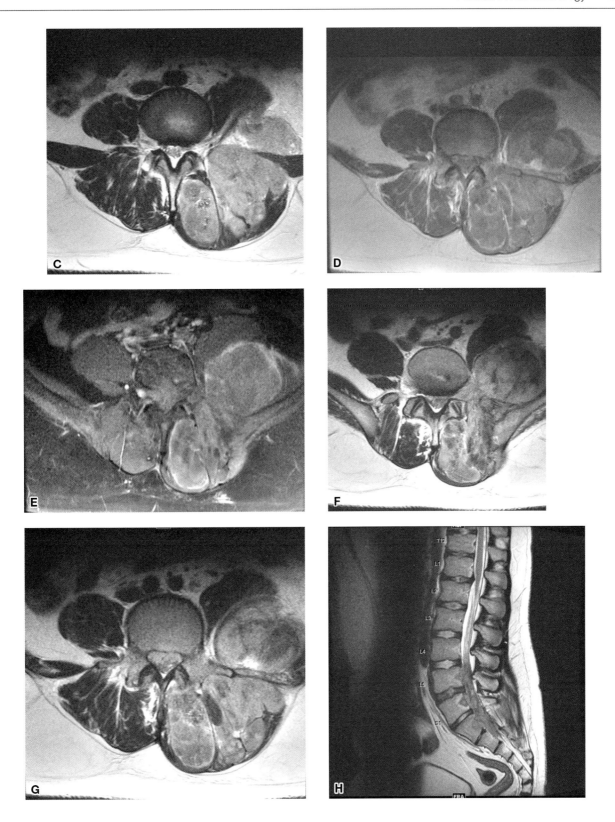

What is the most likely diagnosis?

A. Myelomeningocele
B. Langerhans cell histiocytosis
C. Ewing sarcoma
D. Ependymoma

44 A 14-year-old female presents with back pain.

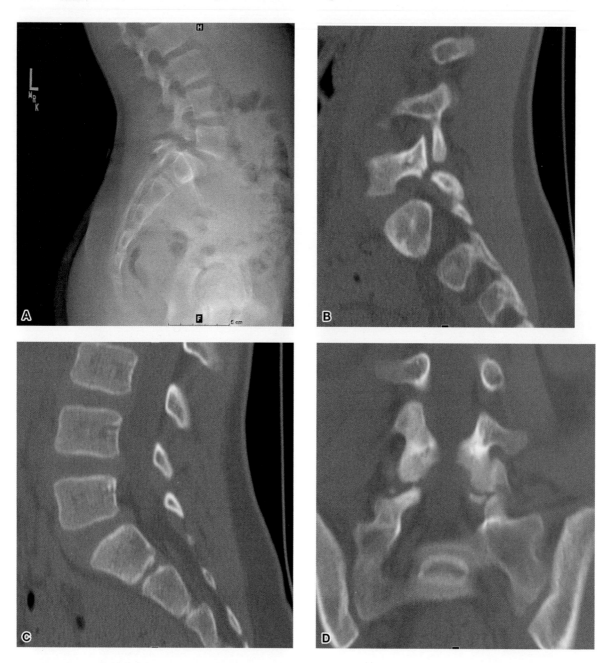

What is the most likely diagnosis?

A. Vertebral hemangioma
B. Spondylolysis
C. Sickle cell disease
D. Gaucher disease

45 A former premature infant presents with a history of anal atresia.

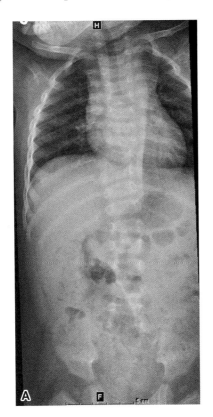
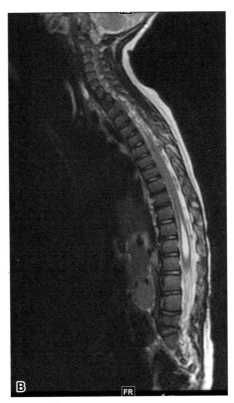

Which of the following CNS abnormalities is most commonly associated with maternal diabetes?

A. Chiari II malformation
B. Diastematomyelia
C. Caudal regression syndrome
D. Chordoma

46 A 17-year-old female presents with a long history of UTI.

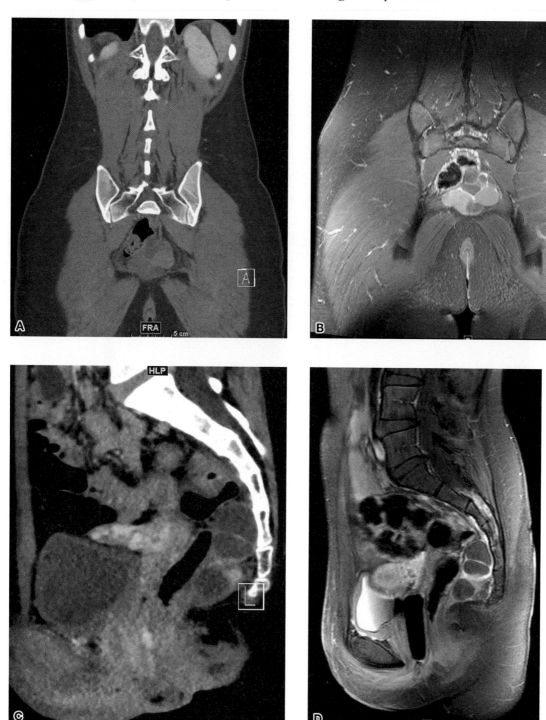

What is the most likely diagnosis?

A. Rhabdomyosarcoma

B. Ovarian torsion

C. Ewing sarcoma

D. Sacrococcygeal teratoma

47 A 14-year-old male presents with neck pain.

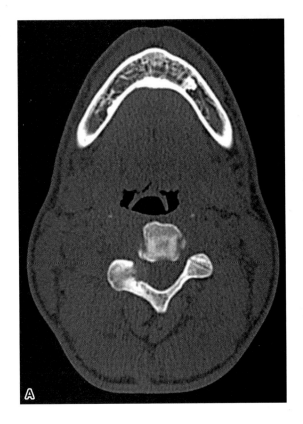

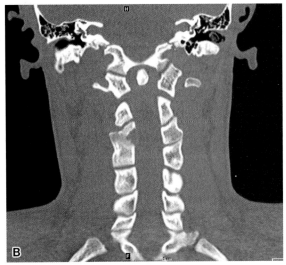

What is the most likely diagnosis?

A. Ewing sarcoma
B. Osteogenic sarcoma
C. Osteoblastoma
D. Metastatic neuroblastoma

ANSWERS AND EXPLANATIONS

Brain

1 **Answer C.** The neonatal head ultrasound images demonstrate an echogenic midline mass superior to the third ventricle. There is dilatation of the lateral ventricles, colpocephaly, and absence of the corpus callosum. Agenesis of the corpus callosum (ACC) is the most common developmental abnormality, resulting from failure of commissuration and can occur for a number of reasons including genetic, metabolic, or vascular abnormalities, but in most cases, the cause is not found. The term "ACC" implies that the entire structure has failed to form, but in other fetuses, the corpus callosum may fail to form in part, leading to the term "hypoplasia of the corpus callosum." In the context of the detection of antenatal malformations, ACC is much more common than hypoplasia of the corpus callosum.

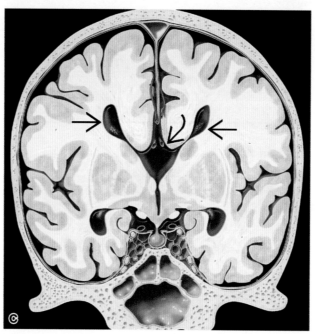

Coronal image shows corpus callosal agenesis with widely spaced lateral ventricles (*straight arrows*). The third ventricle (*curved arrow*) is elevated and is contiguous dorsally with the interhemispheric fissure. (Reprinted with permission from Woodward PJ, Kennedy A, Puchalski MD, et al. *Diagnostic Imaging: Obstetrics.* 3rd ed. Elsevier; 2017:108.)

Imaging findings often include ventriculomegaly, colpocephaly (dilatation of the trigones and occipital horns), and absent cavum septum pellucidum. In the sagittal plane, there is a radial, spoke wheel, or sunray appearance of the gyri from the expected location of the corpus callosum. The echogenic midline mass in this case is consistent with an interhemispheric lipoma. Half of all midline intracranial lipomas are associated with ACC.

References: Barkovich AJ, Raybaud CA. Congenital malformations of the brain and skull. In: Barkovich AJ, Raybaud C, eds. *Pediatric Neuroimaging.* 5th ed. Lippincott Williams & Wilkins; 2012:367-568.

Craven I, Bradburn MJ, Griffiths PD. Antenatal diagnosis of agenesis of the corpus callosum. *Clin Radiol.* 2015;70(3):248-253.

2 **Answer D.** Brain MRI images demonstrate right open lip schizencephaly with a cleft of cerebrospinal fluid (CSF) extending from the pial margin of the right frontoparietal lobe to the ependymal margin of the right lateral ventricle. This schizencephaly cleft is lined by polymicrogyria. Schizencephaly is a rare cortical malformation that manifests as a gray matter–lined cleft extending from the ependyma to the pia mater. This malformation is thought to be the result of an acquired in utero insult affecting the germinal zone prior to neuronal migration.

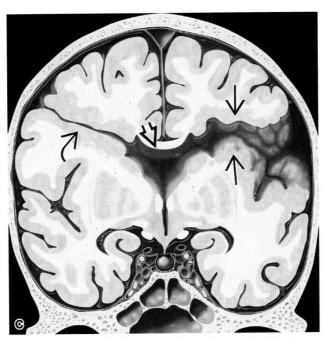

Coronal image shows right closed-lip (*curved arrow*) and left open-lip (*straight arrows*) schizencephaly defects, both lined by gray matter. The cavum septi pellucidi (CSP) is absent (*hollow arrow*). In schizencephaly, the defect extends from the inner table of the skull to the underlying ventricle. (Reprinted with permission from Woodward PJ, Kennedy A, Puchalski MD, et al. *Diagnostic Imaging: Obstetrics.* 3rd ed. Elsevier; 2017:134.)

There are two types of schizencephaly: type 1 or open lip and type 2 or closed lip. Closed-lip MRI findings include irregular tract of gray matter extending from the cortical surface to ventricle. The gray matter lining can appear dysplastic (lumpy/bumpy on margin of cleft or at gray-white interface). Open lip can appear wide and wedge shaped or with nearly parallel walls. The gray matter lining cleft may be harder to discern than in closed lip. The most common signs/symptoms include seizures (more common with unilateral clefts), mild motor deficit ("congenital" hemiparesis), developmental delay, paresis, microcephaly, and spasticity.

Schizencephaly is frequently associated with other cerebral anomalies including:

- Septo-optic dysplasia (SOD)
- Gray matter heterotopia
- Absent septum pellucidum

References: Barkovich AJ, Kjos BO. Schizencephaly: correlation of clinical findings with MR characteristics. *AJNR Am J Neuroradiol.* 1992;13(1):85-94.

Nabavizadeh SA, Zarnow D, Bilaniuk LT, Schwartz ES, Zimmerman RA, Vossough A. Correlation of prenatal and postnatal MRI findings in schizencephaly. *AJNR Am J Neuroradiol.* 2014;35(7):1418-1424.

3 **Answer A.** Head ultrasound and brain MRI demonstrate a monoventricle, large dorsal cyst, fused thalami, and fused anterior cerebral mantle. Alobar holoprosencephaly is the most severe form of holoprosencephaly and consists of complete lack of separation of the cerebral hemispheres with a large posterior monoventricle. Single midline structures such as the falx, interhemispheric fissure, septum pellucidum, and corpus callosum are absent, whereas paired midline structures are fused, including the thalami and basal ganglia. Affected patients suffer from dysmorphic facies, microcephaly, seizures, and developmental delay.

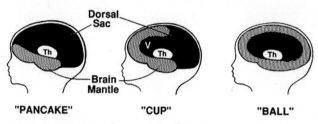

Diagram of three morphologic types of alobar holoprosencephaly (and semilobar holoprosencephaly) in sagittal view. Pancake type: The flattened residual brain mantle at the base of the brain with a correspondingly large dorsal sac. Cup type: This type has more brain mantle but it does not cover the monoventricle. The dorsal sac communicates widely with the monoventricle. Ball type: Brain mantle completely covers the monoventricle, and a dorsal sac may or may not be present. Th, thalami; V, ventricle. (Modified from McGahn JP, Ellis W, Lindfors KK, et al. Congenital cerebrospinal fluid-containing intracranial abnormalities: sonographic classification. *J Clin Ultrasound.* 1988;16:531-544.)

Holoprosencephaly is a spectrum of congenital abnormalities characterized by incomplete separation of the cerebral hemispheres. Abnormalities range from incomplete formation of the falx cerebri and interhemispheric fissure to a complete lack of separation of the cerebral hemispheres with a large monoventricle. There are three types, which include alobar, semilobar, and lobar (SOD).

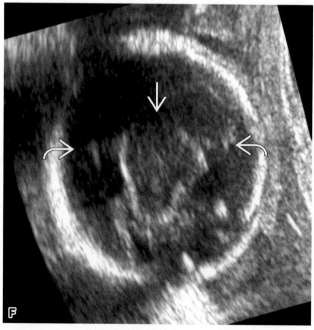

Coronal ultrasound of the brain of a fetus with trisomy 13 shows fused thalami (*straight arrow*) and a monoventricle (*curved arrows*). These are classic features of alobar holoprosencephaly. Chromosomal abnormalities, especially trisomy 13, are common with HPE. (Reprinted with permission from Woodward PJ, Kennedy A, Puchalski MD, et al. *Diagnostic Imaging: Obstetrics.* 3rd ed. Elsevier; 2017:118.)

Midline facial abnormalities in the setting of alobar holoprosencephaly include:

- Cyclopia
- Ethmocephaly (small narrow-set eyes with absence of nose)
- Cebocephaly (small narrow-set eyes with a flattened nose and one nostril)
- Cleft palate and lip
- Solitary maxillary central incisor

Facial malformations of any kind should trigger very careful evaluation of brain. "The face predicts the brain."

References: Barkovich AJ. Congenital malformations of the brain and skull. In: Barkovich AJ, ed. *Pediatric Neuroimaging*. 4th ed. Lippincott Williams & Wilkins; 2005:291-439.

Winter TC. *Diagnostic Imaging: Obstetrics*. 2nd ed. Lippincott Williams & Wilkins; 2011:1-2.

4 **Answer D.** On CT, there is a mildly hypodense nonenhancing sellar and suprasellar lesion. The sellar component of this mass has associated calcification. MRI demonstrates a T1/T2 hyperintense cystic-appearing sellar and suprasellar mass with peripheral enhancement. There is gradient recalled echo (GRE) hypointensity within the sellar component. The lesion causes deformity and displacement upon the optic apparatus. Craniopharyngioma is the most common suprasellar mass in children. Craniopharyngiomas arise from the metaplastic squamous epithelial rests along the hypophysis. They are more common in males. The vast majority arise within the suprasellar cistern; however, they may arise within the sella turcica and occasionally the third ventricle. There is a bimodal age distribution, with children between the ages of 5 and 10 exhibiting the adamantinomatous type and second peak in the fifth and sixth decade. Clinical presentation includes visual disturbances related to compression of the optic chiasm, pituitary hypofunction related to compression of the gland or hypothalamus, and/or symptoms of increased intracranial pressure.

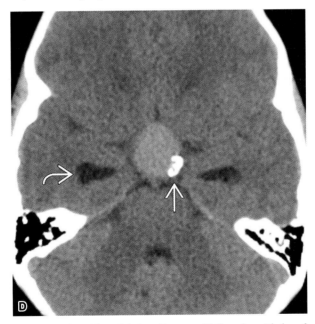

Axial non-enhanced CT (NECT) in a 7-year-old female with headache and vomiting after minor trauma shows a hyperdense cystic craniopharyngioma with wall calcification (*straight arrow*). Note the mild enlargement of the temporal horns (*curved arrow*) caused by obstruction of the lateral ventricles at the foramen of Monro. (Reprinted with permission from Merrow AC Jr. *Diagnostic Imaging: Pediatrics*. 3rd ed. Elsevier; 2017:1062.)

Imaging findings typically include a cystic or solid and cyst mass. Approximately 80% to 90% of all craniopharyngiomas have a cystic component. Smaller lesions may be purely solid. The vast majority have calcification and enhance after administration of IV contrast. Rim enhancement may be seen around the cystic portions of these tumors, and the solid portions typically demonstrate more avid, solid enhancement. The cystic component is frequently hyperintense on T2 and may be hypointense, isointense, or hyperintense on T1.

Reference: Sartoretti-Schefer S, Wichmann W, Aguzzi A, Valavanis A. MR differentiation of adamantinous and squamous-papillary craniopharyngioma. *AJNR Am J Neuroradiol.* 1997;18:77-87.

5 **Answer B.** There is a nonenhancing mass associated with the tuber cinereum. The pituitary stalk and posterior pituitary bright spot are present. This case illustrates the characteristic appearance of a hamartoma of the tuber cinereum. The mass is isointense to gray matter on T1 imaging and sits just anterior to the mammary bodies at the level of the floor of the third ventricle.

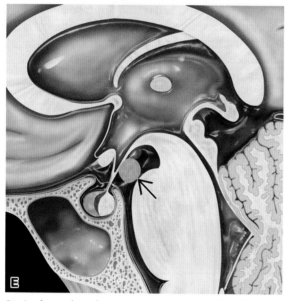

Sagittal graphic shows a classic pedunculated tuber cinereum hamartoma (*arrow*) interposed between the infundibulum anteriorly and mammillary bodies posteriorly. The mass resembles gray matter. (Reprinted with permission from Osborn AG, Salzman KL, Jhaveri MD. *Diagnostic Imaging: Brain.* 3rd ed. Elsevier; 2016:1028.)

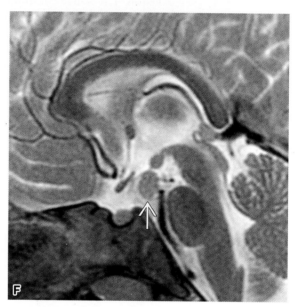

Sagittal T2-weighted MRI in a patient presenting with precocious puberty reveals a pedunculated hypothalamic mass (*arrow*) located between the median eminence and mammillary bodies. (Reprinted with permission from Osborn AG, Salzman KL, Jhaveri MD. *Diagnostic Imaging: Brain.* 3rd ed. Elsevier; 2016:1028.)

Hamartomas are benign nonneoplastic lesions that are likely congenital in origin. Many are symptomatic, but symptoms may be more common in children and typically include gelastic seizures, "fits of laughter," and precocious puberty. Knowledge of this lesion and its radiologic and clinical presentations usually allows the diagnosis to be established in most cases. Atypical imaging findings including marked hyperintensity on T2 or lesion larger than 1.5 cm raise the possibility of hypothalamic glioma.

Reference: Boyko OB, Curnes JT, Oakes WJ, Burger PC. Hamartomas of the tuber cinereum: CT, MR and pathologic findings. *AJNR Am J Neuroradiol.* 1991;12:309-314.

6 **Answer A.** MRI demonstrates a lobulated mixed cystic and solid-enhancing pineal region mass, isointense to gray matter on T2 and T1 images, and containing several small internal foci of GRE hypointensity. There is extension to the left splenium of the corpus callosum and possible involvement of the midbrain. There is associated expansion of the third and lateral ventricles as well as periventricular T2 hyperintensity, consistent with moderate hydrocephalus. There is mild downward displacement of the cerebellar tonsils.

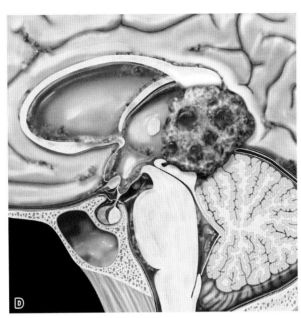

Sagittal graphic shows a large, heterogeneous pineal mass with areas of hemorrhage and necrosis. Note the compression of adjacent structures, hydrocephalus, and diffuse cerebrospinal fluid (CSF) seeding, which is typical of pineoblastoma. (Reprinted with permission from Osborn AG, Salzman KL, Jhaveri MD. *Diagnostic Imaging: Brain.* 3rd ed. Elsevier; 2016:530.)

Tumors of pineal cell origin (pineoblastoma and pineocytoma) comprise only 15% of pineal region masses. Unlike germ cell tumors, which show a marked predilection in males, tumors of pineal cell origin occur equally among men and woman. Tumors of pineal origin frequently calcify. Calcification of the pineal gland in a child under 7 years of age should raise suspicion of tumor. After 7 years of age, the pineal gland begins to show calcification, which increases with age. Parinaud syndrome is a cluster of abnormalities of eye movement and pupil dysfunction with paralysis of upward gaze (downward gaze is usually preserved). This syndrome is associated with young patients with brain tumors in the pineal gland or midbrain.

MRI is most useful in characterizing masses in the pineal region. Tumors arising in the parapineal region in a child are usually gliomas arising from the tectal plate, whereas tumors arising in the parapineal region in adults may represent gliomas or meningiomas arising from the tentorium. Tumors of germ cell origin occur in children as do pineoblastomas, whereas pineocytomas are generally seen in adults.

Reference: Smirniotopoulos JG, Rushing EJ, Mena H. Pineal region masses: differential diagnosis. *Radiographics.* 1992;12:577-596.

7 **Answer B.** Parinaud syndrome is a cluster of abnormalities of eye movement and pupil dysfunction with paralysis of upward gaze (downward gaze is usually preserved). This syndrome is associated with young patients with brain tumors in the pineal gland or midbrain.

8 **Answer B.** On MRI, there is a large, round right cerebellar mass with T2 hyperintensity, internal mural nodules, and peripheral contrast enhancement. There is mass effect on the fourth ventricle and left midline shift. Astrocytomas are the most common brain tumors of childhood, with 60% occurring in the posterior fossa (40% in the cerebellum, 20% in the brain stem). Most of them are juvenile pilocytic astrocytomas (JPAs), which are World Health Organization (WHO) grade 1 benign tumors. Differential diagnosis of cystic cerebellar masses includes hemangioblastomas, which have similar appearance to JPA.

These are more common in young adults and children and are usually part of von Hippel-Lindau disease. Medulloblastoma and ependymomas usually have a shorter clinical history. They are typically centered on the fourth ventricle, isodense or hyperdense on nonenhanced CT, and characteristically not cystic. However, purely solid JPAs do occur.

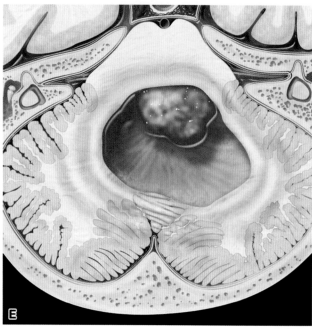

Axial graphic shows the characteristic "cyst with mural nodule" appearance of a posterior fossa pilocytic astrocytoma (PA). These World Health Organization (WHO) grade I tumors commonly arise in the cerebellar hemispheres and compress the fourth ventricle. (Reprinted with permission from Osborn AG, Salzman KL, Jhaveri MD. *Diagnostic Imaging: Brain*. 3rd ed. Elsevier; 2016:452.)

As a rule, JPAs arise from the midline and can extend into the cerebellar hemispheres. Most are large at presentation (>5 cm). The tumor usually consists of a cyst with a solid nodule within the cyst wall. The cyst is most typically adjacent to the tumor (no peripheral enhancement), but in 40%, it may develop within it as a cyst-like necrotic center (peripheral enhancement). The frequency of JPA is equal in boys and girls usually occurring between birth and 9 years of age. The symptoms (headaches, early morning vomiting, ataxia) develop gradually over several months to become persistent and acute.

References: Campbell JW, Pollack IF. Cerebellar astrocytomas in children. *J Neurooncol.* 1996;28:223-231.

Rashidi M, DaSilva VR, Minagar A, Rutka JT. Nonmalignant pediatric brain tumors. *Curr Neurol Neurosci Rep.* 2003;3:200-205.

9 **Answer B.** On CT, there is a heterogeneous soft tissue mass centered at the fourth ventricle with foci of internal calcification. There is lateral and third ventriculomegaly. On MRI, there is an enhancing mass within the posterior fossa in the midline. The mass has restricted diffusion, indicating that the mass is densely cellular. There is also GRE susceptibility, which indicates a component of hemorrhage or mineralization. There is extension of the mass outside the left foramen of Luschka. There is mass effect on the fourth ventricle causing enlargement of the lateral ventricles. There is also periventricular edema. The major differential diagnostic consideration of a midline posterior fossa mass in children is a fourth ventricular ependymoma. These typically expand rather than compress the fourth ventricle. Less commonly, cerebellar astrocytomas may occur in the midline; however, they are typically hemispheric lesions.

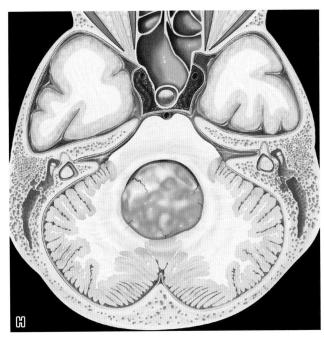

Axial graphic shows a spherical tumor centered in the fourth ventricle, typical of medulloblastoma. (Reprinted with permission from Osborn AG, Salzman KL, Jhaveri MD. *Diagnostic Imaging: Brain.* 3rd ed. Elsevier; 2016:536.)

Medulloblastomas comprise up to one-third of all pediatric posterior fossa tumors. They occur more commonly in boys and arise from the medullary velum of the fourth ventricle from primitive neuroectoderm. In children, they are typically midline masses associated with the inferior vermis. Subarachnoid seeding of the leptomeninges is very common at presentation; therefore, screening of the spine is recommended to exclude spread. On unenhanced CT, medulloblastomas are typically hyperdense relative to brain parenchyma because of their dense cellularity. Calcification, cystic change, and/or hemorrhage may be present in up to 10% to 20% of lesions. On MRI, most medulloblastomas are mildly hypointense to brain parenchyma on T1 and vary in signal intensity on T2 images. These masses avidly enhance after contrast administration. As CSF seeding is common at presentation, imaging with contrast of the whole neuraxis is recommended to identify drop metastases and leptomeningeal spread. Although rare, extraneural spread is reported. Treatment typically consists of surgical resection, radiation therapy, and chemotherapy, with the prognosis strongly influenced by surgical resection, presence of CSF metastases at the time of diagnosis, and expression of the c-erbB-2 (HER2/neu) oncogene.

Reference: Nueller DP, Moore SA, Sato Y, Yuh WTC. MR spectrum of medulloblastoma. *Clin Imaging.* 1992;16:250-255.

10 **Answer A.** CSF seeding is common in the setting of medulloblastoma; therefore, imaging with contrast of the whole neuraxis is recommended to identify drop metastases and leptomeningeal spread.

11 **Answer C.** Fetal MRI demonstrates bilateral ventriculomegaly. The septum pellucidum is absent. There is a small and upward tilted vermis and large posterior fossa CSF intensity space, which is continuous with the fourth ventricle. Postnatal MRI demonstrates marked lateral ventriculomegaly with moderate third ventricular enlargement and a large posterior fossa cyst. There is partial agenesis of the cerebellar vermis with upward tilted vermian remnant. There are bilateral small cerebellar hemispheres.

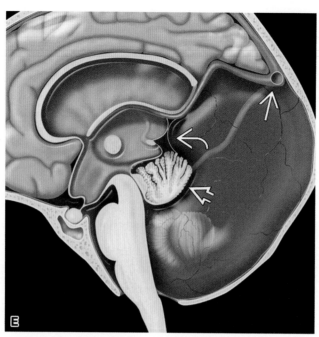

Sagittal graphic of classic Dandy-Walker malformation shows an enlarged posterior fossa, elevated torcular herophili (*straight arrow*), superior rotation of hypoplastic cerebellar vermis (*hollow arrow*), an overexpanded fourth ventricle with a thin wall (*curved arrow*), and a dilated ventricle (hydrocephalus). (Reprinted with permission from Osborn AG, Salzman KL, Jhaveri MD. *Diagnostic Imaging: Brain.* 3rd ed. Elsevier; 2016:26.)

The Dandy-Walker complex (which includes Dandy-Walker malformation [DWM] and its variants) is a congenital anomaly believed to be related to an in utero insult to the fourth ventricle leading to complete or partial outflow obstruction of CSF. As a result, there is cyst-like dilatation of the fourth ventricle, which protrudes between the cerebellar hemispheres to prevent their fusion, and there is incomplete formation of all or part of the inferior vermis. DWMs are associated with hydrocephalus in 75% of cases. In addition, a significant number of patients are associated with supratentorial anomalies including dysgenesis of the corpus callosum, migrational anomalies, and encephaloceles. The radiologic hallmark of DWM is communication of a retrocerebellar cyst with the fourth ventricle.

Reference: Barkovich AJ, Kjos BO, Norman D, Edwards MS. Revised classification of posterior fossa cysts and cyst-like malformations based on the results of multiplanar MR imaging. *AJR Am J Roentgenol.* 1989;153:1289-1300.

12 **Answer D.** MRI demonstrates a hypoplastic superior cerebellar vermis and dysplastic inferior cerebellar vermis. There is a dysmorphic fourth ventricle, which has "batwing" appearance. There is a hypoplastic cerebellar vermis with hypoplasia of the superior cerebellar peduncle resembling the "molar tooth sign" in the midbrain. There is an elongated and thinned superior cerebellar peduncle and interpeduncular fossa. The size of the brain stem is smaller than the normal appearance. There is a retrocerebellar mega cisterna magna with supracerebellar extension. There is partial agenesis of the septum pellucidum.

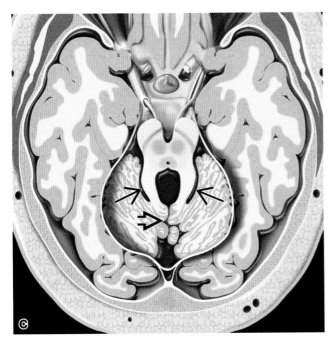

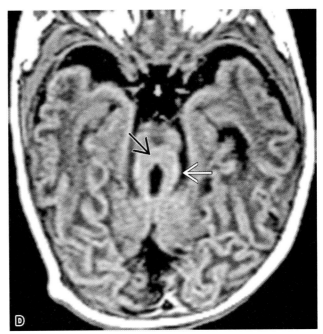

Axial graphic depicts Joubert malformation. Thickened superior cerebellar peduncle (*arrows*) around the elongated fourth ventricle forms the classic "molar tooth" seen in this anomaly. Note the cleft cerebellar vermis (*hollow arrow*). (Reprinted with permission from Osborn AG, Salzman KL, Jhaveri MD. *Diagnostic Imaging: Brain*. 3rd ed. Elsevier; 2016:36.)

Axial T1-weighted MRI at the midbrain/pons junction (isthmus) shows the fourth ventricle pointed anteriorly (*white arrow*), explaining the sagittal thinning of the isthmus. It is flanked on both sides by thick, elongated, in-plane superior cerebellar peduncles (*black arrow*), forming the "molar tooth." (Reprinted with permission from Osborn AG, Salzman KL, Jhaveri MD. *Diagnostic Imaging: Brain*. 3rd ed. Elsevier; 2016:36.)

Joubert syndrome (JS) is a very rare, autosomal recessive condition. It is characterized by agenesis of cerebellar vermis, abnormal eye movements with nystagmus, episodes of hyperpnea and apnea, delayed generalized motor development, retinal coloboma and dystrophy, and, sometimes, multicystic kidney disease. A spectrum of cerebellar developmental anomalies are categorized into complete or incomplete cerebellar agenesis, medial aplasia/hypoplasia, and lateral aplasia/hypoplasia. These anomalies in cerebellar development may result in prominent CSF spaces or CSF collections/cystic dilatation of the fourth ventricle (giant cisterna magna, DWMs) in the posterior fossa. The predominant abnormality in JS is aplasia or hypoplasia of the vermis, particularly the superior portion. These patients have dysplastic cerebellar tissue including heterotopic and dysplastic cerebellar nuclei; abnormal development of the inferior olivary nuclei; and incomplete formation of the pyramidal decussation. It is an autosomal recessive disorder.

The characteristic appearance of JS includes:

- Diminutive vermis
- Enlarged fourth ventricle that is "batwing" shaped
- Superior cerebellar peduncles that are vertically oriented and elongated in the anteroposterior (AP) direction
- Separation or disconnection of the cerebellar hemispheres, which are apposed by not fused in the midline

Reference: Friede RL, Boltshauser E. Uncommon syndromes of cerebellar vermis aplasia. I: Joubert syndrome. *Dev Med Child Neurol*. 1978;20:758-763.

13 **Answer D.** There is an absent septum pellucidum and dysmorphic appearance of the lateral ventricles. The corpus callosum is present but is dysmorphic. Right cerebral gray matter–lined cleft extends to the right lateral ventricle, compatible with closed-lip schizencephaly. There is extensive polymicrogyria in the left parietal occipital lobe and right occipital, parietal, and temporal lobes. The cerebellar vermis appears small and dysplastic. The optic nerves and chiasm appear small.

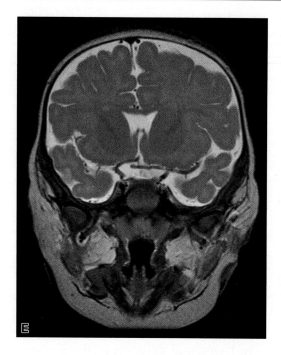

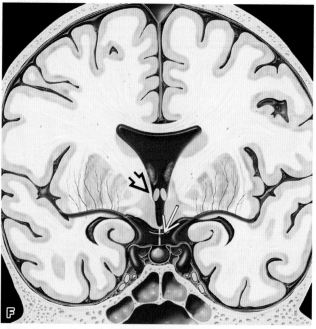

Coronal graphic depicts flat-roofed anterior horns and the absence of a midline septum pellucidum. The anterior horns are draped inferiorly around the fornices (*hollow arrow*) and the optic chiasm (*arrow*) is small. (Reprinted with permission from Osborn AG, Salzman KL, Jhaveri MD. *Diagnostic Imaging: Brain*. 3rd ed. Elsevier; 2016:52.)

SOD, also known as de Morsier syndrome, is a condition characterized by optic nerve hypoplasia and absence of septum pellucidum and, in two-thirds of patients, hypothalamic-pituitary dysfunction. It is best thought of as being part of the holoprosencephaly spectrum. Clinical presentation of SOD is varied and mostly dependent on whether or not it is associated with schizencephaly (~50% of cases). This association is used to define two forms of the condition:

- Not associated with schizencephaly
  - Visual apparatus more severely affected
    - Hypothalamic-pituitary dysfunction present in 60% to 80% of patients
    - May present as hypoglycemia in the neonatal period
    - Small pituitary gland with hypoplastic or absent infundibulum and ectopic posterior pituitary seen as focus of T1 high signal intensity in median eminence of hypothalamus
    - Olfactory bulbs may be absent (Kallmann syndrome)
  - Associated with schizencephaly
    - Optic apparatus less severely affected
    - Cortical anomalies: polymicrogyria and cortical dysplasia
    - May be etiologically different
    - Sometimes referred to as SOD plus
  - In addition, a number of other associations are recognized including:
    - Rhombencephalosynapsis
    - Chiari II malformation
    - Aqueductal stenosis (AS)

MRI is the modality of choice for assessing SOD. Imaging may demonstrate a "point down" appearance of the lateral ventricular frontal horns on coronal images, absent septum pellucidum, hypoplastic pituitary stalk, hypoplastic optic chiasm/optic nerves, and globes.

References: Barkovich AJ, Fram EK, Norman D. Septo-optic dysplasia: MR imaging. *Radiology*. 1989;171(1):189-192.

Sener RN. Septo-optic dysplasia associated with cerebral cortical dysplasia (cortico-septo-optic dysplasia). *J Neuroradiol*. 1996;23(4):245-247.

14 **Answer B.** There are multiple calcified subependymal nodules and cortical thickening in all lobes of the brain. There are enhancing tubers in the left frontal lobe. There are enhancing subependymal nodules at the right foramen of Monro. Tuberous sclerosis was classically described as presenting in childhood with a triad (Vogt triad) of:

- Seizures: absent in one-quarter of individuals
- Mental retardation: up to half have normal intelligence
- Adenoma sebaceum: only present in about three-quarters of patients

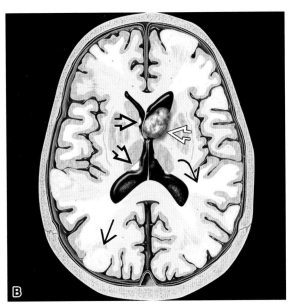

Axial graphic of typical brain involvement in tuberous sclerosis complex shows a giant cell astrocytoma (*black hollow arrows*) in the left foramen of Monro, subependymal nodules (*white hollow arrow*), radial migration lines (curved arrow), and cortical/subcortical tubers (straight arrow). (Reprinted with permission from Osborn AG, Salzman KL, Jhaveri MD. *Diagnostic Imaging: Brain.* 3rd ed. Elsevier; 2016:96.)

Tuberous sclerosis has a significant number of manifestations, involving many organ systems. The most common manifestations are:

- Cortical or subependymal tubers and white matter abnormalities
- Renal angiomyolipomas (AMLs)
- Cardiac rhabdomyoma
- Cutaneous findings: adenoma sebaceum

After the neurological manifestations of tuberous sclerosis, renal manifestations are the second most common clinical feature; four types of lesions can occur: autosomal dominant polycystic kidney disease lesions, isolated renal cyst(s), AMLs, and renal cell carcinomas.

Cortical/subcortical tubers are commonly located in the frontal lobe and demonstrate high T2 and low T1 with only 10% of tubers showing enhancement. The tubers frequently calcify after 2 years of age. The subependymal hamartomas are often associated with calcification. Lesion enhancement is variable and is not a useful feature in distinguishing them from subependymal giant cell astrocytomas (SEGAs). SEGAs' peak occurrence is 8 to 18 years of age and tends to be large and demonstrates growth. These lesions tend to have intense enhancement. The white matter abnormalities demonstrate variable appearance, with nodular, ill-defined, cystic, and band-like lesions seen. One way to differentiate tuberous sclerosis from multiple sclerosis is that radial bands are thought to be relatively specific for tuberous sclerosis.

References: Goh S, Butler W, Thiele EA. Subependymal giant cell tumors in tuberous sclerosis complex. *Neurology.* 2004;63(8):1457-1461.

Takanashi J, Sugita K, Fujii K, et al. MR evaluation of tuberous sclerosis: increased sensitivity with fluid-attenuated inversion recovery and relation to severity of seizures and mental retardation. *AJNR Am J Neuroradiol.* 1995;16(9):1923-1928.

15 Answer A. After the neurological manifestations of tuberous sclerosis, renal manifestations are the second most common clinical feature; four types of lesions can occur: autosomal dominant polycystic kidney disease lesions, isolated renal cyst(s), AMLs, and renal cell carcinomas.

16 Answer C. Head ultrasound demonstrates that the lateral ventricles are moderately enlarged and very little extra-axial fluid is seen. The fourth ventricle is decompressed. Brain MRI demonstrates moderate to marked ventriculomegaly with enlargement of the lateral and third ventricles. The fourth ventricle is normal in size. The cerebral aqueduct is incompletely visualized and appears narrow. AS is the most common cause of congenital obstructive hydrocephalus but can also be seen in adults as an acquired abnormality. Antenatal ultrasound can show features of fetal hydrocephalus with a near-normal posterior fossa. There can be secondary thinning of the cortical mantle as well as secondary macrocephaly. MRI demonstrates enlargement of the lateral and third ventricles. The aqueduct may show narrowing and funneling superiorly. The fourth ventricle is classically not dilated. One must exclude causes of secondary obstruction such as aqueductal or tectal plate tumor. An MRI CSF flow study is helpful, and the absence of a flow void signal intensity on sagittal T2 images at the aqueductal level has been suggested as a sign of AS.

References: McMillan JJ, Williams B. Aqueduct stenosis. Case review and discussion. *J Neurol Neurosurg Psychiatry.* 1977;40(6):521-532.

Stoquart-El Sankari S, Lehmann P, Gondry-Jouet C, et al. Phase-contrast MR imaging support for the diagnosis of aqueductal stenosis. *AJNR Am J Neuroradiol.* 2009;30(1):209-214.

17 Answer A. MRI images demonstrate a mass in the caudal aspect of the fourth ventricle. This rounded mass has high T1 signal, isointense T2 signal, areas of low signal on GRE, and homogeneous enhancement. Differential consideration for a mass centered in the fourth ventricle include:

Medulloblastoma	Arises from vermis or roof of fourth ventricle (superior medullary velum)
	Small round blue cells: hyperdense on CT
	50% have CSF dissemination at diagnosis.
	Solid, enhancing mass within fourth ventricle
	Hydrocephalus in >90%
Ependymoma	Arises from floor of fourth ventricle
	"Plastic" tumor squeezes out lateral recesses and foramen of Magendie.
	Intratumoral cysts and hemorrhage common
	Two-thirds are infratentorial within fourth ventricle.
	Heterogeneous and enhancing mass
Pilocytic astrocytoma	Cyst with enhancing mural nodule
	Typically cerebellar hemisphere rather than intraventricular
	60% are cerebellar; 30% optic nerve/chiasm
Brain stem glioma	Intrinsic to brain stem, not fourth ventricle
	May be dorsally exophytic, project posteriorly into fourth ventricle
Subependymoma	Inferior fourth ventricle, obex (60%)
	Middle-aged and older adults
	T2 hyperintense lobular mass
	No or mild enhancement is typical.
Choroid plexus papilloma	40% involve fourth ventricle (posterior medullary velum), cerebellopontine angle (CPA), and foramina of Luschka
	Fourth ventricle common location in adults
	Lateral ventricle more common in child
	Lobular and vibrantly enhancing mass

There are three types of choroid plexus tumor (CPT):

- Choroid plexus papilloma (CPP) (WHO grade I)
- Atypical choroid plexus papilloma (aCPP) (grade II)
- Choroid plexus carcinoma (CPCa) (grade III)

Classic imaging appearance of CPP is a child with enhancing lobulated (cauliflower-like) mass in atrium of lateral ventricle. CPPs occur in proportion to amount of choroid plexus. CPP is typically located in the following locations:

- 50% in lateral ventricle (usually atrium)
- 40% in fourth ventricle and/or foramina of Luschka
- 5% in third ventricle (roof)

References: Jaiswal AK, Jaiswal S, Sahu RN, et al. Choroid plexus papilloma in children: diagnostic and surgical considerations. *J Pediatr Neurosci.* 2009;4(1):10-16.

Smith A, Smirniotopoulos J, Horkanyne-Szakaly I. From the radiologic pathology archives: intraventricular neoplasms: radiologic-pathologic correlation. *Radiographics.* 2013;33(1):21-43.

18 **Answer D.** There is mid to posterior sagittal synostosis as well as synostosis of the right lambdoid suture resulting in some scaphocephaly and asymmetric posterior brachycephaly. There is also likely synostosis of the transverse occipital suture/synchondrosis between the occipital portion of the basiocciput and the squamosal occipital bone. Craniostenosis or craniosynostosis refers to premature closure of one or more of the cranial sutures. Isolated premature closure of the sagittal suture is most common. Unilateral or bilateral premature closure of the coronal suture is the next most common followed by premature closure of the metopic suture. Depending on which suture prematurely fuses, there are characteristic deformities of the skull and orbits. For example, premature closure of the sagittal suture results in limited transverse growth of the skull, namely, dolichocephaly or scaphocephaly, which is an increased anterior-posterior dimension. Plagiocephaly refers to premature closure of a single coronal or lambdoid suture. In the majority of cases, plagiocephaly is seen with closure of a single coronal suture, resulting in elevation of the lesser wing of the sphenoid bone leading to the "harlequin" appearance of the orbit.

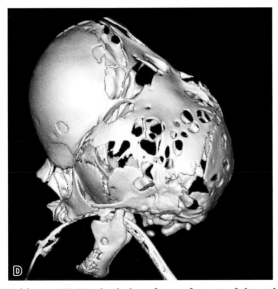

Sagittal bone CT 3D shaded surface reformat of the calvarium in a 1-day-old with Carpenter syndrome shows an abnormal head shape and frontal bossing with facial hypoplasia and premature closure of the squamosal, coronal, lambdoid, and sagittal sutures. (Reprinted with permission from Osborn AG, Salzman KL, Jhaveri MD. *Diagnostic Imaging: Brain.* 3rd ed. Elsevier; 2016:1112.)

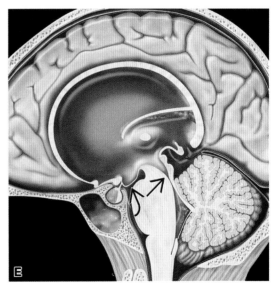

Sagittal graphic shows obstructive hydrocephalus with markedly enlarged lateral and third ventricles, stretched (thinned) corpus callosum, and a funnel-shaped cerebral aqueduct (*straight arrow*) related to distal obstruction. Note the normal size of the fourth ventricle and the herniation of the floor of the third ventricle (*curved arrow*) from the hydrocephalus. (Reprinted with permission from Osborn AG, Salzman KL, Jhaveri MD. *Diagnostic Imaging: Brain.* 3rd ed. Elsevier; 2016:1006.)

Craniosynostosis is usually an isolated abnormality although it can be associated with a variety of syndromes. Such conditions include Apert syndrome, hypophosphatasia, Crouzon disease (craniofacial dysostosis), and Treacher Collins syndrome (mandibulofacial dysostosis).

Reference: Mafee MF, Valvassori GE. Radiology of the craniofacial anomalies. *Otolaryngol Clin North Am.* 1981;14:939-988.

19 **Answer B.** There is a mass within and expanding the left midanterior nasal cavity. The mass is noted to extend superiorly to the level of the cribriform plate. This mass is hypointense on T1 and hyperintense on T2. There is no internal enhancement within the mass. Nasal encephaloceles are in most cases a form of neural tube defect particularly common in Southeast Asia. They are herniation of cranial content through a bony defect in the anterior skull base into the nasal area. Nasal encephaloceles usually present at birth with symptoms of obstruction or other complications. It presents as an external swelling on the nose. The swelling is usually soft, with normal overlying skin, and increases in size on coughing/straining. Symptomatic patients usually present with obstruction or rhinorrhea. Nasal encephaloceles are typically identified in association with a discernible cranial bone defect. Best imaging practices include multiplanar MRI to delineate soft tissues and intracranial relationships and bone CT to define osseous anatomy (except nasofrontal region in infants).

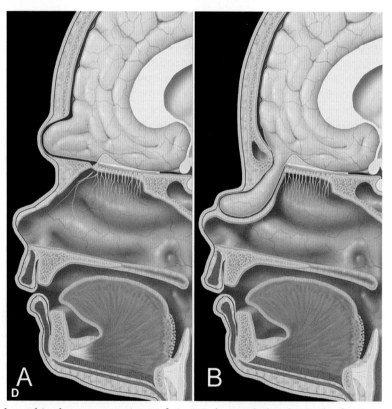

Sagittal graphic shows two variants of sincipital encephalocele. In the frontonasal type (A), the brain extends through the frontonasal suture into the glabellar region. In the nasoethmoidal type (B), the encephalocele extends through the foramen cecum into the nasal cavity. (Reprinted with permission from Osborn AG, Salzman KL, Jhaveri MD. *Diagnostic Imaging: Brain.* 3rd ed. Elsevier; 2016:1116.)

Reference: Tirumandas M, Sharma A, Gbenimacho I, et al. Nasal encephaloceles: a review of etiology, pathophysiology, clinical presentations, diagnosis, treatment, and complications. *Childs Nerv Syst.* 2013;29(5):739-744.

20 **Answer B.** There is an 11-mm-wide crescent-shaped hyperdense extra-axial hematoma overlying the left posterior convexity parietal region. Extradural hematoma (EDH), also known as an epidural hematoma, is a collection of blood that forms between the inner surface of the skull and outer layer of the dura, which is called the periosteal layer. They are commonly associated with a history of trauma and associated skull fracture. The source of bleeding is usually a torn meningeal artery (most commonly, the middle meningeal artery). EDHs are typically biconvex in shape and can cause a mass effect with herniation. They are usually limited by cranial sutures, but not by venous sinuses. Both CT and MRI are suitable to evaluate EDHs. When the blood clot is evacuated promptly (or treated conservatively when small), the prognosis of EDHs is generally good.

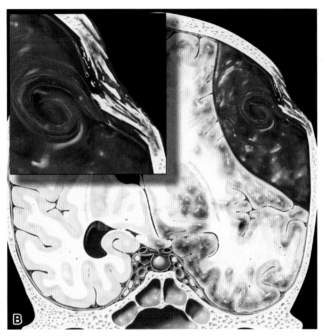

Coronal graphic illustrates swirling acute hemorrhage from a laceration of the middle meningeal artery by an overlying skull fracture. The epidural hematoma displaces the dura inward as it expands. (Reprinted with permission from Osborn AG, Salzman KL, Jhaveri MD. *Diagnostic Imaging: Brain*. 3rd ed. Elsevier; 2016:148.)

Reference: Irie F, Le Brocque R, Kenardy J, et al. Epidemiology of traumatic epidural hematoma in young age. *J Trauma*. 2011;71(4):847-853.

21 **Answer D.** US demonstrates an anechoic, vascular structure at the level of the tentorium with mild mass effect on the right lateral ventricle. MRI and magnetic resonance angiography (MRA) demonstrate prominent galenic/transfalcine perimesencephalic vein with associated hypogenesis of the corpus callosum posteriorly. Vein of Galen aneurysmal malformations (VGAMs), probably better termed as median prosencephalic arteriovenous fistula, are uncommon intracranial anomalies that tend to present dramatically during early childhood with features of a left-to-right shunt and high-output cardiac failure. These malformations account for <1% to 2% of all intracranial vascular malformations but are the cause of 30% of cerebral vascular malformations presenting in the pediatric age group. It is also the most common antenatally diagnosed intracranial vascular malformation. There may be an increased male predilection.

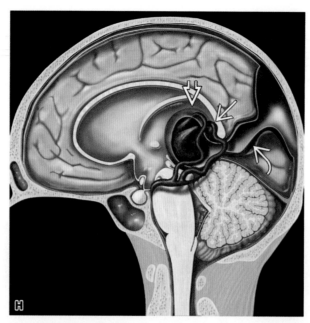

Sagittal graphic depicts classic vein of Galen malformation. Enlarged posterior choroidal arteries (*straight arrow*) drain into a dilated median prosencephalic vein (MPV) of Markowski (*hollow arrow*). The MPV drains into the superior sagittal sinus via an embryonic falcine sinus (*curved arrow*). (Reprinted with permission from Osborn AG, Salzman KL, Jhaveri MD. *Diagnostic Imaging: Brain*. 3rd ed. Elsevier; 2016:406.)

References: Bhattacharya JJ, Thammaroj J. Vein of Galen malformations. *J Neurol Neurosurg Psychiatry*. 2003;74(suppl 1):i42-i44.

Nicholson AA, Hourihan MD, Hayward C. Arteriovenous malformations involving the vein of Galen. *Arch Dis Child*. 1989;64(12):1653-1655.

22 **Answer A.** Angiography remains the gold standard in full characterization of the lesion. It enables to individually catheterize feeding vessels. Venous drainage is via the median prosencephalic vein (MPV), the straight sinus (if present), and then out via the transverse/sigmoid sinuses. By definition, there should be no drainage to other components of the deep venous system. Prior to endovascular intervention, prognosis was dismal, with 100% mortality without treatment and 90% mortality following surgical attempts. Ideally, embolization is deferred until 6 months of age for choroidal VGAM and later for mural types, to allow the cavernous sinus to mature. If cardiac failure is refractory to medical management, embolization may be performed sooner. Both venous and arterial embolization are possible, depending on the number of feeders, and controversy persists in regard to the optimum approach.

23 **Answer A.** US demonstrates bilateral ventriculomegaly, bilateral periventricular hyperechogenicity with shadowing consistent with calcification, and bilateral complex but predominantly cystic changes in both germinal matrices consistent with subacute hemorrhage. The lenticulostriate arteries are hyperechogenic consistent with vasculopathy. MRI demonstrates moderate dysmorphic ventriculomegaly, periventricular calcifications, and subependymal cysts, including prominent bilateral subependymal cysts near the foramen of Monro. There is abnormal gyration pattern with bilateral polymicrogyria as well as frontal predominant undersulcation.

Congenital cytomegalovirus (CMV) infection results from intrauterine fetal infection by CMV. CMV is the most common cause of intrauterine infection and most common cause of congenital infective and brain damage. Antibodies to CMV are seen in 30% to 60% of pregnant women, but only 2.5% have a primary infection during pregnancy, and this can result in fetal infection in approximately 30% of cases. The vast majority (90%) of infected babies are asymptomatic at birth, but some may go on to develop symptoms after 6 to 9 months.

US imaging findings include fetal intracranial calcification: mainly periventricular calcification (hyperechogenic foci), considered one of the most common features; fetal hydrocephalus; heterogeneous appearing brain parenchyma; microcephaly; and intraventricular adhesions.

MR brain imaging findings include:

- Microcephaly
- Migrational abnormalities: lissencephaly, pachygyria, and schizencephaly
- White matter lesions: predominantly parietal or posterior white matter involvement with spared rim in immediately periventricular and subcortical white matter
- Ventriculomegaly and subarachnoid space enlargement
- Delayed myelination
- Periventricular and temporal pole cysts

References: Ceola AF, Angtuaco TL. US case of the day. Congenital cytomegalovirus infection. *Radiographics*. 1999;19(5):1385-1387.

Malinger G, Lev D, Zahalka N, et al. Fetal cytomegalovirus infection of the brain: the spectrum of sonographic findings. *AJNR Am J Neuroradiol*. 2003;24(1):28-32.

24 **Answer A.** Chest radiography demonstrates bilateral healing rib fractures. Noncontrast head CT demonstrated intermediate-density extra-axial (subdural) fluid at the frontal convexities and hyperdense extra-axial (subdural) hemorrhage along the posterior interhemispheric fissure and at the apex. The presence of skull fractures and/or intracranial hemorrhage particularly in infants in the absence of known trauma to explain such injuries should raise the suspicion of child abuse. Head injury is the leading cause of morbidity and mortality in these abused children. Brain injury may be the result of direct trauma, aggressive shaking, or strangulation/suffocation. There is little or no evidence of external trauma.

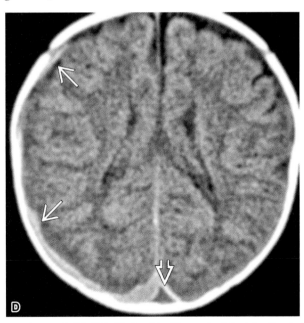

Axial non-enhanced CT (NECT) in this 12-week-old with rib, skull, and humerus fractures and a duodenal hematoma shows a moderate subdural hematoma over the right cerebral hemisphere (*solid arrows*), with a small amount of subdural blood on the left, causing a pseudo "empty delta" sign of the sagittal sinus (*hollow arrow*). (Reprinted with permission from Osborn AG, Salzman KL, Jhaveri MD. *Diagnostic Imaging: Brain*. 3rd ed. Elsevier; 2016:188.)

The most common type of intracranial hemorrhage in the setting of child abuse is subdural hematoma although subarachnoid, epidural, intraventricular, and cortical hemorrhages are also manifestations of nonaccidental trauma.

Bilateral retinal hemorrhages are highly suggestive of child abuse. Complex skull fractures and cerebral infarction are also diagnostic harbingers of child abuse.

Reference: Sato Y, Yuh WTC, Smith WL. Head injury in child abuse: evaluation with MR imaging. *Radiology*. 1989;173:653-657.

25 **Answer B.** Images demonstrate two lytic lesions in the left parietal region and one at the apical parietal region. The skeleton is the most commonly involved organ system in Langerhans cell histiocytosis (LCH) and is by far the most common location for single-lesion LCH, often referred to as eosinophilic granuloma (EG). Patients may have one or, less commonly, many lesions. The most common locations are the skull and long bones:

- Skull: approximately 50%
- Pelvis: 23%
- Femur: 17%
- Ribs: 8% (most common in adults)
- Humerus: 7%
- Mandible: 7%
- Spine

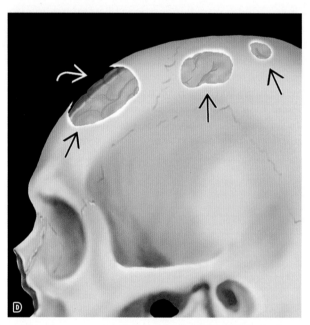

Lateral graphic demonstrates three sharply defined lytic lesions (*straight arrows*) of the membranous calvarium with geographic destruction. Note the beveled margins of the bony lysis (*curved arrow*). (Reprinted with permission from Osborn AG, Salzman KL, Jhaveri MD. *Diagnostic Imaging: Brain*. 3rd ed. Elsevier; 2016:1152.)

Skull radiographic imaging findings include:

- Solitary or multiple punched-out lytic lesions without sclerotic rim
- Double-contour or beveled-edge appearance may be seen due to greater involvement of the inner versus the outer table (hole within a hole) sign
- Button sequestrum representing residual bone
- Geographic skull

Prognosis is excellent when disease is confined to the skeleton, especially if it is a solitary lesion, with the majority of such lesions spontaneously resolving by fibrosis within 1 to 2 years.

Reference: David R, Oria RA, Kumar R, et al. Radiologic features of eosinophilic granuloma of bone. *AJR Am J Roentgenol*. 1989;153(5):1021-1026.

26 **Answer C.** MRI demonstrates multifocal areas of fluid-attenuated inversion recovery (FLAIR) hyperintensity throughout the cerebral white matter, as well as left optic nerve thickening/hyperintensity, and extraocular muscle thickening. Acute disseminated encephalomyelitis (ADEM) is an immune-mediated demyelinating disease related to an antecedent viral infection or vaccination. The cause is believed to be an allergic or autoimmune (cell-mediated) response against the myelin basic protein because of cross-reaction with viral proteins. ADEM has most commonly been associated with measles; however, it has also been associated with chickenpox, rubella, mumps, and other viral agents.

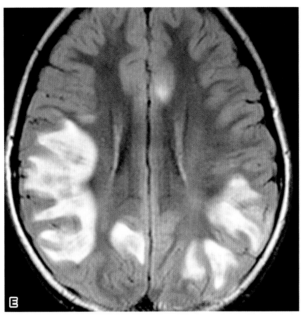

Axial fluid-attenuated inversion recovery (FLAIR) MR shows peripheral, confluent areas of hyperintensity predominantly involving subcortical white matter in this child with acute disseminated encephalomyelitis (ADEM). The bilateral but asymmetric pattern is typical of ADEM. (Reprinted with permission from Osborn AG, Salzman KL, Jhaveri MD. *Diagnostic Imaging: Brain*. 3rd ed. Elsevier; 2016:764.)

Both clinically and on MRI, ADEM may appear identical to the initial presentation of multiple sclerosis. Patients may present with symptoms and focal neurologic deficits typically within 2 to 3 weeks following a viral illness. In addition to focal neurologic deficits, unlike multiple sclerosis, ADEM is not infrequently associated with seizures. ADEM more commonly involves white matter especially in the subcortical region; however, gray matter may also be involved. MRI typically demonstrates multiple hyperintense foci on T2. These lesions may or may not enhance. ADEM is a monophasic process; therefore, no new lesions should develop after 6 months following initial presentation. The diagnosis of ADEM can usually be made by clinical history and CSF analysis.

Reference: Mader I, Stock KW, Ettlin T, Probst A. Acute disseminated encephalomyelitis: MR and CT features. *AJNR Am J Neuroradiol*. 1996;17:104-109.

27 **Answer C.** There is a well-circumscribed and heterogeneously enhancing extradural mass extending dorsally from the posterior sphenoid body and clivus. The mass is T2 bright and has some internal areas of mixed signal and areas of mineralization. Chordomas arise in locations where notochordal remnants are found. They occur most commonly at the sacrum although not infrequently found at the clivus or upper cervical spine. They are considered benign neoplasms; however, they grow quite invasively especially at the skull base where they can invade the neural foramen and cavernous sinus or extend into the middle cranial fossa.

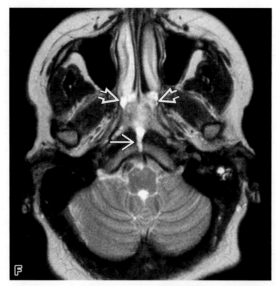

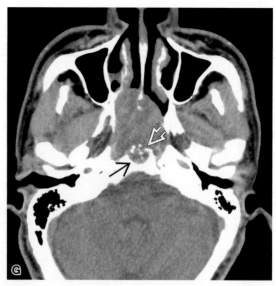

Axial T2-weighted MRI reveals focal midline anterior clival defect (*straight arrow*), representing path of primitive notochord. Tract must be respected with nasopharyngeal component to avoid local recurrence. Note hyperintense mass obstructs posterior nasal cavity bilaterally (*hollow arrows*). (Reprinted with permission from Koch BL, Hamilton BE, Harnsberger HR, et al. *Diagnostic Imaging: Head and Neck.* 3rd ed. Elsevier; 2017:360.)

Axial contrast-enhanced CT (CECT) demonstrates a large nasopharyngeal extraosseous chordoma filling the airway. Notice the anterior clival midline scalloping in the area of the medial basal canal (*straight arrow*). Characteristic bone fragments (*hollow arrow*) are visible in the posterior midline of the tumor. (Reprinted with permission from Koch BL, Hamilton BE, Harnsberger HR, et al. *Diagnostic Imaging: Head and Neck.* 3rd ed. Elsevier; 2017:360.)

On CT, a calcified matrix may be present and regions of bony erosion or destruction are best visualized. On MRI, the signal characteristics of chordoma are variable. These tumors are typically hypointense on T1 and hyperintense on T2. Most chordomas enhance. The differential considerations include chondrosarcoma, metastatic disease, multiple myeloma, and lymphoma.

Reference: Myers SP, Hirsch WJ Jr, Curtin HD, Barnes I, Sekhar LN, Sen C. Chordomas of the skull base: MR features. *AJNR Am J Neuroradiol.* 1992;13:1627-1636.

Head and Neck

28 Answer B. The lateral neck radiograph demonstrates abnormal thickening of the prevertebral soft tissues. Please note that the lateral neck position in this case is suboptimal due to the neck in flexion. The pediatric neck should be positioned in extension for the lateral radiograph since neutral or flexion position can lead to false-positive prevertebral soft tissue thickening due to redundancy of the soft tissues. It may be difficult to obtain correct radiographic positioning due to neck stiffness at the time of presentation.

CT is excellent at evaluating the neck soft tissues in an emergency setting when there is potential narrowing of the patient's airway and inability to obtain optimal radiographic positioning. CT imaging of the neck should be performed with intravenous contrast to differentiate fluid masses (abscess) from phlegmonous thickening (retropharyngeal cellulitis). It is important to note that CT imaging can lead to false-positive and false-negative results with respect to detecting pus. Therefore, surgical exploration may need to be carried out on the basis of clinical presentation.

29 Answer B. Neck radiograph demonstrates abnormal thickening of the prevertebral soft tissues. CT demonstrates a low-density collection with incomplete peripheral enhancement in the left parapharyngeal space consistent with a retropharyngeal abscess. Retropharyngeal abscesses are most frequently encountered in children, with 75% of cases occurring before the age of 5 years and often in the first year of life. This is likely due to the combination of prominent retropharyngeal nodal tissue and frequency of middle ear and nasopharyngeal infections. There may be a slight male predilection. Presentation is variable. In some instances, children present with nonspecific symptoms including generalized irritability, fever, and decreased appetite.

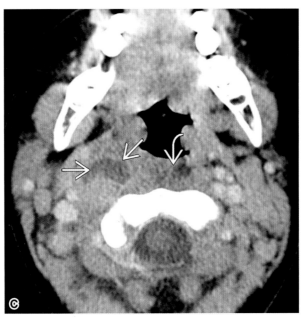

Axial contrast-enhanced CT (CECT) in a child while on antibiotics shows more focal low density in the anterior aspect of right retropharyngeal node (*straight arrows*) and more prominent peripheral enhancement of node. Retropharyngeal edema (*curved arrow*) is also seen without evidence of defined retropharyngeal abscess. (Reprinted with permission from Koch BL, Hamilton BE, Harnsberger HR, et al. *Diagnostic Imaging: Head and Neck*. 3rd ed. Elsevier; 2017:166.)

Radiographs demonstrate soft tissue swelling posterior to the pharynx, with a widening of the prevertebral soft tissues. This appearance cannot be distinguished from a prevertebral abscess, and careful evaluation of the vertebral bodies and disc spaces is important. CT is excellent at evaluating the neck, and timeliness is essential given potential narrowing of the airway. CT imaging should be obtained with IV contrast to allow differentiation of fluid collections from phlegmonous thickening (retropharyngeal cellulitis). It is important to note, however, that CT has an insignificant rate of both false-positive (10%) and false-negative (13%) rates with respect to detecting pus, and as such, surgical exploration may need to be carried out on the basis of clinical presentation. Treatment is similar in principle to that of other infected collections usually requiring both surgical drainage (usually performed via a transoral route) and intravenous antibiotics. In some instances, antibiotics alone may suffice, when collections are small.

With a prompt diagnosis, appropriate antibiotics, and drainage when necessary, almost all patients recover uneventfully. Serious complications in developed nations with prompt access to imaging and antibiotic are uncommon; however, complacency needs to be avoided as retropharyngeal abscess can lead to potentially life-threatening complications.

References: Coulthard M, Isaacs D. Retropharyngeal abscess. *Arch Dis Child*. 1991;66(10):1227-1230.

Craig FW, Schunk JE. Retropharyngeal abscess in children: clinical presentation, utility of imaging, and current management. *Pediatrics*. 2003;111(6 pt 1):1394-1398.

30 **Answer A.** There is unilateral right-sided choanal atresia with a fluid level along the right nasal cavity. The left side is normal. Choanal atresia refers to a lack of formation of the choanal openings. It can be unilateral or bilateral. Approximately two-thirds of cases are unilateral. It frequently presents in neonates where it is one of the most common causes of nasal obstruction. There is a recognized female predilection. Unilateral choanal atresias present late and can be asymptomatic or present with rhinorrhea, whereas bilateral atresias can present with neonatal respiratory distress (infants are obligate nose breathers). Another finding is failure to pass a nasogastric tube.

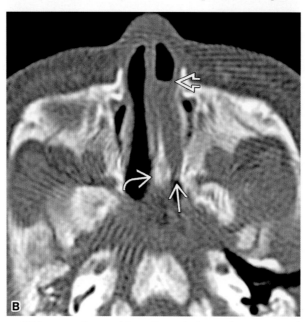

Axial bone CT in a newborn with unilateral choanal atresia on the left demonstrates membranous atresia (*straight arrow*) and fluid layers (*hollow arrow*) in the left nasal cavity. Note the associated thickening of the vomer (*curved arrow*) posteriorly. (Reprinted with permission from Merrow AC Jr. *Diagnostic Imaging: Pediatrics*. 3rd ed. Elsevier; 2017:1148.)

Structurally, there are two main types:

- Osseous: 90%
- Membranous: 10%

Syndromic associations include:

- CHARGE syndrome
- Crouzon syndrome
- DiGeorge syndrome
- Amniotic band syndrome
- Fetal alcohol syndrome
- Treacher Collins syndrome

Other associations include:

- Intestinal malrotation
- Craniosynostosis
- Congenital heart disease

Axial CT scans are the best modality and can demonstrate:

- Unilateral or bilateral posterior nasal narrowing with an obstruction
- Airway <3 mm (measurement done at the reference level of the pterygoid plates in the axial plane)
- Air-fluid level above the obstruction point
- Thickening of the vomer
- Medial bowing of posterior maxillary sinus

Treatment options include endoscopic perforation (for membranous types) and full choanal reconstruction.

References: Hengerer AS, Brickman TM, Jeyakumar A. Choanal atresia: embryologic analysis and evolution of treatment, a 30-year experience. *Laryngoscope.* 2008;118(5):862-866.

Tadmor R, Ravid M, Millet D, et al. Computed tomographic demonstration of choanal atresia. *AJNR Am J Neuroradiol.* 1984;5(6):743-745.

31 **Answer D.** MRI demonstrates a heterogeneously enhancing mass originating in the posterior nasal cavity in the region of the sphenopalatine foramen extending into the medial aspect of the pterygopalatine fossa. This mass extends superiorly through the floor of the sphenoid into the left sphenoid sinus. There is involvement of the anterior left vidian canal within the sphenoid. The mass extends anteriorly into the nasal cavity and posteriorly into the nasopharynx.

Juvenile nasopharyngeal angiofibromas (JNAs) are rare benign but locally aggressive vascular tumors. JNAs occur almost exclusively in males and usually in adolescence. They account for only 0.5% of all head and neck tumors but are the most common of benign nasopharyngeal neoplasms. The presentation is typically with obstructive symptoms, epistaxis, and chronic otomastoiditis because of obstruction of the Eustachian tube.

CT is particularly useful at delineating bony changes. Typically, a lobulated nonencapsulated soft tissue mass is demonstrated centered on the sphenopalatine foramen (which is often widened) and usually bowing the posterior wall of the maxillary antrum anteriorly. There is marked contrast enhancement following administration of contrast, reflecting the prominent vascularity.

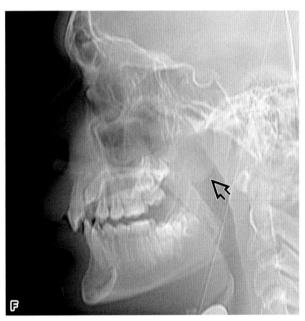

Lateral radiograph of teenage boy with epistaxis shows a rounded mass projecting down into the nasopharynx (*hollow arrow*). Although displacement of the posterior wall of the maxillary sinus is the classic radiographic finding of juvenile nasopharyngeal angiofibroma (JNA), it is rarely encountered. (Reprinted with permission from Merrow AC Jr. *Diagnostic Imaging: Pediatrics.* 3rd ed. Elsevier; 2017:1152.)

References: Duvall AJ, Moreano AE. Juvenile nasopharyngeal angiofibroma: diagnosis and treatment. *Otolaryngol Head Neck Surg.* 1988;97(6):534-540.

Kania RE, Sauvaget E, Guichard JP, et al. Early postoperative CT scanning for juvenile nasopharyngeal angiofibroma: detection of residual disease. *AJNR Am J Neuroradiol.* 2005;26(1):82-88.

32 **Answer A.** Angiography is often useful both in defining the feeding and in preoperative embolization. Supply of these tumors is usually via:

- External carotid artery (majority)
- Internal maxillary artery

- Ascending pharyngeal artery
- Palatine arteries
- Internal carotid artery: less common, usually in larger tumors
- Sphenoidal branches
- Ophthalmic artery

33 **Answer B.** There are mildly enhancing mineralized T2 hypointense masses present within the bilateral globes, which are fairly symmetric in appearance. There is no extension into the surrounding intraorbital structures. Retinoblastomas are the most common intraocular neoplasm found in childhood. Presentation is most frequently with leukocoria or loss of red eye reflex. Overall, approximately 30% to 40% are bilateral and often synchronous. The bilateral occurrence is even higher in inherited forms and tends to occur at a younger age. They are generally characterized by a heterogeneous retinal mass with calcifications, necrotic components, and increased vascularization on Doppler ultrasound/enhancement on CT/MRI. MRI is the modality of choice for pretreatment staging on retinoblastoma. Prognosis depends on the stage. Overall, the cure rate has risen to over 90% in first world nations.

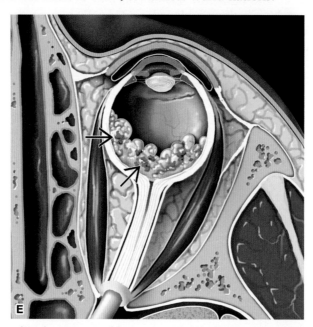

Axial graphic depicts retinoblastoma, with lobulated tumor extending through the limiting membrane into the vitreous. Punctate calcifications (*arrows*) are characteristic. (Reprinted with permission from Merrow AC Jr. *Diagnostic Imaging: Pediatrics*. 3rd ed. Elsevier; 2017.)

References: de Graaf P, Barkhof F, Moll AC, et al. Retinoblastoma: MR imaging parameters in detection of tumor extent. *Radiology*. 2005;235(1):197-207.

Kaufman LM, Mafee MF, Song CD. Retinoblastoma and simulating lesions. Role of CT, MR imaging and use of Gd-DTPA contrast enhancement. *Radiol Clin North Am*. 1998;36(6):1101-1117.

34 **Answer B.** In the left neck, there is a slightly lobulated, oblong slightly T2 hyperintense, minimally enhancing lesion in the left paracervical, submandibular, and carotid spaces.

Also notable, there is a slightly asymmetric morphology of the thymic gland with prominence on the right. Signal characteristics of this gland are similar to the lesion in the left neck.

Ectopic thymus can occur anywhere along the caudal descent of the thymopharyngeal duct (migration of the thymus from the third and fourth branchial pouches to the anterior mediastinum) and also found rarely in the posterior mediastinum and dermis. Ectopic thymic tissue may manifest as a neck mass, which can be mistaken for a pathologic process.

Also, as the thymopharyngeal duct undergoes atrophy, thymic remnants may develop into cysts. Because the parathyroid glands similarly arise from the third and fourth pharyngeal pouches, ectopic parathyroid glands, and hence parathyroid adenomas, may appear anywhere near or within the thyroid or thymus.

Reference: Nasseri F, Eftekhari F. Clinical and radiologic review of the normal and abnormal thymus: pearls and pitfalls. *Radiographics*. 2010;30(2):413-428.

35 **Answer A.** In the region of the right parotid gland, there is a rounded fluid density. There is surrounding thick enhancement with overlying soft tissue swelling. Given the patient's age, differential considerations include an infected or inflamed branchial cleft cyst. Acute inflammation of parotid gland in a child can be caused by:

- Bacterial: Localized bacterial infection ± abscess
  - Usually because of ascending infection
  - May result from adjacent cellulitis
  - *Staphylococcus aureus* (50% to 90%) > *Streptococcus, Haemophilus, E. coli*, and anaerobes
  - Neonatal suppurative parotitis may be bilateral because of bacteremia.
    - More common in premature infants, males
- Viral: Usually from systemic viral infection
  - Mumps paramyxovirus most common cause (so-called epidemic parotitis)
  - Also influenza, parainfluenza, coxsackie A and B, enteric cytopathic human orphan (ECHO), and lymphocytic choriomeningitis viruses
  - CMV and adenovirus reported with HIV infection
- Calculus induced: Ductal obstruction by sialolith
- Autoimmune: Acute episode of chronic disease
  - Sjögren syndrome
  - Mikulicz syndrome
  - Sicca syndrome, acute phase
- Juvenile recurrent parotitis (JRP): Intermittent idiopathic episodes of parotid inflammation
  - Recurrent episodes mimic mumps.
  - Patient often has unilateral symptoms but bilateral imaging abnormalities.
  - Sialographically mimics Sjögren syndrome.

Top differential considerations:

- Infected first branchial cleft anomaly
- Parotid infantile hemangioma
- Salivary gland neoplasms
- Parotid sialosis
- Benign lymphoepithelial lesions of HIV
- Parotid sarcoidosis

References: Francis CL, Larsen CG. Pediatric sialadenitis. *Otolaryngol Clin North Am*. 2014;47(5):763-778.

Spiegel R, Miron D, Sakran W, Horovitz Y. Acute neonatal suppurative parotitis: case reports and review. *Pediatr Infect Dis J*. 2004;23(1):76-78.

36 **Answer A.** On US, in the midline at the suprasternal region, just below the level of thyroid, is a hypoechoic rounded mass with posterior acoustic enhancement and internal echogenic debris. On MRI, there is a T2 hyperintense cystic neck lesion with rim enhancement extending between the hyoid bone and laryngeal prominence.

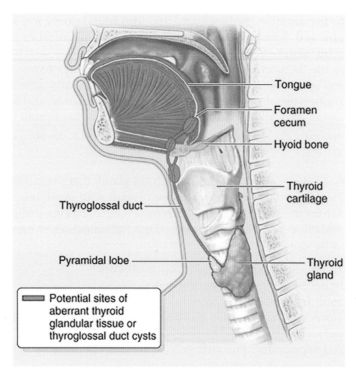

Thyroglossal duct vestiges. (From Moore KL, Dalley AF, Agur AM. *Clinically Oriented Anatomy.* 7th ed. Wolters Kluwer Health; 2014:1041.)

Thyroglossal duct cysts (TGDCs) are the most common congenital neck cysts. They are typically located in the midline and are the most common midline neck mass in young patients. TGDCs typically present during childhood (90% before the age of 10) or remain asymptomatic until they become infected, in which case they can present at any time. TGDCs account for 70% of all congenital neck anomalies and are the second most common benign neck mass, after lymphadenopathy. Presentation is typically either as a painless rounded midline anterior neck swelling or, if infected, as a red warm painful lump. It may move with swallowing and classically elevates on tongue protrusion.

The cysts can occur anywhere along the course of the thyroglossal duct, although infrahyoid location is most common:

- Suprahyoid: 20% to 25% (less common in adults ~5%)
- At the level of hyoid bone: approximately 30% (range 15% to 50%)
- Infrahyoid: approximately 45% (range 25% to 65%)

Typically, they are located in the midline with those off-midline characteristically located next to the thyroid cartilage. Nearly all TGDCs are located within 2 cm of the midline, with more inferior lesions tending to be off-midline. Ectopic thyroid tissue may be present.

Unless infected, they are painless, fluctuant masses, which spread the strap muscles. The fluid is usually anechoic and the walls are thin, without internal vascularity. However, in some cases, the internal fluid may contain debris. This is particularly the case in an adult patient where cysts may be complex heterogeneous masses. If there is associated infection, there may be surrounding inflammatory change.

References: Ahuja AT, King AD, King W, et al. Thyroglossal duct cysts: sonographic appearances in adults. *AJNR Am J Neuroradiol.* 1999;20(4):579-582.

Meuwly JY, Lepori D, Theumann N, et al. Multimodality imaging evaluation of the pediatric neck: techniques and spectrum of findings. *Radiographics.* 2005;25(4):931-948.

37 **Answer B.** Extensive multiloculated bilateral transspatial mixed venolymphatic malformation demonstrating innumerable small fluid-filled cysts involving the face and neck with extension inferiorly to the anterior chest wall and superior mediastinum. Percutaneous sclerotherapy for treatment of bilateral neck lymphatic malformation was performed. The neck radiograph demonstrates retained contrast from the procedure.

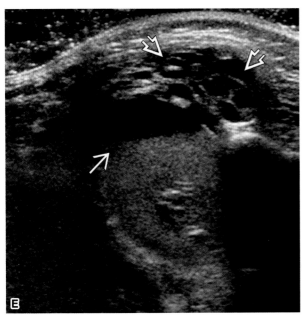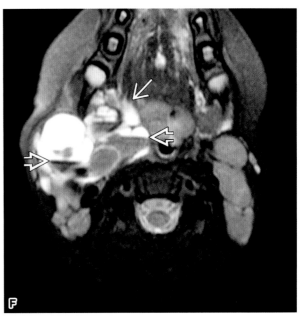

Transverse ultrasound in a 2-year-old boy who presented with sudden onset of neck mass shows a multiloculated lymphatic malformation with fluid-fluid level in the largest microcyst (*straight arrow*) and smaller microcysts anteriorly (*hollow arrows*). (Reprinted with permission from Koch BL, Hamilton BE, Harnsberger HR, et al. *Diagnostic Imaging: Head and Neck*. 3rd ed. Elsevier; 2017:580.)

Axial T2-weighted fat-suppressed (FS) MR in the same child shows better advantage of the deeper extent of the lesion (*straight arrow*) with multiple fluid-fluid levels (*hollow arrows*) secondary to layering blood products, with cysts of varying sizes. (Reprinted with permission from Koch BL, Hamilton BE, Harnsberger HR, et al. *Diagnostic Imaging: Head and Neck*. 3rd ed. Elsevier; 2017:580.)

Lymphatic malformations are benign vascular lesions that arise from embryological disturbances in the development of the lymphatic system. They encompass a wide spectrum of related abnormalities, including cystic lymphatic lesions, angiokeratoma, destructive lymphatic malformations that occur in bones (Gorham-Stout syndrome), lymphatic and chylous leak conditions, and lymphedema. Symptoms of lymphatic malformations are related to the anatomical location of these lesions, as well as to the extent of involvement of the local anatomical structures.

Lymphatic malformations can be seen in any anatomic region but are more commonly seen in lymphatic-rich areas, such as the head and neck (45% to 52%), axilla, mediastinum, groin, and retroperitoneum. These malformations are thought to be the result of abnormal development of the embryonic lymphatics or lymphatic jugular sacs, with failure of these structures to connect or drain into the venous system. In some patients, ectatic adjacent veins can be seen in association with a cystic lymphatic lesion. There are three morphologic types of cystic lymphatic lesions: macrocystic, microcystic, and combined. Histologically, cystic lymphatic malformations are composed of vascular spaces filled with eosinophilic and protein-rich fluid. Hemorrhage within the cystic spaces is common, indicating recent trauma or spontaneous intralesional bleeding.

Large cystic lymphatic lesions can be diagnosed in utero using ultrasound as early as the beginning of the second trimester, but lesions are more commonly noted at birth; the vast majority are evident by 2 years of age. Unlike hemangiomas, lymphatic malformations persist throughout life, grow proportionately with the size of the patient, and do not undergo involution as does hemangioma. The prenatal diagnosis of cervical lymphatic malformations has significant clinical implications. They may be associated with airway obstruction, and prenatal diagnosis can influence the mode, timing, and place of delivery. The term "cystic hygroma" should not be applied to typical lymphatic malformation masses for two reasons. Firstly, the -oma suffix suggests a neoplasm, which it is not. Secondly, this term is prevalent in the obstetric vernacular to denote posterior cervical cystic lesions that are associated with severe, often lethal, chromosomal anomalies. However, it is crucial to distinguish "hygroma" from typical lymphatic malformations seen postnatally, because the latter is not associated with chromosomal abnormalities or syndromes.

CT or MRI can clearly demonstrate the anatomic extent of cystic lesions and their relationship to soft tissues, muscle, and vascular structures.

Reference: Elluru RG, Balakrishnan K, Padua HM. Lymphatic malformations: diagnosis and management. *Semin Pediatr Surg.* 2014;23(4):178-185.

38 **Answer C.** There is a round hypoechoic heterogeneous fusiform lesion within the right sternocleidomastoid (SCM) muscle. The lesion has internal vascularity similar to the adjacent musculature. Fibromatosis colli is a rare form of infantile fibromatosis that occurs within the SCM muscle. Presentation is usually with torticollis and is most frequently related to birth trauma (e.g., forceps delivery) or malposition in the womb. Ultrasound is the imaging modality of choice. The SCM is diffusely enlarged in a fusiform manner, with resultant shortening when the head is turned away from the affected side (mastoid process drawn inferiorly toward the ipsilateral head of clavicle). Echogenicity of the SCM may vary. Color Doppler may reveal a high-resistance waveform. The enlarged area often moves synchronously with the rest of the SCM muscle on real-time sonography. It is a self-limiting condition and usually resolves within 4 to 8 months and is treated conservatively with physiotherapy.

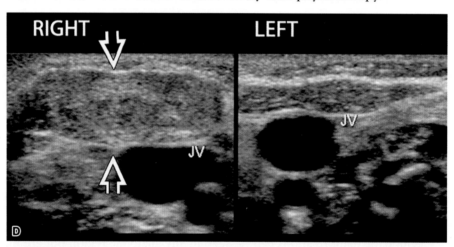

Transverse ultrasound displayed in side-by-side view compares the mid-muscle belly of the sternocleidomastoid just anterior to the jugular vein (JV). The right sternocleidomastoid (*arrows*) is 2 to 3× thicker than the left. (Reprinted with permission from Merrow AC Jr. *Diagnostic Imaging: Pediatrics.* 3rd ed. Elsevier; 2017:1204.)

References: Crawford SC, Harnsberger HR, Johnson L, et al. Fibromatosis colli of infancy: CT and sonographic findings. *AJR Am J Roentgenol.* 1988;151(6):1183-1184.

Patrick LE, O'Shea P, Simoneaux SF, et al. Fibromatoses of childhood: the spectrum of radiographic findings. *AJR Am J Roentgenol.* 1996;166(1):163-169.

Spine

39 **Answer D.** Fetal MRI demonstrates ventriculomegaly with the lateral ventricles measuring up to 14 mm in maximum dimension bilaterally at the level of the atria (10 mm and above is considered enlarged). There is a small posterior fossa with low-lying hindbrain elements. There is a large dorsal neural arch dysraphic defect starting near the T8-T9 level and extending from the lower thoracic to midlumbar spine associated with a fluid-filled sac. Spinal cord and neural elements course along the dorsal aspect of the thoracolumbar dysraphic defect.

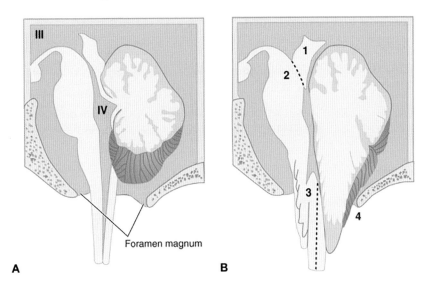

Chiari malformation. Midsagittal section. A: Normal cerebellum, fourth ventricle, and brain stem. B: Abnormal cerebellum, fourth ventricle, and brain stem showing the common congenital anomalies: (1) beaking of the tectal plate, (2) AS, (3) kinking and transforaminal herniation of the medulla into the vertebral canal, and (4) herniation and unrolling of the cerebellar vermis into the vertebral canal. An accompanying meningomyelocele is common. (Reprinted from Fix JD. BRS neuroanatomy. Baltimore, MD: Williams & Wilkins; 1996:72, with permission.)

Chiari II malformation, also known as Arnold-Chiari malformation, is a relatively common congenital malformation of the spine and posterior fossa characterized by myelomeningocele (lumbosacral spina bifida aperta) and a small posterior fossa with descent of the brain stem and cerebellar tonsils. The presentation can be divided according to the age of the individual (although most will have lifelong sequelae) as follows:

- Neonatal
  - Myelomeningocele
  - Brain stem dysfunction resulting in cranial nerve palsies
  - Neurogenic bladder
- Child
  - Musculoskeletal
  - Hydrocephalus
- Young adult
  - Syrinx and scoliosis

Classical signs described on ultrasound include the lemon sign and the banana cerebellum sign. There may also be evidence of fetal ventriculomegaly because of obstructive effects as a result of downward cerebellar herniation. Additionally, many of the associated malformations (e.g., corpus callosal dysgenesis) may be identified. MRI is the modality of choice for detecting and characterizing the full constellation of findings associated with Chiari II malformations:

Posterior fossa

- Small posterior fossa with a low attachment of the tentorium and low torcula
- Brain stem appears "pulled" down with an elongated and low-lying fourth ventricle.

- Tectal plate appears beaked: inferior colliculus is elongated and points posteriorly, with resulting angulation of the aqueduct, which results in AS and hydrocephalus.
- Cerebellar tonsils and vermis are displaced inferiorly through foramen magnum, which appears crowded.

Spine

- Spina bifida aperta/myelomeningocele
- Tethered cord

References: Curnes JT, Oakes WJ, Boyko OB. MR imaging of hindbrain deformity in Chiari II patients with and without symptoms of brainstem compression. *AJNR Am J Neuroradiol.* 1989;10(2):293-302.

el Gammal T, Mark EK, Brooks BS. MR imaging of Chiari II malformation. *AJR Am J Roentgenol.* 1988;150(1):163-170.

40 **Answer B.** Radiographs demonstrate relative shortening of the long bones, including the femurs, shortening of the ribs, flaring of the physis of the long bones, brachydactyly, narrowing of the lumbar interpedicular distance, bullet-shaped vertebral bodies, widening of the intervertebral disc spaces, and disproportionate length of the fibula relative to the tibia. There is rounding of the bilateral iliac wings. There is a trident appearance of the iliac spines. Lack of ossification in the bilateral femoral heads is consistent with hypertrophy of the cartilages. MR evaluation of the brain demonstrates a somewhat horizontal orientation of the clivus, suggesting skull base dysplasia, which can be seen in achondroplasia. There is narrowing of the foramen magnum at the cervicomedullary junction.

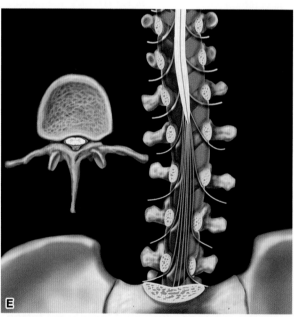

Axial and coronal graphics show spinal canal stenosis and narrowing of the interpedicular distance from L1 to L5. (Reprinted with permission from Merrow AC Jr. *Diagnostic Imaging: Pediatrics.* 3rd ed. Elsevier; 2017:946.)

Achondroplasia is a congenital genetic disorder resulting in rhizomelic dwarfism and is the most common skeletal dysplasia. There are numerous classical radiographic signs. The skull and spine findings include:

Skull

- Relatively large cranial vault with small skull base
- Prominent forehead with depressed nasal bridge
- Narrowed foramen magnum

- Cervicomedullary kink
- Relative elevation of the brain stem resulting in a large suprasellar cistern and vertically oriented straight sinus
- Communicating hydrocephalus (because of venous obstruction at sigmoid sinus)

Spine

- Posterior vertebral scalloping
- Progressive decrease in interpedicular distance in lumbar spine
- Gibbus: thoracolumbar kyphosis with bullet-shaped/hypoplastic vertebra (not to be confused with Hurler syndrome)
- Short pedicle canal stenosis
- Laminar thickening
- Widening of intervertebral discs
- Increased angle between sacrum and lumbar spine

There is often a danger of cervical cord compression because of narrowing of the foramen magnum. Treatment varies and is usually orthopedic, particularly to correct kyphoscoliosis as well as neurosurgical to decompress the foramen magnum or shunt hydrocephalus. Overall prognosis is good, with near-normal life expectancy in heterozygous individuals. When homozygous, the condition is usually fatal because of respiratory compromise.

References: Kao SC, Waziri MH, Smith WL, et al. MR imaging of the craniovertebral junction, cranium, and brain in children with achondroplasia. *AJR Am J Roentgenol.* 1989;153(3):565-569.

Wang H, Rosenbaum AE, Reid CS, et al. Pediatric patients with achondroplasia: CT evaluation of the craniocervical junction. *Radiology.* 1987;164(2):515-519.

41 **Answer D.** There is moderate thoracic kyphosis measuring approximately 60 degrees. There is exaggeration of the normal lumbar lordosis. There is mild anterior wedging and loss of height of multiple contiguous thoracic vertebral bodies. Scheuermann disease, also known as juvenile kyphosis, juvenile discogenic disease, or vertebral epiphysitis, is a common condition, which results in kyphosis of the thoracic or thoracolumbar spine. There is a strong hereditary predisposition (perhaps autosomal dominant) with a high degree of penetrance and variable expressivity and occurs in the thoracic spine in up to 75% of cases, followed by the thoracolumbar spine combined and occasionally lumbar and rarely cervical spine.

To apply the label of classical Scheuermann disease, one needs to meet a number of criteria (Sorensen classification):

- Thoracic spine kyphosis >40 degrees (normal 25 to 40 degrees)
- Thoracolumbar spine kyphosis >30 degrees (normal 0 degrees)

and

- At least three adjacent vertebrae demonstrating wedging of >5 degrees

The condition is associated with Schmorl nodes, limbus vertebrae, scoliosis (~25%), and spondylolisthesis.
Other signs include:

- Vertebral end-plate irregularity because of extensive disc invagination
- Intervertebral disc space narrowing, more anteriorly

References: Blumenthal SL, Roach J, Herring JA. Lumbar Scheuermann's. A clinical series and classification. *Spine.* 1987;12(9):929-932.

Summers BN, Singh JP, Manns RA. The radiological reporting of lumbar Scheuermann's disease: an unnecessary source of confusion amongst clinicians and patients. *Br J Radiol.* 2008;81(965):383-385.

42 **Answer A.** There are multiple cervical spine anomalies with fusion at multiple levels as well as markedly abnormal morphology throughout the spine. There is elevation of the left scapula. Klippel-Feil syndrome (KFS) is a complex heterogeneous entity that results in cervical vertebral fusion. Two or more nonsegmented cervical vertebrae are usually sufficient for diagnosis. There is a recognized female predilection. The classic clinical triad of a short neck, low hairline, and restricted neck motion is considered to be present in <50% of patients with this syndrome.

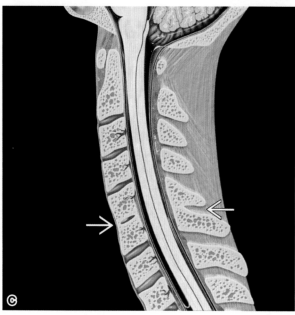

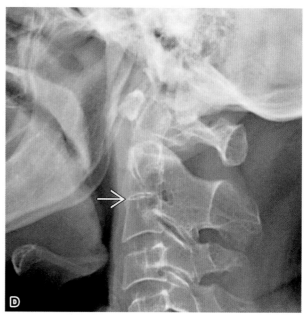

Sagittal graphic (Klippel-Feil syndrome [KFS] type 2) shows congenital fusion (*arrows*) of the C5 to C6 vertebrae and spinous processes, with characteristic rudimentary disc space and distinctive "waist" typical of congenital fusion. (Reprinted with permission from Ross JS, Moore KR. *Diagnostic Imaging: Spine*. 3rd ed. Elsevier; 2016:136.)

Lateral radiograph (Klippel-Feil syndrome [KFS] type 2) demonstrates typical C2/3 congenital segmentation failure ("fusion") with characteristic rudimentary disc space (*arrow*) and fusion of the facets and spinous processes. The disc space appearance helps distinguish from post-cervical fusion. (Reprinted with permission from Ross JS, Moore KR. *Diagnostic Imaging: Spine*. 3rd ed. Elsevier; 2016:136.)

Associations and imaging findings

- Sprengel deformity of the shoulder
- Anomalies of the aortic arch and branching vessels, for example, carotid and subclavian arteries
- Spinal scoliosis
- Intervertebral disc herniation
- Cervical spondylosis
- Renal abnormalities, for example, unilateral renal agenesis
- Vertebral fusion
- AP narrowing of the vertebral bodies (wasp-waist sign)
- Hemivertebrae
- Spina bifida

Reference: Ulmer JL, Elster AD, Ginsberg LE, et al. Klippel-Feil syndrome: CT and MR of acquired and congenital abnormalities of cervical spine and cord. *J Comput Assist Tomogr*. 1993;17(2):215-224.

43 **Answer C.** There is a large cellular-appearing left paraspinal soft tissue mass, which extends into the posterior paraspinal musculature and into the left lower pelvis displacing the left psoas anteriorly and extending into the iliac vessels and psoas muscles. The lesion extends through the neural foramina on the left from L5 through S2-S3 and into the left lateral and ventral epidural space filling the spinal canal and effacing the CSF with displacement of the nerve roots posteriorly into the right from the level of L4-L5 through S3. There is also involvement of the right neural foramen at L5-S1.

Ewing sarcoma is a small, round cell tumor, which accounts for one-quarter of all primary bone tumors during childhood. It has a peak incidence during the second decade and is very rare after 30 years of age. Typical complaints of patients with Ewing sarcoma are pain and swelling of the affected bone. The most commonly affected bones are the femur, pelvis, and other long bones of the extremities. Vertebrae are affected in <5% of the cases and may present with nerve root or spinal cord compression. The prognosis is usually poor.

Ewing sarcoma is the second most common highly malignant primary bone tumors of childhood after osteosarcoma, typically arising from medullary cavity with invasion of the Haversian system and typically occurs in children and adolescents between 10 and 20 years of age. It is rare in African Americans. Ewing sarcoma is a small round blue cell tumor with regular-sized primitive-appearing cells. It is closely related to the soft tissue tumors peripheral primitive neuroectodermal tumor (pPNET), Askin tumor, and neuroepithelioma, which collectively are referred to as Ewing sarcoma family of tumors (ESFT). Ewing sarcoma of the spine is a rare condition that appears with a clinical triad of local pain, neurological deficit, and palpable mass.

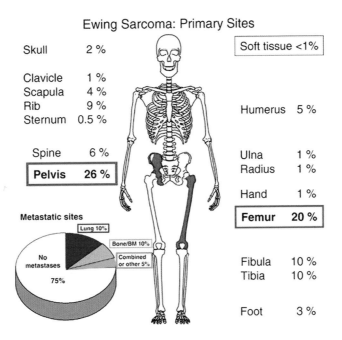

As far as location within long bones, the tumor is almost always metadiaphyseal or diaphyseal:

Middiaphysis: 33%
Metadiaphysis: 44%
Metaphysis: 15%
Epiphysis: 1% to 2%

References: Dini LI, Mendonca R, Gallo P. Primary Ewing's sarcoma of the spine. *Arq Neuropsiquiatr.* 2006;64(3-A):654-659.

Goktepe AS, Alaca R, Mohur H, Coskun U. Paraplegia: an unusual presentation of Ewing's sarcoma. *Spinal Cord.* 2002;40(7):367-369.

44 **Answer B.** There is spondylolysis at L5 with associated 8 mm grade 2 anterolisthesis of L5 on S1.

Spondylolysis is a defect in the pars interarticularis of the neural arch, the portion of the neural arch that connects the superior and inferior articular facets. It is commonly known as pars interarticularis defect or more simply as pars defect. Spondylolysis is present in approximately 5% of the population and higher in the adolescent athletic population. Spondylolysis is commonly asymptomatic. Symptomatic patients often have pain with extension and/or rotation of the lumbar spine. Approximately 25% of individuals with spondylolysis have symptoms at some time. It is a common cause of low back pain in adolescents and in particular athletes.

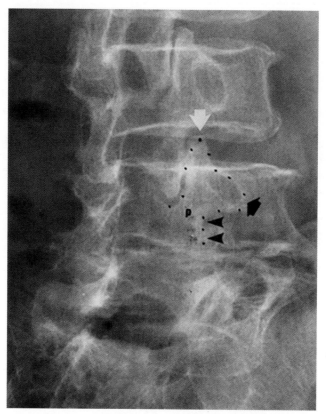

The "Scotty dog." On the oblique radiograph of the lumbar spine, the appearance of the posterior elements is commonly referred to as resembling the side view of a "Scotty dog." In this oblique radiograph, the "Scotty dog" is outlined by *dots*. The superior articular process (*white arrow*) represents the dog's ear; the pedicle (*black arrow*), the dog's muzzle; the inferior articular process (*small arrows*), the dog's front leg; and the pars interarticularis (p), the dog's neck.

Spondylolysis is believed to be caused by repeated microtrauma, resulting in stress fracture of the pars interarticularis. A dysplastic pars is usually present. Genetics are also believed to be a factor. It is more common in men than in women. Traumatic pars defects result from high-energy trauma where there is hyperextension of the lumbar spine and are rare in a congenitally normal vertebra.

Location

• 90% of cases of spondylolysis occur at the L5 level and 10% occur at L4 level
• Unilateral or bilateral

Associations

• 65% of patients with spondylolysis will progress to spondylolisthesis
• Spina bifida occulta

Imaging features

- Scotty dog sign: on oblique radiographs, a break in the pars interarticularis can have the appearance of a collar around the dog's neck.
- Inverted Napoleon hat sign

Surgery is only considered in rare circumstances as most cases respond to conservative management.

References: Jinkins JR, Matthes JC, Sener RN, et al. Spondylolysis, spondylolisthesis, and associated nerve root entrapment in the lumbosacral spine: MR evaluation. *AJR Am J Roentgenol.* 1992;159(4):799-803.

Syrmou E, Tsitsopoulos PP, Marinopoulos D, et al. Spondylolysis: a review and reappraisal. *Hippokratia.* 2010;14(1):17-21.

45 **Answer C.** Spine radiograph and MRI demonstrate midthoracic and lower lumbar segmentation/formation anomalies. There is a hydrosyringomyelia of the low-lying conus medullaris. Caudal regression syndrome (CRS) represents a spectrum of structural defects of the caudal region. Malformations vary from isolated partial agenesis of the coccyx to lumbosacral agenesis. In an antenatal setting, there are associations with maternal diabetes (type I or type II) and polyhydramnios.

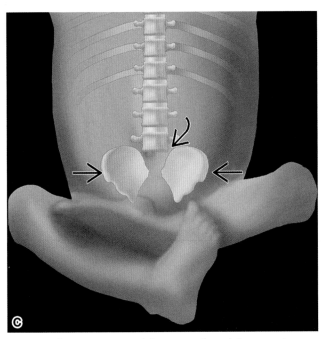

Graphic illustrates several features of caudal regression sequence (CRS) including abnormal lower extremity position with muscle wasting, shortened spine (*curved arrow*), and medial position of iliac wings (*straight arrows*). (Reprinted with permission from Woodward PJ, Kennedy A, Puchalski MD, et al. *Diagnostic Imaging: Obstetrics.* 3rd ed. Elsevier; 2017:244.)

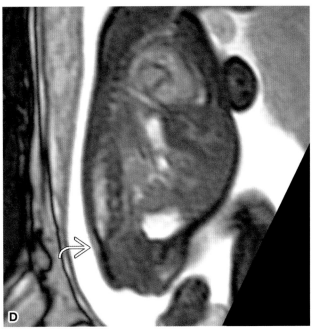

Sagittal T2-weighted MRI identified caudal regression sequence (CRS), with abrupt tapering of the lumbar spine (*curved arrow*). This patient had VACTERL, which is associated with CRS. After delivery, x-rays also showed hemivertebrae. (Reprinted with permission from Woodward PJ, Kennedy A, Puchalski MD, et al. *Diagnostic Imaging: Obstetrics.* 3rd ed. Elsevier; 2017:247.)

Imaging appearances can significantly vary depending on the severity of regression. In general, the following may be seen:

- Lumbosacral vertebral body dysgenesis/hypogenesis
- Level of atresia/dysgenesis is usually below L1 and often limited to sacrum.
- Truncated, blunt spinal cord terminating above the expected level
- Severe canal narrowing rostral to last intact vertebra

References: Singh SK, Singh RD, Sharma A. Caudal regression syndrome—case report and review of literature. *Pediatr Surg Int.* 2005;21(7):578-581.

Stroustrup Smith A, Grable I, Levine D. Case 66: caudal regression syndrome in the fetus of a diabetic mother. *Radiology.* 2004;230(1):229-233.

46 **Answer D.** There is a mixed cystic solid heterogeneous mass in the presacral space closely associated with the sacrum, distal sigmoid colon, and rectum. There are heterogeneous cystic components of the mass, with several T1 hypointense and T2 hyperintense cysts and several T1 and T2 intermediate intensity cysts, possibly representing cysts containing hemorrhage or proteinaceous material.

Sacrococcygeal teratoma (SCT) refers to a teratoma arising in the sacrococcygeal region. The coccyx is almost always involved. It is the most common congenital tumor in the fetus and neonate. The tumor is composed of all three germ cells (i.e., ectoderm, mesoderm, and endoderm).

Pathology-based classification:

* Benign (mature): most common
* Malignant (immature)

Location-based classification system according to the American Academy of Pediatric Surgery Section Survey:

* Type I: developing only outside the fetus (can have small presacral component); accounts for the majority of cases
* Type II: extrafetal with intrapelvic presacral extension
* Type III: extrafetal with abdominopelvic extension
* Type IV: tumor developing entirely in the fetal pelvis

An SCT can be benign or malignant depending on whether it is mature or immature. The majority, however, tend to be benign. Those presenting in older infants tend to have a higher malignant potential, which those presenting in utero have a poor prognosis because of complications.

Complications include:

* High-output cardiac failure from arteriovenous shunting: which in turn can cause hydrops fetalis
* Ureteric obstruction
* Gastrointestinal tract obstruction
* Compression of underlying nerves: giving urinary/fecal incontinence
* Anemia
* Dystocia
* Tumor rupture

References: Avni FE, Guibaud L, Robert Y, et al. MR imaging of fetal sacrococcygeal teratoma: diagnosis and assessment. *AJR Am J Roentgenol.* 2002;178(1):179-183.

Danzer E, Hubbard AM, Hedrick HL, et al. Diagnosis and characterization of fetal sacrococcygeal teratoma with prenatal MRI. *AJR Am J Roentgenol.* 2006;187(4):W350-W356.

47 **Answer C.** There is an expansile, mixed lytic/sclerotic lesion involving the right C3 lamina. Osteoblastomas are rare and benign primary bone tumors. They may be locally aggressive and tend to affect the axial skeleton more often than their histologic relative, osteoid osteoma. Patients typically present around the second to third decades of life. With spinal lesions, a painful scoliosis is a common presenting symptom. Otherwise, it presents with an insidious onset of dull pain, worse at night, with minimal response to salicylates in only 7% of patients (unlike osteoid osteoma). The area will characteristically be swollen and tender with a decreased range of motion.

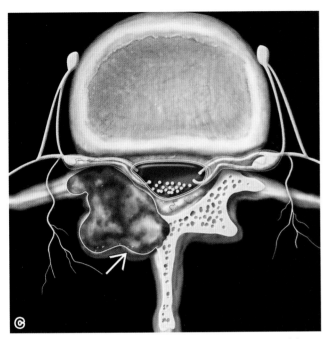

Axial graphic shows expansile, highly vascular osteoblastoma (*arrow*) arising in the right lamina and impinging on exiting nerve root. (Reprinted with permission from Ross JS, Moore KR. *Diagnostic Imaging: Spine*. 3rd ed. Elsevier; 2016:712.)

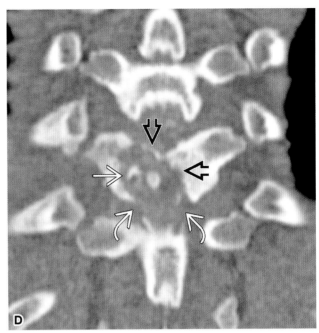

Coronal bone CT shows expansile osteoblastoma (*hollow arrows*) of right lamina. Matrix (*straight arrow*) mimics "rings and arcs" of chondroid matrix. Cortical breakthrough (*curved arrows*) is evident at inferior tumor margin. (Reprinted with permission from Ross JS, Moore KR. *Diagnostic Imaging: Spine*. 3rd ed. Elsevier; 2016:712.)

Osteoblastoma is histologically similar to an osteoid osteoma except that it is much larger. The tumor is bone and osteoid forming and is comprised of osteoblasts. There is high associated vascularity.

Location

- Spinal column: often involves the posterior column
- Cervical spine
- Sacrum
- Metaphysis and distal diaphysis of the long bones

Osteoblastomas can have a wide range of radiographic patterns. Lesions are typically larger than 2 cm. On radiography, lesions tend to be expansile and predominantly lytic with a rim of reactive sclerosis. There may be surrounding sclerosis or periostitis in up to 50% of cases.

References: Atesok KI, Alman BA, Schemitsch EH, et al. Osteoid osteoma and osteoblastoma. *J Am Acad Orthop Surg.* 2012;19(11):678-689.

Kroon HM, Schurmans J. Osteoblastoma: clinical and radiologic findings in 98 new cases. *Radiology.* 1990;175(3):783-790.

Shaikh MI, Saifuddin A, Pringle J, et al. Spinal osteoblastoma: CT and MR imaging with pathological correlation. *Skeletal Radiol.* 1999;28(1):33-40.

1 A 9-day-old presents with a history of congenital stridor. An upper GI was performed (Fig. A). The most likely diagnosis is:

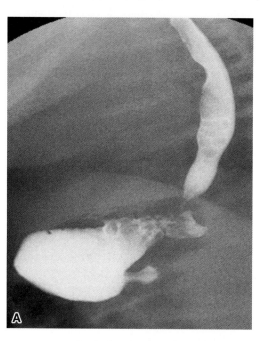 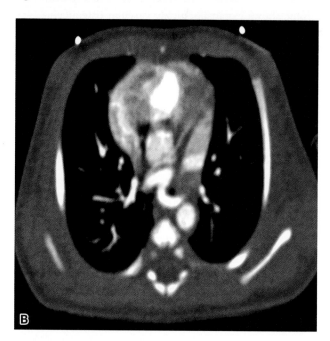

A. Pulmonary artery sling
B. Right arch with aberrant left subclavian
C. Tracheomalacia
D. Esophageal stenosis

2 Which of the following would reduce the dose to the child when performing the upper GI examination?

A. Use of an antiscatter grid
B. Reducing the magnification
C. Increasing the source to skin distance
D. Increasing the pulse rate

3 Concerning the diagnosis in Question 1, a type II is classified as having the following characteristic:

A. Carina in a normal location at the level of T4 to T5
B. Low carina at the level of T6
C. High carina at the level of T3
D. Tracheal bronchus

4 A right and left renal angiogram was performed on a 15-year-old female. What is the most likely diagnosis?

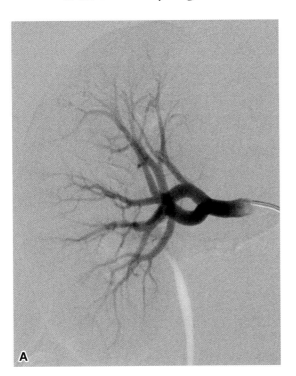

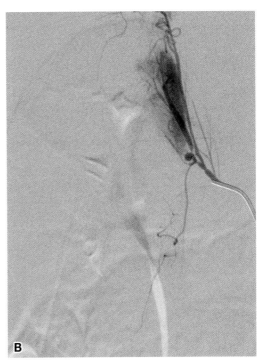

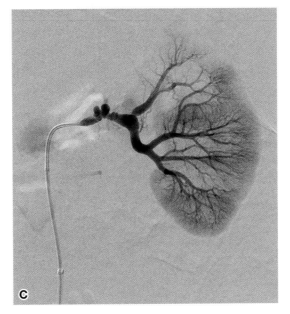

A. Autosomal dominant polycystic kidney disease
B. Atherosclerosis
C. Fibromuscular dysplasia
D. Segmental arterial mediolysis

5 Of the following choices, what is the most common presenting sign of the disease in Question 4?

A. Chest pain
B. Headache
C. No presenting signs or symptoms
D. Hypertension

6 The most common subtype of this disease in Question 4 is the following:

A. Medial
B. Perimedial
C. Intimal
D. Serosal

7 The indications for percutaneous intervention in a patient with the disease in Question 4 include which of the following?

A. Resistant hypertension
B. Intolerance to hypertensive medications
C. Renal impairment
D. Noncompliance with hypertensive medications
E. A and C only
F. All of the above

8 A 2-day-old presents with a history of a two-vessel cord and Williams syndrome. Which of the following is *true*?

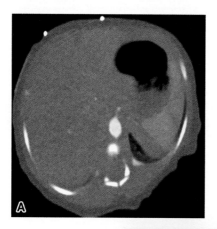
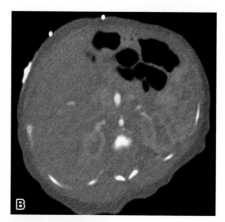
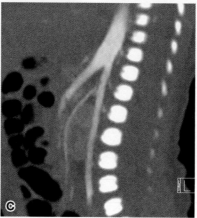

A. The infrarenal aorta is decreased in caliber.
B. The infrarenal aorta is enlarged in caliber.
C. The superior mesenteric artery is normal in caliber.
D. The superior mesenteric artery is decreased in caliber.

9 In the pediatric population, which is the first-line imaging modality to evaluate the disorder shown in Question 8?

A. Ultrasound with Doppler
B. Contrast-enhanced MRI
C. Contrast-enhanced CT
D. Subtraction angiography

10 A commonly occurring collateral pathway to supply the lower extremities in the disorder shown in Question 8 is:

A. Intercostal arteries to inferior mesenteric artery to hemorrhoidal arteries to external iliac arteries
B. Intercostal arteries to inferior mesenteric artery to infrarenal abdominal aorta
C. Superior mesenteric artery to inferior mesenteric artery to hemorrhoidal arteries to external iliac arteries
D. Superior mesenteric artery to inferior mesenteric artery to infrarenal abdominal aorta

11 An 18-month-old with elevated liver function tests presents for MRI following abnormality noted on recent abdominal sonogram. The following axial and volume-rendered images were obtained.

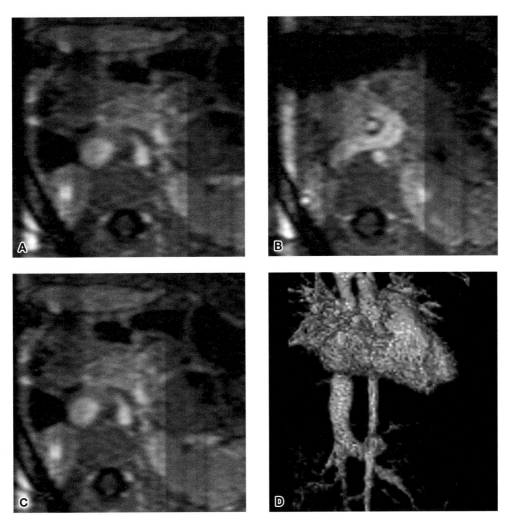

The most likely explanation for the prominent vessel extending below the SMA axis is:

A. Arteriovenous fistula
B. Aneurysmal dilatation of the left renal vein
C. Congenital portosystemic shunt
D. Interrupted IVC

12 What is the most likely classification of the abnormality shown in Question 11?

A. Type 1
B. Type 2
C. Type 3
D. Type 4

13 Type 1 congenital extrahepatic portosystemic shunts are associated with which of the following?

A. Conserved portal vein supply
B. Hepatoblastoma
C. Congenital heart disease
D. Male predilection

14 A 17-year-old underwent a contrast-enhanced CT angiogram of the chest.

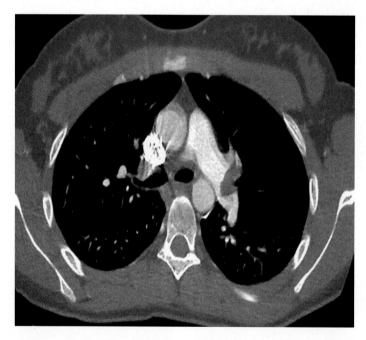

What is the most common symptom in older children presenting with this diagnosis?

A. Shortness of breath
B. Chest pain
C. Hemoptysis
D. Syncope
E. Tachypnea

15 What is the most common risk factor for the diagnosis in Question 14 in a child?

A. Septicemia
B. Dehydration
C. Malignancy
D. Congenital thrombophilia
E. Central venous catheter

16 Which of the following is a chronic complication of children following the diagnosis in Question 14?

A. Left ventricular dysfunction
B. Vascular dissection
C. Pneumonia
D. Pulmonary hypertension

17 An 8-year-old underwent a contrast-enhanced MRI of the chest.

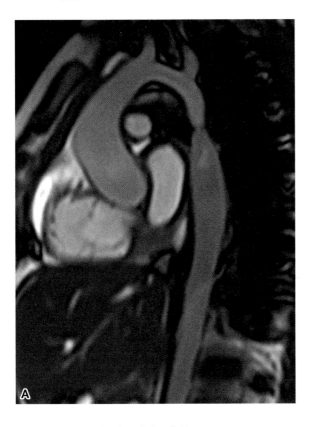
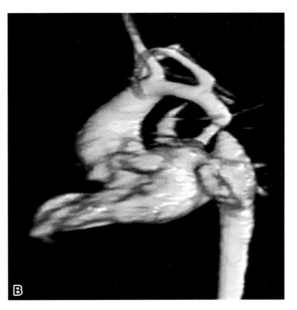

Which of the following is *true* concerning this diagnosis?

A. Female predominance
B. Clinically presents with lower body hypertension
C. Bicuspid aortic valve that is seen in <10% of affected patients
D. Can be associated with cerebral artery aneurysms

18 Which of the following is the advantage of imaging the disorder in Question 17 with MRI in comparison to CT?

A. Increased spatial resolution
B. Multiplanar imaging capability
C. Ability to quantify collateral flow
D. Improved diagnostic accuracy

19 What is the preferred technique in neonates and infants for repair of the condition in Question 17?

A. End-to-end anastomosis
B. Left subclavian flap anastomosis
C. Extra-anatomic bypass
D. Angioplasty

20 A 10-year-old with a history of tracheomalacia underwent a contrast-enhanced CT evaluation of the chest.

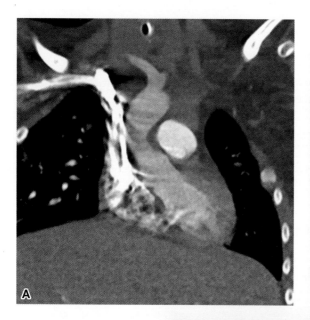
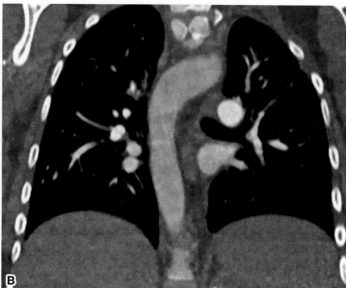
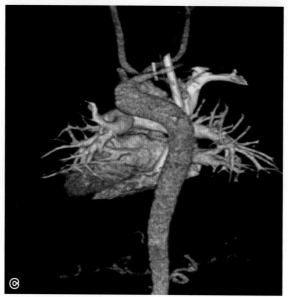

What is the diagnosis?

A. Double aortic arch
B. Left aortic arch with aberrant right subclavian artery
C. Right aortic arch with an aberrant left subclavian artery
D. Circumflex aortic arch

21 Is the abnormality in Question 20 a vascular ring?

A. Yes, the vascular ring is completed by the ligamentum.

B. Yes, the vascular ring is completed by a vessel passing adjacent to the trachea and esophagus.

C. No, the ligamentum is on the contralateral side and does complete the vascular ring.

D. No, there is no vessel passing adjacent to the trachea and esophagus to complete the vascular ring.

22 Which of the following is *true* concerning aortic arch anomalies?

A. Circumflex aortic arch is usually an isolated anomaly.

B. Right aortic arch with aberrant left subclavian artery is commonly associated with congenital heart disease.

C. Right dominant double aortic arch is usually an isolated anomaly.

D. Left dominant double aortic arch is commonly associated with congenital heart disease.

23 A 5-month-old with a history of high fever underwent a contrast-enhanced MRA.

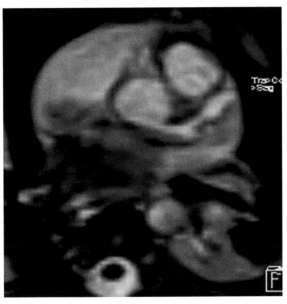

What is the most likely diagnosis?

A. Anomalous left coronary artery

B. Henoch-Schönlein Purpura

C. Kawasaki disease

D. Polyarteritis nodosa

E. Takayasu arteritis

24 Additional finding of the disorder in Question 23 is which of the following?

A. Diffuse lymphadenopathy

B. Hydrops of the gallbladder

C. Atrial myxoma

D. Extrapleural sequestration

25 Initial imaging evaluation of the coronary arteries in the disorder is performed using which modality?

A. MRI/MRA

B. CT angiography

C. Echocardiography

D. Conventional angiography

26 A teenager presenting with a history of solitary right kidney and hypertension underwent a contract-enhanced CT of the abdomen and pelvis.

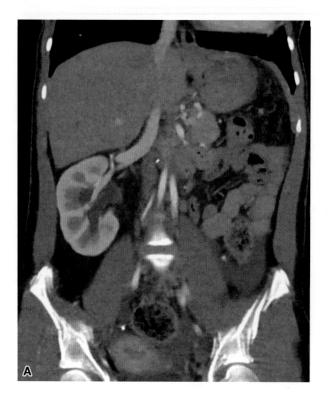 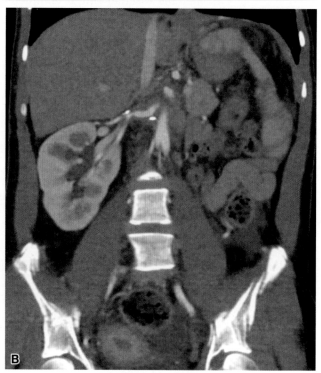

What is the cause of this patient's hypertension?

A. Aortic coarctation
B. Pheochromocytoma
C. Renal parenchymal disease
D. Renal artery stenosis

27 The patient in Question 26 also presents with lower extremity venous insufficiency. What is the cause of the venous insufficiency?

A. Duplicated inferior vena cava
B. Renal vein stenosis
C. Congenital absence of the inferior vena cava
D. Retroaortic right renal vein

28 Which of the following statements concerning the embryogenesis of the inferior vena cava is *true*?

A. Persistence of the right and left supracardinal veins leads to the development of a double inferior vena cava.
B. Regression of the right vitelline vein and persistence of the left vitelline vein lead to the development of a left inferior vena cava.
C. Regression of the hemiazygos vein leads to azygos continuation of the inferior vena cava.
D. Persistence of the ventral limb of the embryonic left renal vein leads to a circumaortic left renal vein.

ANSWERS AND EXPLANATIONS

1 **Answer A.** A pulmonary artery sling causes an anterior impression on the esophagus (arrow in A) and a posterior impression on the trachea due to the left pulmonary artery passing between the trachea and esophagus (arrow in B). The left pulmonary artery arises from the posterior aspect of the right pulmonary artery. This condition occurs because of the obliteration of the primitive left sixth aortic arch.

A right arch with an aberrant left subclavian artery would produce a posterior impression on the esophagus, not an anterior impression.

Tracheomalacia is a condition where there is flaccidity of the airway wall and supporting cartilage. On imaging, there is collapse of the tracheal lumen most pronounced during expiration or coughing. This condition is associated with vascular rings such as a pulmonary artery sling but is not demonstrated on this image.

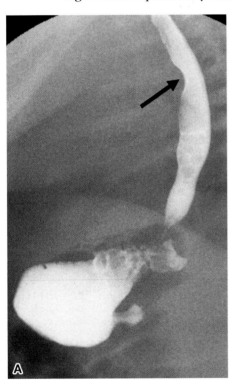
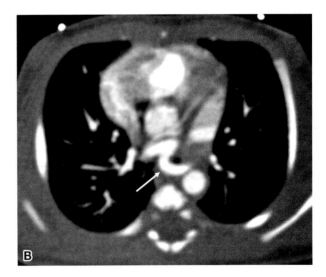

References: Lee EY, Dorkin H, Vargas SO. Congenital pulmonary malformations in pediatric patients: review and update on etiology, classification, and imaging findings. *Radiol Clin North Am.* 2011;49(5):921-948.

Yedururi S, Guillerman P, Chung T, et al. Multimodality imaging of tracheobronchial disorders in children. *Radiographics.* 2008;28(3):e29.

2 **Answer B.** When the magnification increases, the field of view becomes smaller. Unfortunately, when the field of view becomes smaller and the magnification increases, the dose also increases. Reducing the magnification or enlarging the field of view will therefore decrease the radiation dose.

The antiscatter grid attenuates scattered radiation. Given that detection of this scattered radiation decreases image quality, it is often necessary to use the grid in larger patients. With placement of the grid, the primary dose of radiation must be increased to replace the scattered dose at the image receptor. In pediatric patients, the smaller body produces less scatter, and therefore, use of a grid only minimally improves image quality. Children under the age of 3 to 5 years generally can be imaged without the grid with similar image quality.

Decreasing the source to skin distance (SSD) will decrease the dose to the child. The inverse square law states that the intensity of radiation of the beam is inversely proportional to the square of the SSD. Because of this, decreasing the SSD will decrease the dose to the child, and increasing the SSD will increase the dose to the child.

The pulse rate is the number of fluoroscopic images created per second. Increasing the pulse rate would increase the number of images per second and therefore increase the dose. Decreasing the pulse rate would decrease the number of images per second and decrease the dose.

Reference: Hernanz-Schulman M, Strauss K, Bercha IH. Fluoroscopy and radiation safety content for radiologists. http://www.imagegently.org/Portals/6/Radiologists/Background 4radiologists.pdf

3 **Answer B.** A type II pulmonary artery sling is characterized by a low position of the carina at the level of T6. A type II pulmonary artery sling is associated with long-segment tracheal stenosis, a T-shaped carina, and a bridging bronchus.

Types of Pulmonary Artery Slings	
Type 1	Position of carina: *normal* (T4-T5)
Type 2	Position of the carina: *low* (T6)
	Associated with long-segment tracheal stenosis, T-shaped carina, bridging bronchus

Reference: Lee EY, Dorkin H, Vargas SO. Congenital pulmonary malformations in pediatric patients: review and update on etiology, classification, and imaging findings. *Radiol Clin North Am.* 2011;49(5):921-948.

4 **Answer C.** Right and left renal angiograms demonstrate a normal right main renal artery but an early upper pole branch with irregular narrowing and a small aneurysm (arrow in A). The left main renal artery also has an irregular stenosis and two small aneurysms (arrows in B). These findings are most compatible with fibromuscular dysplasia, particularly in this age group. Fibromuscular dysplasia is a nonatherosclerotic disease involving medium-sized vessels, most commonly the renal, extracranial carotid, and vertebral arteries. Percutaneous transluminal renal angioplasty is the treatment of choice for renal fibromuscular dysplasia.

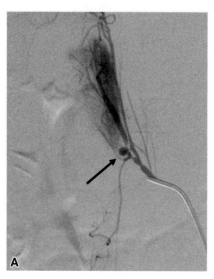
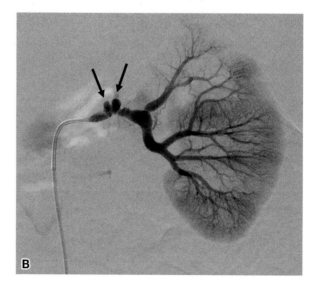

References: Meuse MA, Turba UC, Sabri SS, et al. Treatment of renal artery fibromuscular dysplasia. *Tech Vasc Interv Radiol.* 2010;13:126-133.

O'Connor SC, Gornik HL. Recent developments in the understanding and management of fibromuscular dysplasia. *J Am Heart Assoc.* 2014;3(6):e001259.

Varennes L, Tahon F, Kastler A, et al. Fibromuscular dysplasia: what the radiologist should know: a pictorial review. *Insights Imaging.* 2015;6(3):295-307.

5 **Answer D.** The most common presenting sign of fibromuscular dysplasia is hypertension followed by headache.

Most Common Presenting Signs and Symptoms of Fibromuscular Dysplasia	
Presenting Symptom	**%**
Hypertension	64
Headache	52
Pulsatile tinnitus	28
Dizziness	26
Cervical bruit	22
Neck pain	22

Reference: O'Connor SC, Gornik HL. Recent developments in the understanding and management of fibromuscular dysplasia. *J Am Heart Assoc.* 2014;3(6):e001259.

6 **Answer A.** The most common histopathologic subtypes of fibromuscular dysplasia are medial (60% to 70%), perimedial (10% to 20%), and intimal fibromuscular dysplasia (1% to 2%). This classification is based on the most affected arterial layer. Both medial and perimedial fibromuscular dysplasia tend to develop stenosis and aneurysms, whereas intimal fibrodysplasia develops smooth focal or tubular narrowing.

Types of Fibromuscular Dysplasia		
Type	**Frequency**	**Pathology**
Medial	60-70%	Rarefaction of smooth muscles cells replaced by fibrosis
Perimedial	15-25%	Excessive elastic tissue external to the media
Intimal	1-2%	Circumferential intimal thickening with proliferation of subendothelial connective tissue

References: Meuse MA, Turba UC, Sabri SS, et al. Treatment of renal artery fibromuscular dysplasia. *Tech Vasc Interv Radiol.* 2010;13:126-133.

Varennes L, Tahon F, Kastler A, et al. Fibromuscular dysplasia: what the radiologist should know: a pictorial review. *Insights Imaging.* 2015;6(3):295-307.

7 **Answer F.** Per the American College of Cardiology, the indications for percutaneous intervention in fibromuscular dysplasia include resistant hypertension, intolerance to antihypertensive medications, noncompliance with antihypertensive medications, and renal impairment. Other reasons for intervention are renal artery dissection and renal artery aneurysm.

References: Meuse MA, Turba UC, Sabri SS, et al. Treatment of renal artery fibromuscular dysplasia. *Tech Vasc Interv Radiol.* 2010;13:126-133.

O'Connor SC, Gornik HL. Recent developments in the understanding and management of fibromuscular dysplasia. *J Am Heart Assoc.* 2014;3(6):e001259.

8 **Answer A.** This patient has narrowing of the infrarenal aorta (arrows) consistent with middle aortic syndrome. The etiologies of this disorder include genetic causes such as Williams syndrome, Alagille syndrome, and neurofibromatosis. Additionally, vasculitis such as Takayasu arteritis and intrauterine infection such as rubella have been associated with this disorder.

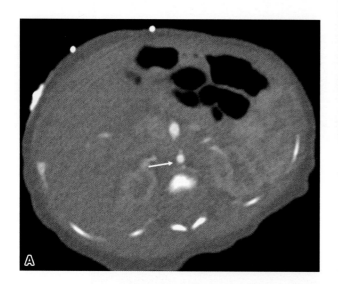
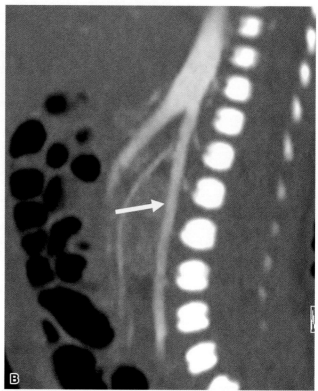

References: Kim SM, Jung IM, Min SI, et al. Surgical treatment of middle aortic syndrome with Takayasu arteritis or midaortic dysplastic syndrome. *Eur J Endovasc Surg.* 2015;50:206-212.

Rumman RK, Nickel C, Matsuda-Abedini M, et al. Disease beyond the arch: a systemic review of middle aortic syndrome in childhood. *Am J Hypertens.* 2015;28:833-846.

9 **Answer A.** Given the lack of ionizing radiation and the ability to perform without sedation, ultrasound with Doppler is the imaging modality of choice to initially evaluate a child with suspected middle aortic syndrome.

10 **Answer C.** The most commonly occurring collateral pathways in abdominal aortoiliac stenosis are

1. Superior mesenteric artery to inferior mesenteric artery to hemorrhoidal arteries to external iliac arteries
2. Intercostal, subcostal, and lumbar arteries to superior gluteal and iliolumbar arteries to internal iliac arteries to external iliac arteries
3. Intercostal, subcostal, and lumbar arteries to circumflex arteries to external iliac arteries

Reference: Sebastia C, Quiroga S, Boye R, et al. Aortic stenosis: spectrum of diseases depicted at multisection CT. *Radiographics.* 2003;23:S79-S91.

11 **Answer C.** There is connection of the splenic and superior mesenteric vein (arrow) to the inferior vena cava consistent with a congenital extrahepatic portosystemic shunt. This is a condition in which the portomesenteric blood drains into a systemic vein, therefore bypassing the liver.

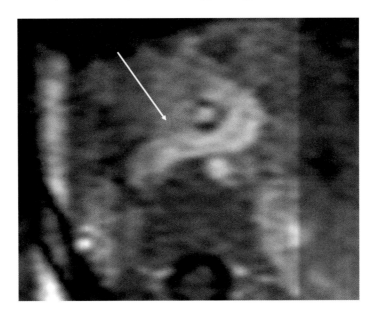

References: Alonso-Gamarra E, Parrion M, Perez A, et al. Clinical and radiologic manifestations of congenital extrahepatic portosystemic shunts: a comprehensive review. *Radiographics*. 2011;32:707-722.

Kobayashi N, Niwa T, Kirikoshi H, et al. Clinical classification of congenital extrahepatic portosystemic shunts. *Hepatol Res*. 2010;40:585-593.

12 **Answer B.** Congenital portosystemic shunts are initially classified as intrahepatic or extrahepatic. In this case, the abnormal connection is extrahepatic. Extrahepatic shunts are classified into type 1 or type 2. In type 1, there is absence of the intrahepatic portal venous supply. Type 1 is subclassified into type 1a where the splenic vein and superior mesenteric vein drain separately into a systemic vein or type 1b where the splenic vein and superior mesenteric vein form a common trunk before draining into a systemic vein. In type 2, the intrahepatic portal venous supply is present but some of the flow is diverted to the systemic circulation. In this case, a portal vein is present, so it is a type 2 extrahepatic portosystemic shunt.

References: Alonso-Gamarra E, Parrion M, Perez A, et al. Clinical and radiologic manifestations of congenital extrahepatic portosystemic shunts: a comprehensive review. *Radiographics*. 2011;32:707-722.

Kobayashi N, Niwa T, Kirikoshi H, et al. Clinical classification of congenital extrahepatic portosystemic shunts. *Hepatol Res*. 2010;40:585-593.

13 **Answer C.** Type 1 congenital extrahepatic portosystemic shunts are characterized by congenital absence of the portal vein and multiple associated anomalies such as polysplenia, congenital heart defects, and malrotation. Additionally, there is a female predilection. Type 2 congenital extrahepatic portosystemic shunts have a portal vein supply, no gender predilection, and fewer associated anomalies.

Reference: Alonso-Gamarra E, Parrion M, Perez A, et al. Clinical and radiologic manifestations of congenital extrahepatic portosystemic shunts: a comprehensive review. *Radiographics.* 2011;32:707-722.

14 Answer B. The axial image demonstrates a pulmonary embolism within the left pulmonary artery extending into the segmental vessels (arrow). Although children may present with all of the listed symptoms, in older children, 84% of cases present with pleuritic chest pain.

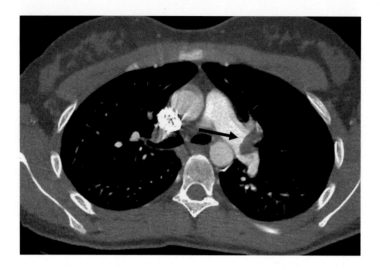

Reference: Thacker PG, Lee EY. Pulmonary embolism in children. *AJR Am J Roentgenol.* 2015;204:1278-1288.

15 Answer E. The most common risk factor for pulmonary embolism in both neonates and older children is a central venous catheter. Additional risk factors in neonates are dehydration, septicemia, and peripartum asphyxia. In older children, other risk factors are malignancy, renal disease, surgery or trauma, and congenital thrombophilia. Up to 98% of children have an identifiable risk factor with 88% having two more risk factors present.

Reference: Thacker PG, Lee EY. Pulmonary embolism in children. *AJR Am J Roentgenol.* 2015;204:1278-1288.

16 Answer D. Chronic complications of a pulmonary embolus in children are recurrence, pulmonary hypertension possibly leading to right heart failure, and complications related to anticoagulation therapy.

Reference: Thacker PG, Lee EY. Pulmonary embolism in children. *AJR Am J Roentgenol.* 2015;204:1278-1288.

17 Answer D. The images demonstrate focal narrowing of the postductal thoracic aorta (arrows) consistent with a coarctation. Coarctation of the aorta is a congenital narrowing of the aorta. There is a male predominance with a male-to-female ratio of 1.5:1. The clinical presentation is upper body hypertension with lower body hypoperfusion. This condition is associated with multiple other anomalies including bicuspid aortic valve, cerebral aneurysms, Turner syndrome, and Noonan syndrome. A bicuspid aortic valve is seen in 20% to 85% of patients with coarctation.

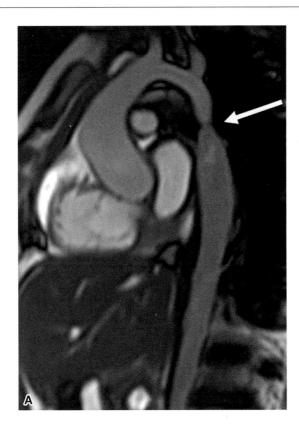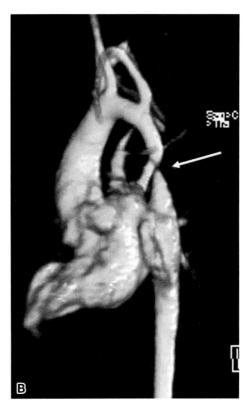

References: Nance JW, Ringel RE, Fishman EK. Coarctation of the aorta in adolescents and adults: a review of clinical features and CT imaging. *J Cardiovasc Comput Tomogr.* 2016;10:1-12.

Sebastia C, Quiroga S, Boye R, et al. Aortic stenosis: spectrum of diseases depicted at multisection CT. *Radiographics.* 2003;23:S79-S91.

18 **Answer C.** MRI has several advantages over CT in imaging coarctation including the lack of ionizing radiation and the ability to use phase contrast imaging to quantify collateral flow and flow and velocity across the area of narrowing. CT has higher spatial resolution and can be acquired more rapidly than MRI. Both modalities have multiplanar imaging capability, and there has been no proven difference in diagnostic accuracy when comparing these modalities.

Reference: Nance JW, Ringel RE, Fishman EK. Coarctation of the aorta in adolescents and adults: a review of clinical features and CT imaging. *J Cardiovasc Comput Tomogr.* 2016;10:1-12.

19 **Answer A.** The preferred method of repair in a neonate or infant is end-to-end anastomosis. This repair has decreased risk of re-coarctation and reintervention with improved outcomes.

Reference: Nance JW, Ringel RE, Fishman EK. Coarctation of the aorta in adolescents and adults: a review of clinical features and CT imaging. *J Cardiovasc Comput Tomogr.* 2016;10:1-12.

20 **Answer D.** A circumflex aortic arch is when the aorta passes to the left trachea but courses posteriorly to the trachea and esophagus when becoming the descending aorta. This is most often associated with an anomalous right subclavian artery, but a normal branching pattern can be seen.

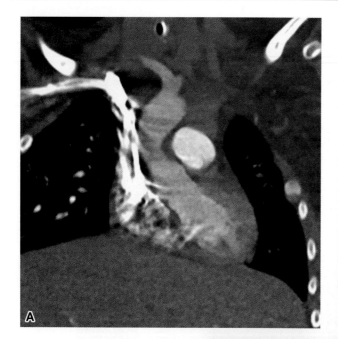

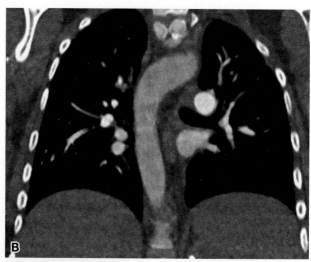

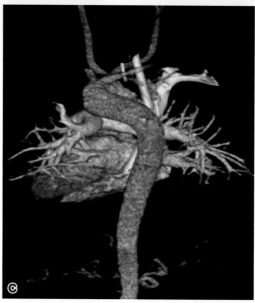

References: Smith BM, Lu JC, Dorfman AL, et al. Rings and slings revisited. *Magn Reson Imaging Clin N Am.* 2015;23:127-135.

Weinberg PM. Aortic arch anomalies. *J Cardiovasc Magn Reson.* 2006;8:633-643.

21 **Answer A.** A circumflex aortic arch always forms a vascular ring. The ring is completed by the right ductus or ligamentum connecting the descending aorta to the pulmonary artery. The ligamentum cannot be visualized on imaging.

References: Smith BM, Lu JC, Dorfman AL, et al. Rings and slings revisited. *Magn Reson Imaging Clin N Am.* 2015;23:127-135.

Weinberg PM. Aortic arch anomalies. *J Cardiovasc Magn Reson.* 2006;8:633-643.

22 **Answer C.** A double aortic arch, whether right dominant, codominant, or left dominant, is usually an isolated anomaly.

Arch Anomaly	Association with Congenital Heart Disease (CHD)
Right aortic arch with aberrant left subclavian artery	Usually isolated
Double aortic arch	Usually isolated
Right aortic arch with mirror image branching pattern	Associated with CHD such as tetralogy of Fallot, truncus arteriosus, and ventricular septal defect (VSD)
Circumflex aortic arch	Associated with CHD such as VSD, double outlet right ventricle, and coarctation

Reference: Smith BM, Lu JC, Dorfman AL, et al. Rings and slings revisited. *Magn Reson Imaging Clin N Am.* 2015;23:127-135.

23 **Answer C.** The image demonstrates aneurysms of the left anterior descending coronary artery (arrow). Given the aneurysms, the most likely diagnosis is Kawasaki disease. Kawasaki disease is a self-limiting vasculitis that occurs in infants and young children. It is characterized by an initial acute phase of up to 14 days and a convalescent phase that lasts months to years. Patients experience a high fever minimally responsive to antipyretics. Conjunctivitis occurs in 85% of children. Additional symptoms include diarrhea, abdominal pain, vomiting, scrotal swelling, and arthritis. Coronary artery aneurysms occur in 20% of untreated children, most of which occur during the convalescent phase.

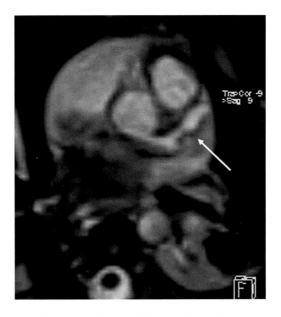

References: Pipitone N, Versari A, Hunder GG, et al. Role of imaging in the diagnosis of large and medium-sized vessel vasculitis. *Rheum Dis Clin North Am.* 2013;39:593-608.

Weiss PF. Pediatric vasculitis. *Pediatr Clin North Am.* 2012;59:407-423.

24 **Answer B.** Although patients with Kawasaki disease have unilateral cervical lymphadenopathy in 25% of cases, diffuse lymphadenopathy is unusual. Hydrops of the gallbladder along with diarrhea, vomiting, and abdominal pain can be seen. During the acute phase, patients may present with valvulitis, pericarditis, or myocarditis. Aneurysms are seen in the coronary arteries but additionally can be seen in visceral vessels such as the mesenteric and renal arteries.

References: Khanna G, Sargar K, Baszis KW. Pediatric vasculitis: recognizing multisystemic manifestations at body imaging. *Radiographics*. 2015;35:849-865.

Weiss PF. Pediatric vasculitis. *Pediatr Clin North Am*. 2012;59:407-423.

25 **Answer C.** Per the American Heart Association, patients with Kawasaki disease should be initially evaluated with echocardiography. This should be followed by reevaluation with echocardiography at 2 weeks and 6 to 8 weeks. Echocardiography has shown to have high sensitivity and specificity for evaluating coronary artery alterations.

Reference: Pipitone N, Versari A, Hunder GG, Salvarani C. Role of imaging in the diagnosis of large and medium-sized vessel vasculitis. *Rheum Dis Clin North Am*. 2013;39:593-608.

26 **Answer D.** The image demonstrates stenosis of the right renal artery (arrow) causing renovascular hypertension. Many patients with renal artery stenosis have comorbid conditions like vasculitis, neurofibromatosis, or syndromes such as Turner or Marfan. Additionally, pediatric patients may have fibromuscular dysplasia as noted in Question 4.

In coarctation of the aorta, there is hypertension within the upper extremities but low blood pressure within the lower extremities.

Pheochromocytomas can cause hypertension due to catecholamine excess, but there is no evidence of a mass in this patient.

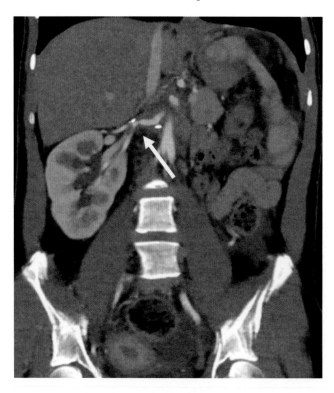

References: Siddiqui MA, Mittal PK, Little BP, et al. Secondary hypertension and complications: diagnosis and role of imaging. *Radiographics*. 2019;39(4):1036-1055.

Vo NJ, Hammelman BD, Racadio JM, Strife CF, Johnson ND, Racadio JM. Anatomic distribution of renal artery stenosis in children: implications for imaging. *Pediatr Radiol*. 2006;36(10):1032-1036.

27 **Answer C.** The image demonstrates absence of the infrarenal inferior vena cava (arrow). Absence of the infrarenal inferior vena cava is due to the failure of the development of the posterior cardinal and supracardinal veins. The suprarenal inferior vena cava is formed by the confluence of the renal veins. In this case the left renal vein is absent given that this patient has left renal agenesis.

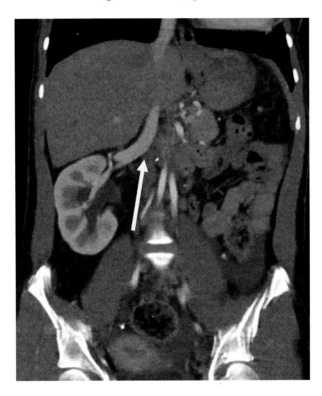

References: Bass JE, Redwine MD, Kramer LA, Huynh PT, Harris Jr JH. Spectrum of congenital anomalies of the inferior vena cava: cross-sectional imaging findings. *Radiographics*. 2000;20(3):639-652.

Li SJ, Lee J, Hall J, Sutherland TR. The inferior vena cava: anatomical variants and acquired pathologies. *Insights Imaging*. 2021;12(1):1-22.

28 **Answer A.** A double inferior vena cava develops due to the persistence of the right and left supracardinal veins. Embryology of additional inferior vena cava anomalies is noted in the table below.

Inferior Vena Cava (IVC) Anomaly	Embryology
Left IVC	Regression of the right supracardinal vein with persistence of the left supracardinal vein
Double IVC	Persistence of both the left and right supracardinal veins
Azygos continuation of the IVC	Failure to form the right subcardinal-hepatic anastomosis, with hypoplasia of the right subcardinal vein
Circumaortic left renal vein	Persistence of the dorsal limb of the embryonic left renal vein and renal collar
Retroaortic left renal vein	Persistence of the dorsal arch of the renal collar but regression of the ventral arch
Absent infrarenal IVC with preservation of the suprarenal segment	Failure of the development of the posterior cardinal and supracardinal veins

References: Bass JE, Redwine MD, Kramer LA, Huynh PT, Harris Jr JH. Spectrum of congenital anomalies of the inferior vena cava: cross-sectional imaging findings. *Radiographics*. 2000;20(3):639-652.

Eldefrawy A, Arianayagam M, Kanagarajah P, Acosta K, Manoharan M. Anomalies of the inferior vena cava and renal veins and implications for renal surgery. *Cent European J Urol*. 2011;64(1):4.

1 Which of the following is a characteristic that distinguishes the right ventricle (RV) from the left ventricle?

A. The RV has an intermediary papillary muscle.
B. The RV has a moderator band.
C. The RV has fibrous continuity of the AV valve and outflow tract.
D. The RV does not have a well-developed infundibulum.

2 A 3-year-old patient with a history of congenital heart disease status post repair presents for a cardiac MRI.

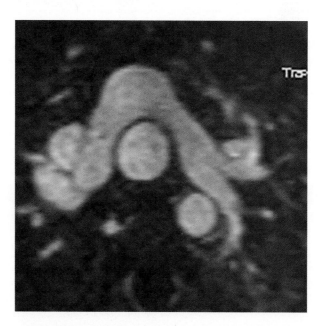

What is this patient's underlying diagnosis?

A. Tetralogy of Fallot
B. Hypoplastic left heart syndrome
C. Total anomalous pulmonary venous return
D. D-transposition of the great arteries

3 Regarding the diagnosis in Question 2, which is *true*?

A. There is ventriculoarterial discordance and atrioventricular discordance.
B. There is ventriculoarterial discordance and atrioventricular concordance.
C. There is ventriculoarterial concordance and atrioventricular discordance.
D. There is ventriculoarterial concordance and atrioventricular concordance.

4 The most common postoperative complication following surgical correction of the diagnosis in Question 1 is:

A. Coronary artery occlusion
B. Pulmonary vein stenosis
C. Mitral insufficiency
D. Aortic stenosis

5 A newborn presents with the following frontal radiograph of the chest.

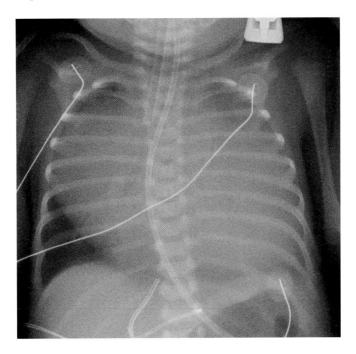

What is the most likely diagnosis?

A. Atrial septal defect
B. Ebstein anomaly
C. Tetralogy of Fallot
D. Total anomalous pulmonary venous return

6 In regard to the diagnosis in Question 5, the pulmonary vascularity is:

A. Increased
B. Normal
C. Decreased

7 The following is a surgical treatment for correction of the disorder in Question 5:

A. Tricuspid valvuloplasty
B. Jatene arterial switch
C. Left subclavian flap repair
D. Unroofing of the coronary artery

8 A 4-year-old patient presents with the following radiograph of the chest.

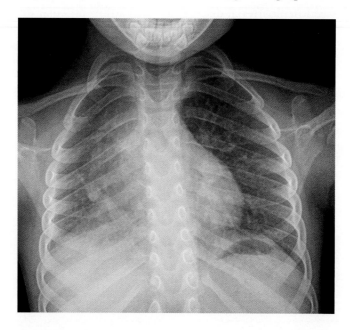

What is the diagnosis?

A. Partial anomalous pulmonary venous return
B. Tetralogy of Fallot with aortopulmonary collateral
C. Ventricular septal defect
D. Atrial septal defect

9 Which of the following is an anomaly commonly associated with the disorder in Question 8?

A. Pleuropulmonary blastoma
B. Horseshoe lung
C. Congenital absence of the pericardium
D. Cor triatriatum

10 In a pediatric patient, what is the next step in imaging the disorder in Question 8?

A. CT angiogram
B. MR angiogram
C. Echocardiogram
D. Cardiac catheterization

11 Balanced gradient echo (A), first-pass perfusion (B), and delayed enhancement (C) imaging were performed on a 7-year-old patient with a history of a cardiac mass.

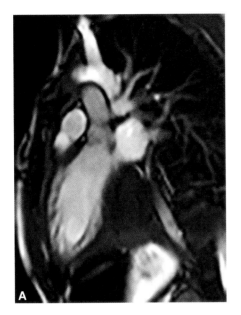
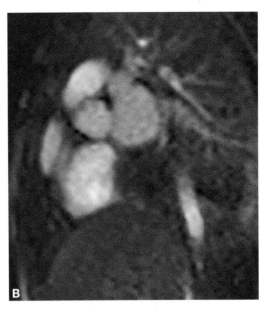

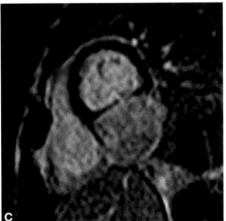

What is the most likely diagnosis?

A. Rhabdomyoma
B. Myxoma
C. Fibroma
D. Lipoma
E. Teratoma

12 What is a typical imaging characteristic of the tumor in Question 11?

A. Strong first-pass perfusion
B. Typical location within the pericardium
C. Hyperenhancement on myocardial delayed enhancement
D. Hypoechoic appearance on echocardiography

13 Which of the following concerning a cardiac fibroma is *true*?

A. It may remain stable for years or regress.
B. Asymptomatic patients are most often treated with chemotherapy.
C. Recurrence following surgery is common.
D. Arrhythmias are uncommon.

14 An MR angiogram of a 10-year-old male with chest pain was performed.

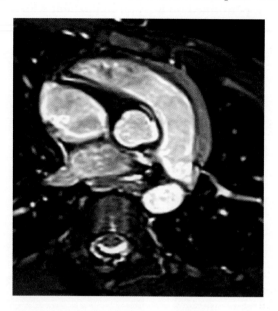

What is the diagnosis?

A. Anomalous left coronary artery from the right coronary cusp
B. Anomalous right coronary artery from the left coronary cusp
C. Anomalous left coronary artery from the pulmonary artery
D. Anomalous right coronary artery from the pulmonary artery
E. Normal coronary anatomy

15 Which imaging modality is commonly used for confirmation of the abnormality in Question 14?

A. Echocardiography
B. Ventilation/perfusion scan
C. ECG-gated CT angiography
D. T1 mapping with myocardial delayed enhancement

16 What defines a high origin of a coronary artery?

A. 1 cm above the aortic annulus
B. 2 cm above the aortic annulus
C. 1 cm above the sinus of Valsalva
D. 2 cm above the sinus of Valsalva
E. 1 cm above the sinotubular junction
F. 2 cm above the sinotubular junction

17 Which of the following is a potentially hemodynamically significant coronary artery anomaly?

A. Duplication of the left or right coronary artery
B. High origin of the coronary artery
C. Interarterial course of a coronary artery
D. Prepulmonic course of a coronary artery
E. Transseptal course of a coronary artery
F. Retroaortic course of a coronary artery

18 A cardiac MRI was performed on a 3-year-old patient with congenital heart disease.

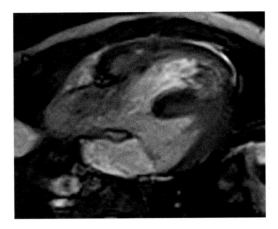

What is the diagnosis?

A. Transposition of the great arteries
B. Total anomalous pulmonary venous return
C. Cor triatriatum
D. Tetralogy of Fallot
E. Hypoplastic left heart syndrome

19 Which of the following is *not* a characteristic of the disorder in Question 18?

A. Overriding aorta
B. Ventricular septal defect
C. Right ventricular hypertrophy
D. Anomalous pulmonary venous return
E. Main and/or branch pulmonary artery obstruction
F. Pulmonary valve atresia

20 The most common coronary anomaly associated with the diagnosis in Question 18 is the following:

A. Right coronary artery from the left anterior descending artery
B. Right coronary artery from the left circumflex artery
C. Right coronary artery from the left main coronary artery
D. Left coronary artery from the right coronary artery

21 Which of the following is *not* a postoperative complication of the disorder in Question 18?

A. Left ventricular dysfunction
B. Right ventricular dysfunction
C. Residual ventricular septal defect
D. Aortic insufficiency
E. Pulmonic insufficiency

22 A 2-day-old patient presents with respiratory distress. Initial chest radiograph was performed.

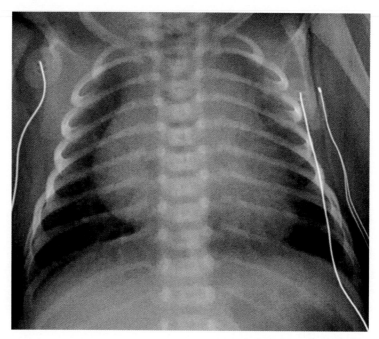

Which of the following is *not* a potential diagnosis for this patient?

A. Truncus arteriosus
B. Tetralogy of Fallot
C. Transposition of the great arteries
D. Hypoplastic left heart syndrome

23 A cardiac MRI was performed. Below is a four-chamber balanced gradient echo image (A) and a sagittal image from an MRA (B).

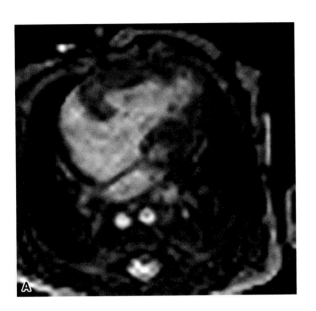
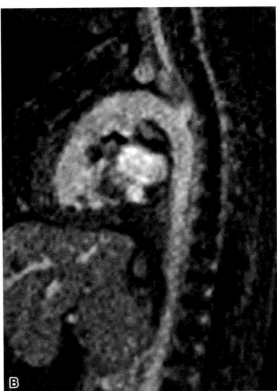

What is the diagnosis?

A. Truncus arteriosus
B. Tetralogy of Fallot
C. Transposition of the great arteries
D. Hypoplastic left heart syndrome

24 In a neonate with the disorder in Question 23, how are the coronary arteries perfused prior to surgical intervention?

A. Left to right flow through the ductus arteriosus during ventricular systole
B. Left to right flow through the ductus arteriosus during ventricular diastole
C. Right to left flow through the ductus arteriosus during ventricular systole
D. Right to left flow through the ductus arteriosus during ventricular diastole

25 Which of the following is *true* in regard to the Norwood procedure for surgical correction of hypoplastic left heart syndrome?

A. Stage 1 of the Norwood procedure is typically the creation of a bidirectional Glenn shunt.
B. Stage 1 of the Norwood procedure is typically performed at 1 month of life.
C. Stage 2 of the Norwood procedure is typically the creation of a Blalock-Taussig shunt.
D. Stage 2 of the Norwood procedure is typically performed at 2 months of life.
E. Stage 3 of the Norwood procedure is typically the creation of a Fontan.
F. Stage 3 of the Norwood procedure is typically performed at 6 months of life.

26 A cardiac examination was performed on a child but was complicated by motion artifact. Which of the following is a technique that can be used to reduce motion artifact when imaging this child?

A. Radial k-space filling
B. Changing the field of view
C. Decreasing the pixel size
D. Gradient moment nulling

27 A teenager with a dilated ascending aorta presents for cardiac MRI. The following images were obtained in the plane of the aortic valve and of the left ventricular tract.

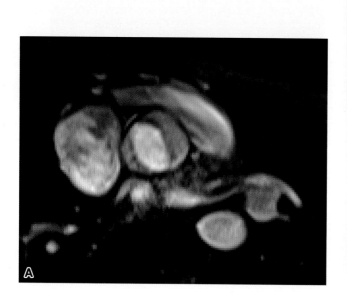
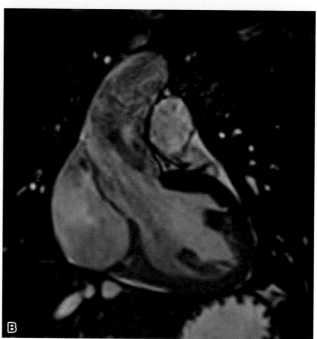

What is the cause of this patient's dilated ascending aorta?

A. Aortic coarctation
B. Ehlers-Danlos syndrome
C. Bicuspid aortic valve
D. Hypertrophic cardiomyopathy

28 Which of the following is a complication of the diagnosis in Question 27?

A. Aortic insufficiency
B. Aortic stenosis
C. Aortic dissection
D. Endocarditis
E. All of the above

ANSWERS AND EXPLANATIONS

1 **Answer B.** The distinguishing features of the morphological right ventricle (RV) are a moderator band, which is a muscular band that extends from the interventricular septum to the base of the anterior papillary muscle. Additionally, the RV has a well-developed infundibulum, septal papillary muscles, and lack of fibrous continuity of the atrioventricular valve and outflow tract.

Reference: Hecht MD, Kim DC, Jacobs JE. Anatomy of the heart at multidetector CT: what the radiologist needs to know. *Radiographics.* 2007;27(6):1569-1582.

2 **Answer D.** The patient is status post arterial switch operation (ASO) and a LeCompte maneuver for transposition of the great arteries (TGA). In this surgery, the coronaries are excised from the aorta and the ascending aorta, and the main pulmonary artery is switched. The LeCompte maneuver involves placing the ascending aorta (asterisk) posterior to the bifurcation of the main pulmonary artery. This maneuver reduces the risk of compression or kinking of the coronary arteries.

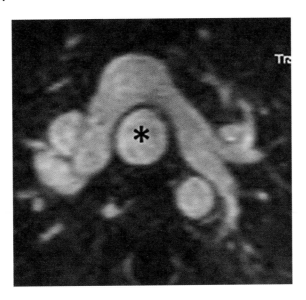

Reference: Gaca AM, Jaggers JJ, Dudley LT, et al. Repair of congenital heart disease: a primer—part 1. *Radiology.* 2008;247:617-631.

3 **Answer B.** In dextro-TGA, there is ventriculoarterial discordance but atrioventricular concordance. The aorta arises from the morphological RV, and the main pulmonary artery arises from the morphological left ventricle. The left atrium enters the left ventricle, and the right atrium enters the RV consistent with atrioventricular concordance. In congenitally corrected or L-TGA, there is atrioventricular and ventriculoarterial discordance.

References: Gaca AM, Jaggers JJ, Dudley LT, et al. Repair of congenital heart disease: a primer—part 1. *Radiology.* 2008;247:617-631.

Warnes CA. Transposition of the great arteries. *Circulation.* 2006;114:2699-2709.

4 **Answer A.** An obstructed coronary artery leading to myocardial ischemia is the most common cause of morbidity and mortality following an ASO for D-TGA. This risk is most common in the initial 3 months following ASO. Additionally, neoaortic root dilatation occurs in nearly all patients post-ASO, and neoaortic valve regurgitation occurs in most patients post-ASO. Less common long-term sequelae are supravalvular pulmonary stenosis and aortic stenosis.

Reference: Villafane J, Lantin-Hermoso MR, Bhatt AB, et al. D-transposition of the great arteries. *J Am Coll Cardiol.* 2014;64:498-511.

5 **Answer B.** The characteristic appearance of Ebstein anomaly on a chest radiograph is marked cardiomegaly with decreased pulmonary vascularity. Although tetralogy of Fallot (TOF) may also present with decreased vascularity on radiograph, it does not typically present with marked cardiomegaly.

In Ebstein anomaly, there is displacement of the septal and posterior leaflets (arrows) of the tricuspid valve into the RV forming an atrialized portion of the RV.

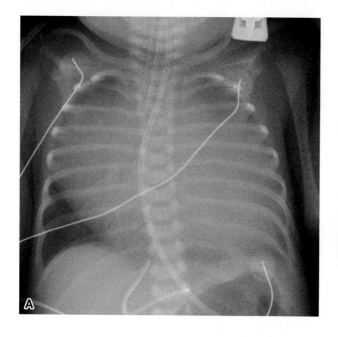 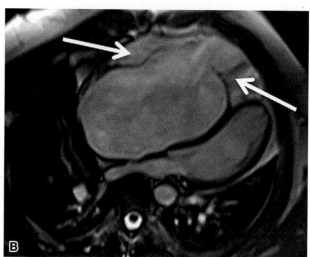

Reference: Epstein ML. Tricuspid atresia, stenosis, and regurgitation. In: Moss AJ, Allen HD, eds. *Moss and Adams' Heart Disease in Infants, Children, and Adolescents: Including the Fetus and Young Adult.* 7th ed. Wolters Kluwer Health/Lippincott Williams & Wilkins; 2008:817-834.

6 **Answer C.** Although the degree of abnormality varies in patients with Ebstein anomaly, the pulmonary vascularity would be typically decreased. During ventricular systole, much of the cardiac output is sent retrograde into the true right atrium rather than antegrade into the true RV and main pulmonary artery.

Reference: Epstein ML. Tricuspid atresia, stenosis, and regurgitation. In: Moss AJ, Allen HD, eds. *Moss and Adams' Heart Disease in Infants, Children, and Adolescents: Including the Fetus and Young Adult.* 7th ed. Wolters Kluwer Health/Lippincott Williams & Wilkins; 2008:817-834.

7 **Answer A.** Management of Ebstein anomaly can be variable depending on the severity of the disease. Biventricular repair involving tricuspid valvuloplasty such as cone reconstruction may be performed. Tricuspid valve replacement is another surgical procedure used in Ebstein anomaly repair. Single ventricle repair involving a bidirectional cavopulmonary anastomosis (Glenn) and/or a total cavopulmonary anastomosis (Fontan) may be needed for a poorly functioning RV.

References: Gaca AM, Jaggers JJ, Dudley T, et al. Repair of congenital heart disease: a primer—part 1. *Radiology*. 2008;247:617-631.

Jinghao Z, Kai L, Yanhui H, et al. Individualized surgical treatments for children with Ebstein anomaly. *Thorac Cardiovasc Surg*. 2017;65(08):649-655.

8 **Answer A.** On the chest radiograph, there is a prominent vessel within the right hemithorax (arrow in Figure A) consistent with an anomalous pulmonary vein draining to the inferior vena cava. This finding is consistent with a right lower lobe anomalous pulmonary venous connection. The pulmonary veins normally drain into the left atrium. In partial anomalous pulmonary venous return (PAPVR), some of the veins drain anomalously into the systemic venous system rather than to the left atrium (arrow in Figure B).

In this case, the right lung is also decreased in size in comparison to the left with elevation of the right hemidiaphragm. This finding in addition to the PAPVR is consistent with hypogenetic lung syndrome or scimitar syndrome. In this syndrome, the right lung partially drains to the inferior vena cava with a variable degree of lung hypoplasia. The right pulmonary artery may be hypoplastic or aplastic.

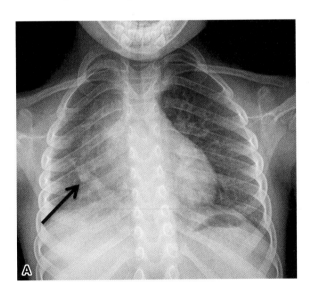 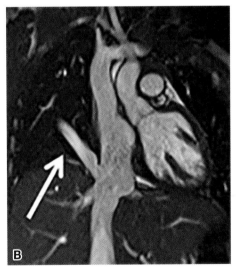

Reference: Konen E, Raviv-Zilka L, Cohen RA, et al. Congenital pulmonary venolobar syndrome: spectrum of helical CT findings with emphasis on computerized reformatting. *Radiographics*. 2003;23:1175-1184.

9 **Answer B.** This patient presents with not only PAPVR but also hypogenetic lung syndrome or scimitar syndrome. Patients with scimitar have associated anomalies including congenital heart disease, particularly sinus venosus atrial septal defects (ASD), bronchogenic cysts, accessory diaphragms, and hernias. Scimitar syndrome is also associated with horseshoe lung where an isthmus of the right lung base extends posteriorly joining the posterobasal segments of the right and left lung.

Reference: Konen E, Raviv-Zilka L, Cohen RA, et al. Congenital pulmonary venolobar syndrome: spectrum of helical CT findings with emphasis on computerized reformatting. *Radiographics*. 2003;23:1175-1184.

10 **Answer C.** A chest radiograph is the initial screening modality used to evaluate patients with suspected PAPVR. Given that it is noninvasive, echocardiogram is the next imaging modality in evaluating pediatric patients with this disorder. If additional imaging is desired, cross-sectional imaging such as MRI/MR angiography (MRA) and CT/CT angiography (CTA) can be performed. MRI is usually preferred given the lack of ionizing radiation and the ability to characterize pulmonary and systemic flow. CT would be preferred if evaluation of the lung parenchyma is desired. Cardiac catheterization is performed for endovascular procedures or if additional hemodynamic data are needed.

Reference: Sung LY, Ting C, Varghese C, Hellinger JC. Scimitar syndrome. In: Reid JR, Paladin A, Davros WJ, et al, eds. *Pediatric Radiology*. Oxford University Press; 2013:105-109.

11 **Answer C.** The most likely diagnosis is a cardiac fibroma. Fibromas are low in signal on balanced gradient echo imaging (arrow), do not demonstrate first-pass perfusion (+), and do demonstrate myocardial delayed enhancement (asterisk). Rhabdomyoma could be considered, but rhabdomyomas do not demonstrate myocardial delayed enhancement.

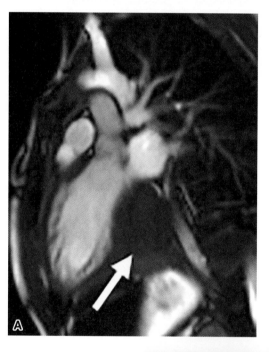
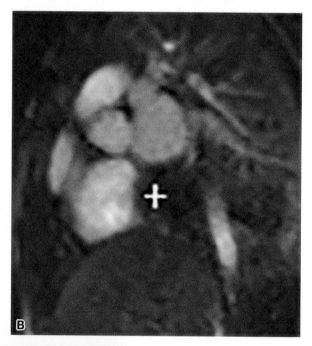
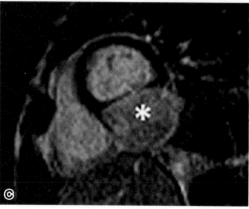

The table below describes characteristics of select pediatric cardiac masses (from Beroukhim et al. 2011).

Tumor	Location	T1	T2	First-Pass Perfusion	Myocardial Delayed Enhancement
Fibroma	Intramyocardial, ventricular septum, or free wall	Variable	Variable	No	Positive
Rhabdomyoma	Intramyocardial or intracavitary	Variable	Bright	No	Negative
Myxoma	Left atrium typically	Variable	Bright	No	Variable
Hemangioma	Variable	Dark	Bright	Strong	Variable but if positive homogenous
Malignant	Variable but infiltrative	Variable	Variable	Variable	Variable but if positive heterogeneous

Reference: Beroukhim RS, Prakash A, Buechel ERV, et al. Characterization of cardiac tumors in children by cardiovascular magnetic resonance imaging. *J Am Coll Cardiol*. 2011;58:1044-1054.

12 **Answer C.** Cardiac fibromas demonstrate strong delayed hyperenhancement on myocardial delayed imaging. They are most often heterogeneous on T1- and T2-weighted imaging. They do not demonstrate first-pass perfusion. The lesions are most often echogenic on echocardiography. Their location is usually intramyocardial involving either the ventricular septum or ventricular free wall.

References: Beroukhim RS, Prakash A, Buechel ERV, et al. Characterization of cardiac tumors in children by cardiovascular magnetic resonance imaging. *J Am Coll Cardiol*. 2011;58:1044-1054.

Grebenc ML, Rosado de Christenson M, Burke AP, et al. Primary cardiac and pericardial neoplasms: radiologic-pathologic correlation. *Radiographics*. 2000;20:1073-1103.

13 **Answer A.** Cardiac fibromas may be stable for years or even regress. Although one-third of patients may be asymptomatic, presenting symptoms may include arrhythmias, heart failure, or sudden death. If patients are symptomatic, these tumors are resected. Patients may even benefit from partial resection of more extensive tumors. Postsurgical recurrence is rare.

Reference: Grebenc ML, Rosado de Christenson M, Burke AP, et al. Primary cardiac and pericardial neoplasms: radiologic-pathologic correlation. *Radiographics*. 2000;20:1073-1103.

14 **Answer B.** The images demonstrate the right coronary artery (arrow) originating for the left coronary cusp consistent with an anomalous right coronary artery. The right coronary artery takes a tangential course to the aortic root and an interarterial course between the right ventricular outflow tract on the aorta.

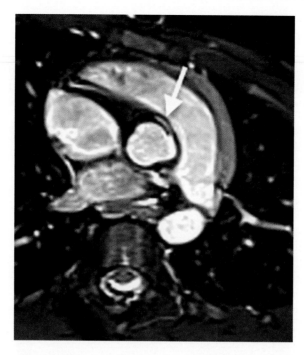

Reference: Shriki JE, Shinbane JS, Rashid MA, et al. Identifying, characterizing, and classifying congenital anomalies of the coronary arteries. *Radiographics*. 2012;32:453-468.

15 **Answer C.** Although history and physical examination are initially used to screen patients for coronary artery anomalies, imaging modalities are needed for detection. Cross-sectional imaging, such as MRA and CTA, are modalities often used to directly visualize the origin of the coronary arteries. Echocardiography can also be used, but this modality is less precise than cross-sectional imaging.

Reference: Angelini P. Novel imaging of coronary artery anomalies to assess their prevalence, the causes of clinical symptoms, and the risk of sudden cardiac death. *Circ Cardiovasc Imaging*. 2014;7:747-754.

16 **Answer E.** A high origin of a coronary artery is defined as greater than or equal to 1 cm above the sinotubular junction of the ascending aorta. This anomaly is not hemodynamically significant but can have significance in patients undergoing aortic valve surgery. Additionally, there is a reported increased incidence of high origin of the right coronary artery in patients with bicuspid aortic valves.

Reference: Shriki JE, Shinbane JS, Rashid MA, et al. Identifying, characterizing, and classifying congenital anomalies of the coronary arteries. *Radiographics*. 2012;32:453-468.

17 **Answer C.** Potentially hemodynamically significant coronary anomalies include the interarterial course of the coronary artery, origin of the coronary artery from the pulmonary artery, and coronary artery fistulas. In an interarterial course, the anomalous coronary artery, either the left coronary from the right cusp or the right coronary from the left cusp, takes a course between the pulmonary artery and the aorta. The interarterial course is more associated with sudden cardiac death. Other features that may increase the risk of sudden cardiac death are a slit-like orifice, acute angle between the anomalous coronary artery and the aorta, and an intramural aortic segment.

References: Biko DM, Chung C, Hitt SM, et al. High-resolution coronary MR angiography for evaluation of patients with anomalous coronary arteries: visualization of the intramural segment. *Pediatr Radiol*. 2015;45:1146-1152.

Shriki JE, Shinbane JS, Rashid MA, et al. Identifying, characterizing, and classifying congenital anomalies of the coronary arteries. *Radiographics*. 2012;32:453-468.

18 **Answer D.** The findings are consistent with tetralogy of fallot (TOF). In the provided image, there is right ventricular hypertrophy (arrow), an overriding aorta (+), and a ventricular septal defect (VSD, asterisk). TOF is the most common cyanotic congenital heart disease. Classically, TOF consists of (1) obstruction of the right ventricular outflow tract, (2) VSD, (3) overriding aorta, and (4) right ventricular hypertrophy.

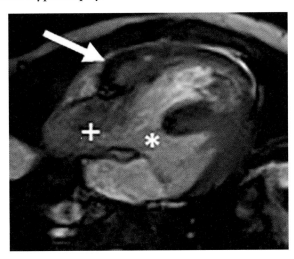

References: Lapierre C, Dubois J, Rypens F, et al. Tetralogy of Fallot: preoperative assessment with MR and CT imaging. *Diagn Interv Imaging*. 2016;97:531-541.

Norton KI, Tong C, Glass RB, Nielsen JC. Cardiac MR imaging assessment following tetralogy of Fallot repair. *Radiographics*. 2006;26:197-211.

19 **Answer D.** As noted in the explanation for Question 17, tetralogy of fallot (TOF) consists of (1) obstruction of the right ventricular outflow tract, (2) VSD, (3) overriding aorta, and (4) right ventricular hypertrophy. The degree of obstruction in TOF is variable, ranging from mild obstruction of the right ventricular outflow tract to main or branch pulmonary artery obstruction, to pulmonary atresia. TOF with pulmonary atresia is the most severe form of this disease.

References: Lapierre C, Dubois J, Rypens F, et al. Tetralogy of Fallot: preoperative assessment with MR and CT imaging. *Diagn Interv Imaging*. 2016;97:531-541.

Norton KI, Tong C, Glass RB, Nielsen JC. Cardiac MR imaging assessment following tetralogy of Fallot repair. *Radiographics*. 2006;26:197-211.

20 **Answer A.** Coronary artery anomalies are present in tetralogy of fallot (TOF) in approximately 5% of cases, with the most common anomaly being the right coronary artery arising from the left anterior descending artery (LAD). This finding is important to report as it may change the surgical approach to this disorder. Additionally, a right aortic arch is seen in 25% of patients, an atrial septal defect (ASD) is seen in 5% of patients, and a left superior vena cava is seen in 11% of patients.

Reference: Lapierre C, Dubois J, Rypens F, et al. Tetralogy of Fallot: preoperative assessment with MR and CT imaging. *Diagn Interv Imaging*. 2016;97:531-541.

21 **Answer D.** Surgical repair in tetralogy of fallot (TOF) involves removing the right ventricular obstruction. This most often involves placement of a transannular patch or conduit in addition to closure of the ventricular septal defect (VSD) and infundibular muscle resection. Postoperative complications of surgical intervention in these patients include residual VSD, pulmonic insufficiency and subsequent right ventricular enlargement and dysfunction, residual pulmonic stenosis, tricuspid insufficiency, right ventricular outflow tract aneurysm, conduit obstruction, and left ventricular dysfunction.

Reference: Norton KI, Tong C, Glass RB, Nielsen JC. Cardiac MR imaging assessment following tetralogy of Fallot repair. *Radiographics*. 2006;26:197-211.

22 **Answer B.** The pulmonary vascularity is increased on the presented radiograph. Truncus arteriosus, transposition of the great arteries (TGA), and hypoplastic left heart syndrome (HLHS) all may present with increased pulmonary vascularity. Given the right ventricular outflow tract obstruction, tetralogy of fallot (TOF) and Ebstein anomaly usually present with decreased or normal vascularity on chest radiograph.

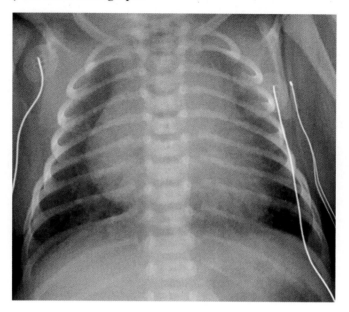

Reference: Ferguson EC, Krishnamurthy R, Oldham SA. Classic imaging signs of congenital cardiovascular abnormalities. *Radiographics*. 2007;27:1323-1334.

23 **Answer D.** Hypoplastic left heart syndrome (HLHS) is a spectrum that involves hypoplasia or absence of the left ventricle with hypoplasia of the ascending aorta. In this case, the left ventricle is severely hypoplastic (arrow) with flow to the aorta supported via the right ventricle consistent with this syndrome. There may be mitral and/or aortic valve stenosis or atresia. The neonate born with this disorder is dependent on the ductus arteriosus for maintenance of systemic perfusion.

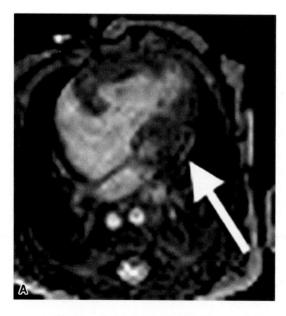
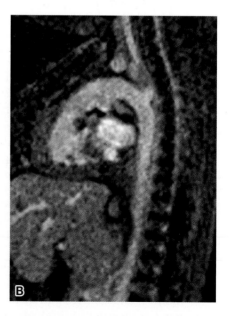

References: Bardo DM, Frankel DG, Applegate KE, et al. Hypoplastic left heart syndrome. *Radiographics*. 2001;21:705-717.

Greenleaf CE, Urencio JM, Salazar JD, et al. Hypoplastic left heart syndrome: current perspectives. *Transl Pediatr*. 2016;5:142-147.

24 **Answer D.** In hypoplastic left heart syndrome (HLHS), the ductus arteriosus must be maintained for systemic perfusion. At birth, the blood flow is right to left across the ductus arteriosus during ventricular systole, which perfuses the systemic circulation. In ventricular diastole, the flow across the ductus arteriosus is left to right. Blood flow is also retrograde into the ascending aorta during ventricular diastole, which perfuses the coronary arteries.

Reference: Bardo DM, Frankel DG, Applegate KE, et al. Hypoplastic left heart syndrome. *Radiographics*. 2001;21:705-717.

25 **Answer E.** The Norwood procedure is a three-stage surgical procedure performed in patients with single ventricle physiology such as hypoplastic left heart syndrome (HLHS). In this staged procedure, the right ventricle becomes the systemic pump. It is designed to protect the pulmonary vascular bed and transition an infant to definitive repair. See the table below.

	Intervention	Typical Age of Surgery
Stage 1	Divide pulmonary artery and create neoaorta. Create Blalock-Taussig shunt (shunt between subclavian artery and ipsilateral pulmonary artery).	First few days of life
Stage 2	Remove Blalock-Taussig shunt. Create bidirectional Glenn shunt (superior vena cava to pulmonary artery anastomosis).	3-6 months
Stage 3	Fontan (inferior vena cava to pulmonary artery anastomosis) Bidirectional Glenn shunt remains.	18 months-4 years

References: Bardo DM, Frankel DG, Applegate KE, et al. Hypoplastic left heart syndrome. *Radiographics*. 2001;21:705-717.

Gaca AM, Jaggers JJ, Dudley LT, Bissett GS. Repair of congenital heart disease: a primer-part 1. *Radiology*. 2008;247:617-631.

26 **Answer A.** There are several techniques to correct ghosting or smearing of an MRI from either voluntary or involuntary patient motion. The use of radial k-space filling as opposed to rectilinear k-space filling is one of these techniques. Using this technique, data are acquired in radial sections, which vary the phase-encoding direction. This disperses the patient motion over radial sections rather than rectilinear sections, which improves image quality. The table below summarizes a few techniques to correct several common MR artifacts caused by motion.

Type of Artifact	MR Techniques for Correction	Explanation
Ghosting and smearing	Radial k-space filling	Data are acquired in radial sections varying the phase-encoding direction and dispersing the patient motion over radial sections
	Cardiac gating	k-space lines acquired during a certain phase of each heart beat
	Respiratory gating	k-space lines acquired during a certain phase of respiration
Pulsatile flow artifact	Gradient moment nulling	Application of gradient pulses to eliminate phase shifts produced by the moving protons
	Saturation pulse	Radiofrequency pulse applied perpendicular or parallel to the imaging plane to eliminate ghosting from moving structures

Reference: Morelli JN, Runge VM, Ai F, et al. An image-based approach to understanding the physics of MR artifacts. *Radiographics*. 2011;31:849-866.

27 **Answer C.** The image demonstrates an elliptical (fish mouth) appearance of the aortic valve consistent with a bicuspid aortic valve (arrow). Bicuspid aortic valve is the most common congenital heart defect, with a prevalence up to 2%. It is typically made of two unequal-sized leaflets, with the larger leaflet having a central raphe that results from fusion of the commissures. The most common pattern of bicuspid aortic valve is fusion of the right and left cusps.

Ehlers-Danlos syndrome (EDS) is a connective tissue disorder that manifests as hypermobility, elastic or doughy skin, and soft tissue or vascular fragility. Ascending aortic dilatation is common in EDS but in this case a bicuspid aortic valve is present.

In hypertrophic cardiomyopathy, there may be dilatation of the ascending aorta due to left ventricular outflow tract obstruction but that is not demonstrated in this case. Aortic coarctation is not a cause of ascending aortic dilatation unless another anatomic disorder is present.

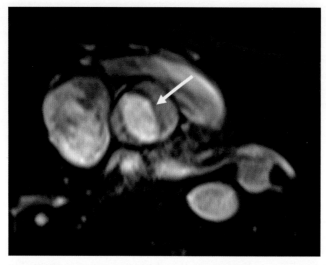

References: Siu SC, Silversides CK. Bicuspid aortic valve disease. *J Am Coll Cardiol.* 2010;55(25):2789-2800.

Ko SM, Song MG, Hwang HK. Bicuspid aortic valve: spectrum of imaging findings at cardiac MDCT and cardiovascular MRI. *AJR Am J Roentgenol.* 2012;198(1):89-97.

28 **Answer E.** Bicuspid aortic valve may be complicated by both aortic insufficiency and aortic stenosis. Aortic stenosis in adults is due to calcification but this is not seen in children. Aortic dilatation is commonly seen with dissections occurring in both the ascending aorta and descending aorta. The prevalence of endocarditis is higher in bicuspid aortic valves than in tricuspid valves, but this complication is low.

References: Siu SC, Silversides CK. Bicuspid aortic valve disease. *J Am Coll Cardiol.* 2010;55(25):2789-2800.

Ko SM, Song MG, Hwang HK. Bicuspid aortic valve: spectrum of imaging findings at cardiac MDCT and cardiovascular MRI. *AJR Am J Roentgenol.* 2012;198(1):89-97.

1 An 11-year-old female presents with chronic visual disturbance. What neurocutaneous syndrome is manifested with these findings?

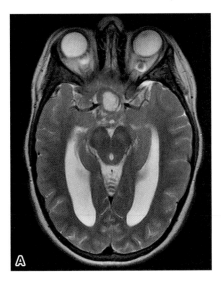
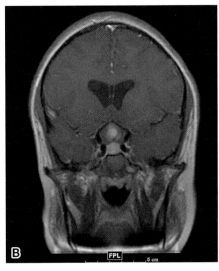
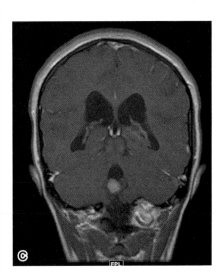

A. Neurofibromatosis type 1
B. Neurofibromatosis type 2
C. Sturge-Weber syndrome
D. Metachromatic leukodystrophy

2 What cutaneous finding is associated with the syndrome affecting the patient in Question 1?

A. Port-wine stain
B. Café au lait spot
C. Facial angiofibroma
D. Vitiligo

3   A 13-year-old female presents with a history of left functional hemispherectomy to alleviate refractory epilepsy. Which syndrome is the likely cause of her seizure disorder?

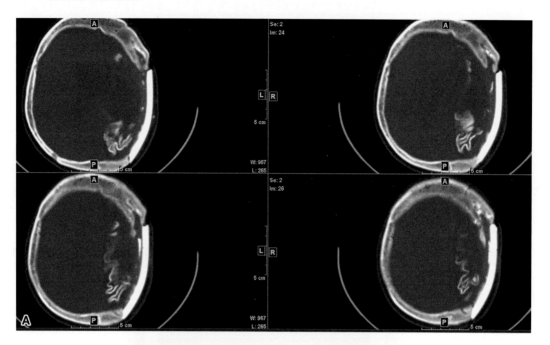

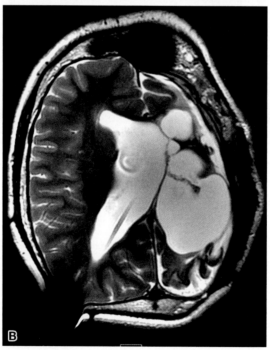

A. Neurofibromatosis type 1

B. Neurofibromatosis type 2

C. Sturge-Weber syndrome

D. Tuberous sclerosis

4   What cutaneous finding is associated with the syndrome affecting the patient in Question 3?

A. Port-wine stain

B. Café au lait spot

C. Facial angiofibroma

D. Vitiligo

5 A newborn presents for a postnatal abdominal radiograph with a history of an abnormal prenatal ultrasound. Which of the following antenatal findings is most associated with this postnatal radiographic finding?

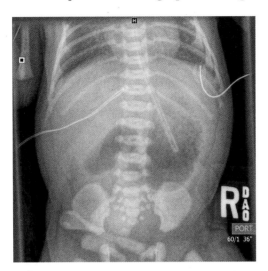

A. Rocker bottom foot
B. Microcephaly
C. Polydactyly
D. Cerebral ventriculomegaly

6 What is the most likely diagnosis for the patient described in Question 5?
A. Trisomy 13
B. Trisomy 18
C. Trisomy 21
D. Trisomy 23

7 A 21-day-old female presents after an abnormal ophthalmic examination. What syndrome is associated with the imaging findings?

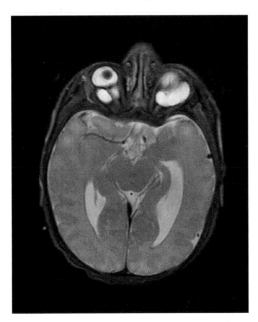

A. Chiari II malformation
B. CHARGE syndrome
C. Tuberous sclerosis
D. Sturge-Weber syndrome

8 A 10-year-old male presents with tall stature and a history of spontaneous pneumothorax. What syndrome does this patient likely have?

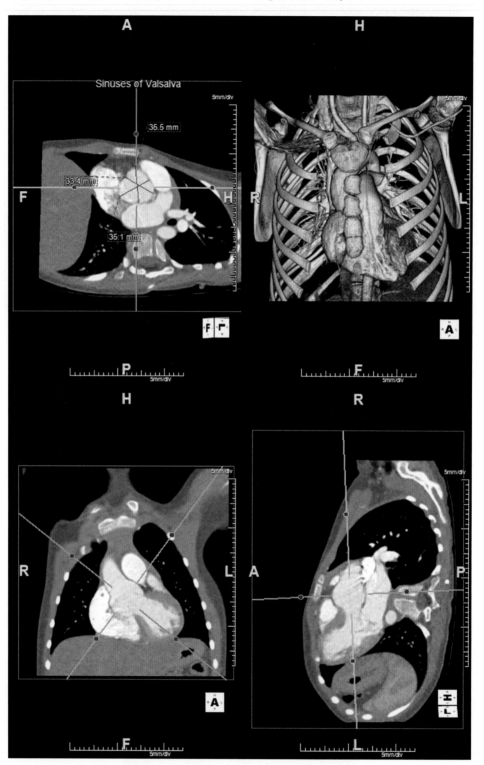

A. Down syndrome

B. Marfan syndrome

C. McCune-Albright syndrome

D. Birt-Hogg-Dubé syndrome

9 What measurement threshold (in millimeters) is used to determine whether intervention is required to correct a dilated or aneurysmal aortic root in the syndrome demonstrated in Question 8?

A. 25
B. 35
C. 45
D. 55

10 A 4-month-old female presents for imaging surveillance. Which of the following syndromes corresponds to this patient's imaging findings?

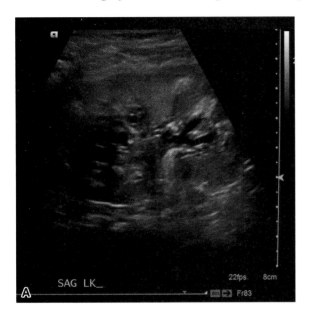
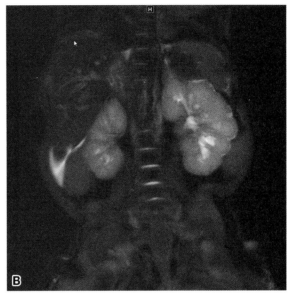

A. von Hippel-Lindau syndrome
B. Neurofibromatosis type 1
C. Neurofibromatosis type 2
D. Beckwith-Wiedemann syndrome

11 Which of the following syndromes are included in the *WT1*-related Wilms tumor (WT) syndromes?

A. Neurofibromatosis type 2
B. von Hippel-Lindau syndrome
C. Denys-Drash syndrome
D. Down syndrome

12 A 26-year-old female presents with a 33-week-old fetus with a neck mass identified on US and MR. Which syndrome is most commonly associated with this fetal neck mass?

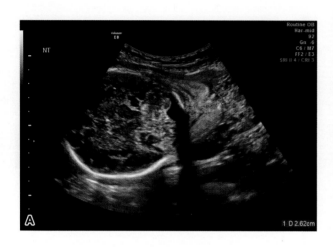

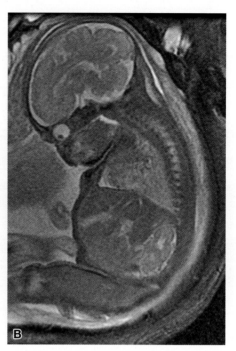

A. Klinefelter syndrome
B. Turner syndrome
C. Patau syndrome
D. Edwards syndrome

13 What is the most appropriate time frame (gestational age in weeks) during pregnancy to perform a nuchal translucency scan to screen for aneuploidy?

A. 8 to 10
B. 11 to 13
C. 14 to 16
D. 17 to 19

14 A 17-year-old female presents with recurrent joint dislocations. Radiographs of her shoulders are shown below. Which of the following syndromes or diseases is most commonly associated with joint laxity and recurrent joint dislocations?

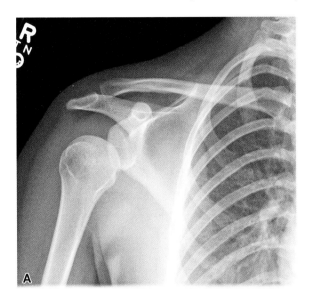

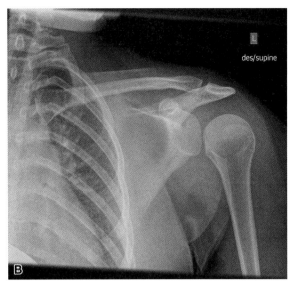

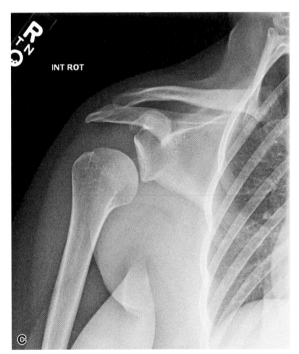

A. Trisomy 21
B. Osteogenesis imperfecta
C. Ehlers-Danlos syndrome
D. Gaucher disease

15 Which of the following is thought to be the inheritance pattern of the most common form of the syndrome or disease demonstrated in Question 14?

A. Autosomal recessive
B. Autosomal dominant
C. X-linked recessive
D. X-linked dominant

16 A 10-month-old with DiGeorge syndrome who is status post thoracic surgery presents for a chest X-ray. Which of the following cardiothoracic abnormalities is most associated with DiGeorge syndrome?

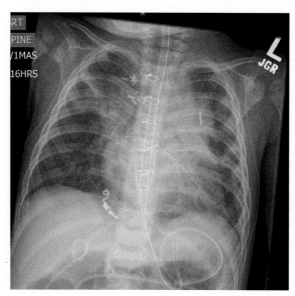

A. Aortic coarctation
B. Tetralogy of Fallot
C. Tricuspid atresia
D. Mitral valve regurgitation

17 Which of the following chromosomal deletions is responsible for DiGeorge syndrome?

A. 13
B. 18
C. 21
D. 22

18 A 17-year-old female with a vascular anomaly presents for an MR examination. Which of the following is the most likely syndrome depicted?

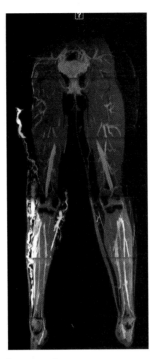

A. Klippel-Trenaunay-Weber syndrome
B. Hemihypertrophy
C. Beckwith-Wiedemann syndrome
D. Maffucci syndrome

19 An 8-year-old female with a history of small bowel transplant presents for a PET/CT scan. What organism has been implicated in this disease process?

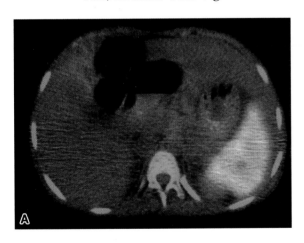
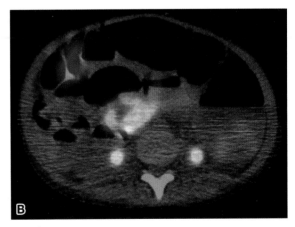

A. Cytomegalovirus
B. *Mycobacterium tuberculosis*
C. *Escherichia coli*
D. Epstein-Barr virus

20 An 8-week-old female presents with multiple congenital anomalies including anal atresia. Given the following imaging abnormalities, what is the most likely diagnosis?

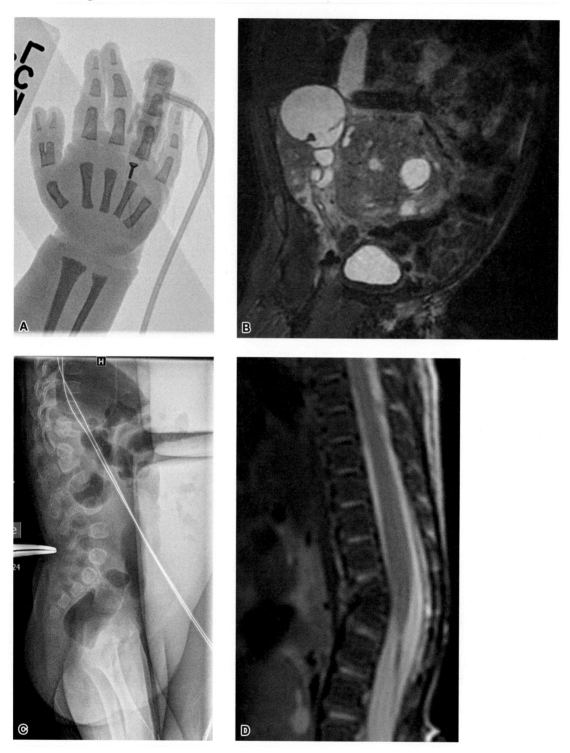

A. VACTERL association
B. Beckwith-Wiedemann syndrome
C. Scheuermann disease
D. Denys-Drash syndrome

21 A 3-year-old patient presents to the emergency room with complaints of a headache. A CT scan of the brain was obtained, and a coronal image is shown below (Image A). This is compared to a coronal image from a limited MR of the brain performed a year before the current study (Image B). What is the next best step in management?

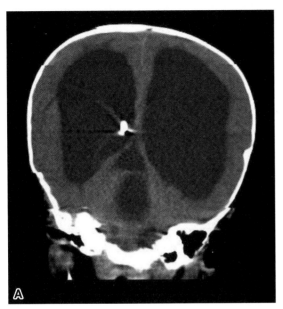

Image A

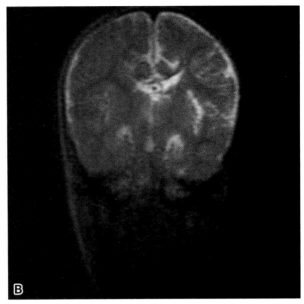

Image B

A. Whole-body MR
B. No further management is needed.
C. Plain film skeletal survey to evaluate for nonaccidental trauma
D. Plain film shunt series

22 A plain film shunt series was subsequently ordered on the patient in question 21 in order to evaluate the integrity of the patient's ventriculoperitoneal shunt catheter. The catheter was noted to be intact, but the distal tip was noted to be kinked (Image A). Because of this finding, an ultrasound exam of the area surrounding the tip was performed and a representative image is shown below (Image B). Concerning the most likely diagnosis, which of the following is true?

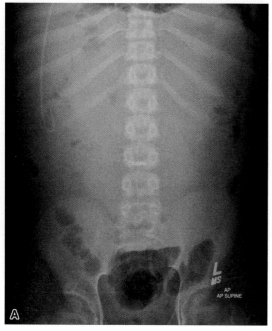

Image A

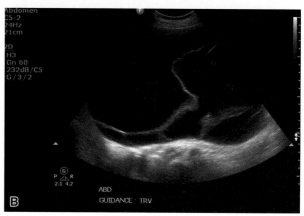

Image B

A. This entity usually develops within the first week after shunting.

B. If infection is present, the wall of the lesion should be excised but the CSF shunt can be left in place.

C. Fine needle aspiration is sometimes used to differentiate this lesion from ascites.

D. The formation of this lesion is a contraindication for future use of the peritoneal cavity in CSF shunting.

23 Regarding transependymal flow of CSF, which of the following is true?

A. It is a form of increased interstitial edema that occurs due to a decrease in intraventricular pressures.

B. CT is more sensitive for the detection of transependymal flow of CSF than MR.

C. Without intervention, this entity ultimately progresses to cerebral atrophy and gliosis.

D. This finding is pathognomonic for CSF shunt malfunction.

24 What is the most specific imaging sign of increased intracranial pressure?

A. Flattening of the posterior globes

B. Low cerebellar tonsils

C. Empty sella

D. Large ventricles

25 What is the most sensitive MRI sign of hydrocephalus?

A. Papilledema

B. Sutural splaying

C. Enlargement of the temporal horns of the lateral ventricles

D. Venous expansion

26 Chest radiographs obtained on a teenage female patient are shown.

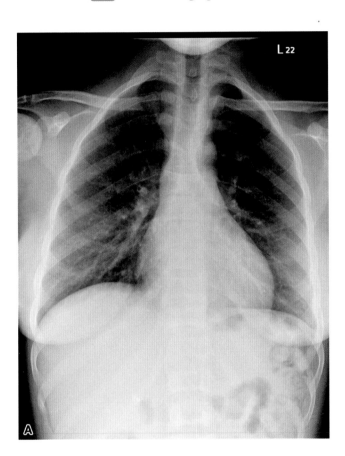
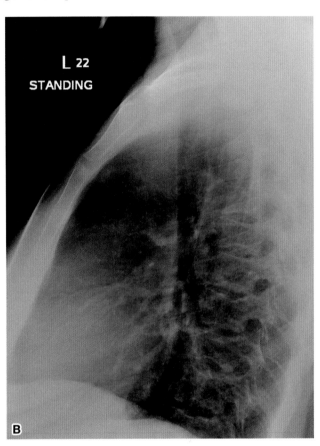

Which of the following conditions does this patient most likely have?

A. Neurofibromatosis type 1

B. Tuberous sclerosis

C. Sickle cell anemia

D. von Hippel-Lindau syndrome

27 A few months later, the same patient described in Question 26 presents with fever, chest pain, and cough. A radiograph obtained on the patient is shown.

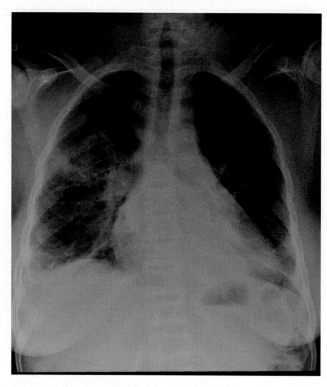

Given the patient's clinical history, which of the following would be the most likely treatment for the patient's symptoms?

A. Oral outpatient antibiotic therapy
B. No treatment is necessary.
C. Antiviral therapy
D. Hydration, transfusion, supplemental oxygen, and analgesia on an inpatient basis

28 Which of the following additional tests would be of most benefit to the patient described in Questions 27 and 28?

A. Transcranial Doppler
B. I-123 MIBG scan
C. Barium enema
D. Voiding cystourethrogram

29 Regarding the imaging evaluation of juvenile idiopathic arthritis (JIA) in children, which of the following is true?

A. There are well-established imaging protocols to evaluate JIA.
B. Radiographs are a good modality for evaluating synovitis.
C. MRI has been shown to detect approximately twice as many erosions as radiographs or ultrasound.
D. Temporomandibular joints are only affected in one of the subtypes of JIA.

30 A sagittal image from an MR examination of the spine performed on a patient with Langerhans cell histiocytosis (LCH) is shown. Regarding LCH, which of the following is true?

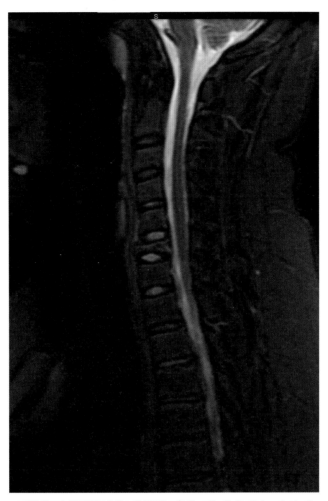

A. Vertebra plana is pathognomonic of this condition.

B. The liver is involved in most cases.

C. The most common clinical manifestation of LCH in the central nervous system is diabetes insipidus.

D. The multifocal multisystem form is the most common subtype.

31 A 16-month-old patient who is status post liver transplantation presents for
a contrast-enhanced CT scan of the abdomen and pelvis. A coronal reconstructed image is shown. Which of the following is the next best step in
management?

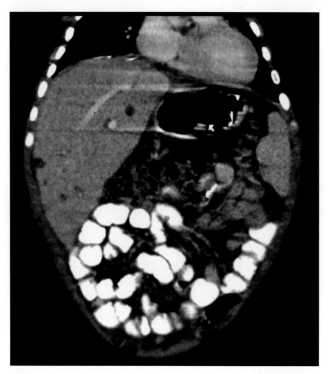

A. Milk scan
B. Tc-99m MAG3 scan
C. Tc-99m HIDA Scan
D. Liver biopsy

32 Which of the following is the most common site of extranodal posttransplant
lymphoproliferative disorder in children?

A. Central nervous system
B. Genitourinary system
C. Gastrointestinal system
D. Thorax

33 A 17-year-old patient with hypertelorism and cleft palate presents for an MR examination. Axial and coronal images from the MR exam are shown. Regarding the most likely etiology, which of the following is true?

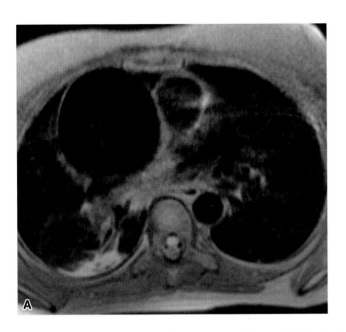 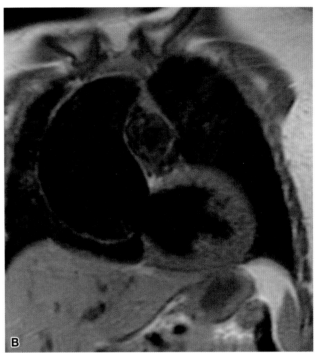

A. Vascular stigmata is usually limited to the thoracic aorta.

B. MRI from head to groin is recommended for affected patients.

C. There is autosomal recessive inheritance.

D. This entity usually has more localized disease than Marfan syndrome.

34 Shown are coronal and axial images from a contrast-enhanced CT scan performed on a patient with abdominal pain who is status post hematopoietic stem cell transplantation.

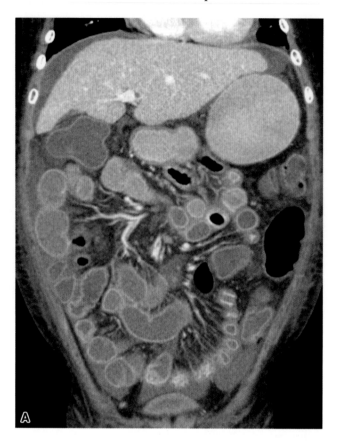

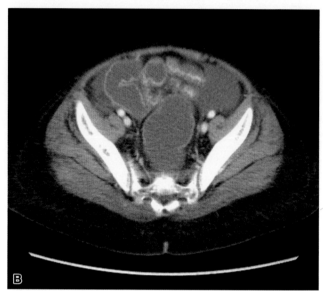

Which of the following is *true* regarding the most likely etiology of the findings?

A. This process is not treatable.

B. Endoscopic biopsy should be performed in all patients to confirm the diagnosis.

C. Abdominopelvic CT is the primary imaging modality to evaluate for potential gastrointestinal findings.

D. Acute disease usually occurs after 100 days following transplant.

35 Which of the following has been found to be the most common extraintestinal imaging finding of graft-versus-host disease affecting the gastrointestinal system?

A. Enlarged and edematous pancreas compatible with pancreatitis

B. Dilated common bile duct

C. Ascites

D. Splenic abscess

ANSWERS AND EXPLANATIONS

1 **Answer A.** There is an enhancing mass at the optic pathway and hypothalamic region consistent with a glioma. There is also an enhancing exophytic mass arising from the right dorsolateral aspect of the medulla, which is also consistent with a glioma. Neurofibromatosis (NF) type 1 (NF1) is a disease characterized by the growth of noncancerous tumors called neurofibromas. These are located on or just underneath the skin as well as in the brain and peripheral nervous system. Neurofibromas may also form in other body parts, including the eyes and orbits.

Ophthalmologic manifestations of NF1 include the following:

- Lisch nodules
- Plexiform neurofibromas
- Choroid hamartomas
- Retinal tumors
- Optic nerve gliomas
- Prominent corneal nerves

An estimated 15% to 40% of children with NF1 have optic nerve glioma or visual pathway gliomas involving the optic nerve, optic chiasm, or optic tract. Some of these lesions are asymptomatic. Bilateral optic nerve gliomas are almost pathognomonic for NF1. Optic nerve gliomas are locally invasive and slow growing with low malignant potential. However, chiasmatic gliomas may invade the hypothalamus and third ventricle, causing obstructive hydrocephalus.

Reference: Listernick R, Charrow J, Greenwald MJ, Esterly NB. Optic gliomas in children with neurofibromatosis type 1. *J Pediatr.* 1989;114(5):788-792.

2 **Answer B.** Flat pigmented lesions of the skin called café au lait spots are hyperpigmented lesions that may vary in color from light brown to dark brown; this is reflected by the name of the condition, which means "coffee with milk." The borders may be smooth or irregular. These spots can grow from birth and can continue to grow throughout the person's lifetime. Having six or more café au lait spots >5 mm in diameter before puberty, or >15 mm in diameter after puberty, is a diagnostic feature of NF1, but other features are required to diagnose NF1.

A port-wine stain (nevus flammeus), also commonly called a firemark, is almost always a birthmark; in rare cases, it can develop in early childhood. It is caused by a vascular anomaly (a capillary malformation in the skin). Port-wine stains are named for their coloration, which is similar in color to port-wine, a fortified red wine from Portugal. Port-wine stains may be part of a syndrome such as Sturge-Weber syndrome or Klippel-Trenaunay syndrome (KTS).

Facial angiofibromas (adenoma sebaceum) is a rash of reddish spots or bumps, which appears on the nose and cheeks in a butterfly distribution. They consist of blood vessels and fibrous tissue. Facial angiofibromas are one of the classic dermatological findings of tuberous sclerosis.

Ataxia telangiectasia can cause features of early aging such as premature graying of the hair. It can also cause vitiligo (an autoimmune disease causing loss of skin pigment resulting in a blotchy "bleach-splashed" look) and warts, which can be extensive and recalcitrant to treatment.

References: Crino PB, Nathanson KL, Henske EP. The tuberous sclerosis complex. *N Engl J Med.* 2006;355(13):1345-1356.

Nowak CB. The phakomatoses: dermatologic clues to neurologic anomalies. *Semin Pediatr Neurol.* 2007;14(3):140-149.

3 **Answer C.** CT demonstrates pial and leptomeningeal vascular calcifications. MRI redemonstrates postsurgical changes of left-sided craniotomy and hemispherectomy with distortion of the left lateral ventricle and a small left cerebral hemisphere. There is left cerebral atrophy and gyriform susceptibility along the residual left cerebral hemisphere. Sturge-Weber syndrome, or encephalotrigeminal angiomatosis, is a phakomatosis characterized by facial port-wine stains and pial angiomas. The diagnosis is usually suspected with the presence of congenital facial cutaneous hemangioma (also known as port-wine stain or facial nevus flammeus). This feature is almost always present and usually involves the ophthalmic division (V1) of the trigeminal nerve. If the V1 territory of the trigeminal nerve is not involved, Sturge-Weber syndrome is unlikely. The differential is a combination of that for multiple intracranial calcifications, cerebral hemiatrophy, and leptomeningeal enhancement, and therefore includes the following:

- Cerebral arteriovenous malformation (AVM)
- Infection (including TORCH infection)
- Neurocysticercosis
- PHACE (*p*osterior fossa anomalies, *h*emangioma, *a*rterial anomalies, *c*ardiac anomalies, and *e*ye anomalies) syndrome
- Healed cortical infarct
- Radiotherapy
- Gobbi syndrome

References: Comi AM. Update on Sturge-Weber syndrome: diagnosis, treatment, quantitative measures, and controversies. *Lymphat Res Biol.* 2007;5(4):257-264.

Griffiths PD. Sturge-Weber syndrome revisited: the role of neuroradiology. *Neuropediatrics.* 1996;27(6):284-294.

4 **Answer A.** A port-wine stain (nevus flammeus), also commonly called a firemark, is almost always a birthmark; in rare cases, it can develop in early childhood. It is caused by a vascular anomaly (a capillary malformation in the skin). Port-wine stains are named for their coloration, which is similar in color to port-wine, a fortified red wine from Portugal. Port-wine stains may be part of a syndrome such as Sturge-Weber syndrome or Klippel-Trenaunay syndrome (KTS).

Flat pigmented lesions of the skin called café au lait spots are hyperpigmented lesions that may vary in color from light brown to dark brown; this is reflected by the name of the condition, which means "coffee with milk." The borders may be smooth or irregular. These spots can grow from birth and can continue to grow throughout the person's lifetime. Having six or more café au lait spots >5 mm in diameter before puberty, or >15 mm in diameter after puberty, is a diagnostic feature of NF1, but other features are required to diagnose NF1.

Facial angiofibroma (adenoma sebaceum) is a rash of reddish spots or bumps, which appears on the nose and cheeks in a butterfly distribution. They consist of blood vessels and fibrous tissue. Facial angiofibroma is one of the classic dermatological findings of tuberous sclerosis.

Ataxia telangiectasia can cause features of early aging such as premature graying of the hair. It can also cause vitiligo (an autoimmune disease causing loss of skin pigment resulting in a blotchy "bleach-splashed" look) and warts, which can be extensive and recalcitrant to treatment.

References: Crino PB, Nathanson KL, Henske EP. The tuberous sclerosis complex. *N Engl J Med.* 2006;355(13):1345-1356.

Nowak CB. The phakomatoses: dermatologic clues to neurologic anomalies. *Semin Pediatr Neurol.* 2007;14(3):140-149.

5 **Answer D.** The abdominal radiograph demonstrates two lucent regions in the upper abdomen (double bubble) consistent with duodenal atresia in the setting of trisomy 21. The two bubbles represent the stomach lumen and the duodenal bulb, respectively. Down syndrome (or trisomy 21) is the most common trisomy and the commonest chromosomal disorder. It is a major cause of intellectual disability and has numerous multisystem manifestations.

Antenatal "soft markers" for aneuploidy include:

- Nuchal fold thickness >6 mm
- Hypoplastic nasal bone
- Echogenic intracardiac focus
- Echogenic bowel
- Shortened humerus
- Shortened femur
- Single umbilical artery
- Renal pyelectasis

Structural abnormalities include:

- Cardiac
- Atrioventricular septal defect (AVSD)
- Abdominal
- Duodenal atresia
- Esophageal atresia
- Central nervous system (CNS)
- Cerebral ventriculomegaly
- Craniofacial/calvarial
- Short maxilla
- Mild brachycephaly

Reference: Smith-Bindman R, Hosmer W, Feldstein VA, et al. Second-trimester ultrasound to detect fetuses with Down syndrome: a meta-analysis. *JAMA*. 2001;285(8):1044-1055.

6 **Answer C.** Aneuploidy refers to an abnormal number of chromosomes and is a type of chromosomal abnormality. There are a large number of potential aneuploidic anomalies. The most common three aneuploidies encountered in the obstetric and pediatric population include trisomy 21 (most common), trisomy 18, and trisomy 13. The double bubble demonstrated on the abdominal radiograph in Question 5 is most consistent with duodenal atresia in the setting of trisomy 21. Trisomy 13, also called Patau syndrome, presents with heart defect, brain, or spinal cord abnormalities, microphthalmia, polydactyly, cleft lip/palate, and hypotonia. Trisomy 18, also called Edwards syndrome, presents with intrauterine growth restriction (IUGR), low birth weight, heart defects, abnormal head shape, micrognathia, and clenched fists with overlapping fingers. Trisomy 23 is also known as XXY male syndrome, and Klinefelter syndrome is associated with male infertility, gynecomastia, small testes, and reduced facial and body hair.

Reference: Estroff JA. Imaging clues in the prenatal diagnosis of syndromes and aneuploidy. *Pediatr Radiol*. 2012;42(suppl 1):S5-S23.

7 **Answer B.** There is bilateral microphthalmia and retro-ocular cyst-like structures consistent with colobomas. The bilateral olfactory apparatus is absent. CHARGE syndrome is an acronym that classically describes a combination of head and neck, cardiac, CNS, and genitourinary disorders:

C: Coloboma
H: Heart defects (congenital heart disease)
A: Atresia (choanal)
R: Retardation (mental)
G: Genital hypoplasia
E: Ear abnormalities/deafness

Coloboma is a collective term encompassing any focal discontinuity in the structure of the eye. Colobomas are due to failure of closure of the choroidal fissure posteriorly. Typically, colobomas are bilateral, small, and are not accompanied by other deeper abnormalities. It occurs along the inferomedial aspect of the globe and optic nerve. On CT or MRI, the affected globe is usually small with a focal posterior defect in the globe with vitreous herniation. A retrobulbar fluid-density cyst may be present.

References: Simmons JD, LaMasters D, Char D. Computed tomography of ocular colobomas. *AJR Am J Roentgenol.* 1983;141(6):1223-1226.

Tellier AL, Cormier-Daire V, Abadie V, et al. CHARGE syndrome: report of 47 cases and review. *Am J Med Genet.* 1998;76(5):402-409.

8 Answer B. CT angiography of the chest demonstrates a dilated aortic root/ascending aorta measuring up to 3.6 cm at the sinuses of Valsalva. Marfan syndrome is a multisystem connective tissue disease with autosomal dominant inheritance of a defect in the fibrillin 1 gene. The affected patients are tall with long disproportionate extremities, pectus excavatum deformity, and arachnodactyly and may also experience upward and lateral optic lens dislocation. Cardiovascular disease is common, particularly aortic root dilatation and dissection, which is the most common cause of sudden death in these patients.

Cardiovascular complications are predominantly due to cystic medial necrosis of the vessels and are the most frequent cause of death. Aortic root dilatation and myxomatous degeneration of the mitral valve resulting in mitral valve regurgitation are the two most common cardiac manifestations. Among the total number of patients with aortic root aneurysms, those with a diagnosis of Marfan syndrome dominate the younger age range but they are nevertheless a minority of all patients with ascending aortic aneurysms. They are prone to acute dissection, and prior to the introduction of prophylactic root replacement, this was the cause of death in two-thirds of all patients and often at a young age.

References: Ha HI, Seo JB, Lee SH, et al. Imaging of Marfan syndrome: multisystemic manifestations. *Radiographics.* 2007;27(4):989-1004.

Treasure T, Takkenberg JJ, Pepper J. Surgical management of aortic root disease in Marfan syndrome and other congenital disorders associated with aortic root aneurysms. *Heart.* 2014;100(20):1571-1576.

9 Answer C. Current guidelines for the management of valvular heart disease state that irrespective of the presence and severity of aortic valve regurgitation, surgery should be considered in patients with Marfan syndrome with risk factors (family history of dissection, size increase 2 mm/year in repeated examinations) and who have aortic root disease with a maximum ascending aortic diameter of ≥45 mm.

Reference: Treasure T, Takkenberg JJ, Pepper J. Surgical management of aortic root disease in Marfan syndrome and other congenital disorders associated with aortic root aneurysms. *Heart.* 2014;100(20):1571-1576.

10 Answer D. Ultrasonography (US) demonstrates a mixed solid cystic mass in the upper left kidney. MRI demonstrates an enlarged left kidney containing a collection of multiple cysts within the medulla of the upper pole, as well as multiple peripheral subcortical cysts. Left nephrectomy was performed, and pathology demonstrated a focus of Wilms tumor (WT) present in a background of nephroblastomatosis. Beckwith-Wiedemann syndrome (BWS) is a congenital overgrowth disorder. The syndrome is characterized by omphalocele, macroglossia, gigantism, neonatal hypoglycemia, hemihypertrophy, hepatosplenomegaly, nephromegaly, cardiac anomalies, adrenal cytomegaly, pancreatic islet cell hyperplasia, facial nevus flammeus, and ear lobe creases. There is a high risk (about 10%) of the development of embryonal neoplasms, particularly WT in a child with BWS, especially those with hemihypertrophy.

References: Andrews MW, Amparo EG. Wilms' tumor in a patient with Beckwith-Wiedemann syndrome: onset detected with 3-month serial sonography. *AJR Am J Roentgenol.* 1993; 160(1):139-140.

Choyke PL, Siegel MJ, Oz O, et al. Nonmalignant renal disease in pediatric patients with Beckwith-Wiedemann syndrome. *AJR Am J Roentgenol.* 1998;171(3):733-737.

11 **Answer C.** The *WT1*-related WT (Wilms tumor) syndromes are a group of hereditary disorders caused by alterations in a gene known as *WT1*. This group of disorders includes:

- WAGR (**W**ilms tumor–**A**niridia–**G**enitourinary malformation–**R**etardation) syndrome
- Denys-Drash syndrome (DDS)
- Frasier syndrome (FS)
- Genitourinary anomalies (abnormalities of the reproductive and urinary systems)

Patients with DDS may have the following clinical features:

- Higher risk of developing WT (the risk is estimated to be >90%)
- Abnormal or undermasculinized reproductive organs in boys
- Normal or abnormal female reproductive organs
- Higher risk of developing a gonadoblastoma (a tumor of the developing reproductive organs, including the ovaries and testes)
- End-stage renal (kidney) disease: patients may develop renal failure, often in association with a condition known as diffuse mesangial sclerosis.

In addition to the *WT1*-related WT syndromes, there are several other genetic conditions associated with the development of WT. Some of these conditions include the following:

- BWS (Beckwith-Wiedemann Syndrome)
- Li-Fraumeni syndrome
- NF1 (Neurofibromatosis type 1)
- Sotos syndrome
- Fanconi anemia
- Bloom syndrome
- Simpson-Golabi-Behmel syndrome
- Perlman syndrome
- Trisomy 18

Patients with these conditions have a greater risk of developing a malignant tumor of the kidney known as WT or nephroblastoma. WT is the most common type of kidney cancer affecting children. Very rarely, WT can occur in adults.

Reference: Lowe LH, Isuani BH, Heller RM, et al. Pediatric renal masses: Wilms tumor and beyond. *Radiographics.* 2000;20(6):1585-1603.

12 **Answer B.** US demonstrates an echogenic soft tissue mass at the posterior neck. MR was performed to assess for pulmonary lymphangiectasia in the setting of genetically proven Turner syndrome. The cystic hygroma is demonstrated (white arrows).

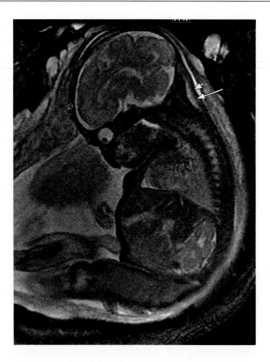

Cystic hygromas can occur as an isolated finding or in association with other birth defects as part of a syndrome. They result from environmental factors, genetic factors, or unknown factors.

Environmental causes for cystic hygroma include:

- Maternal viral infections, such as parvovirus of fifth disease
- Maternal substance abuse, such as abuse of alcohol

Genetic syndromes with cystic hygroma as a clinical feature:

- The majority of prenatally diagnosed cystic hygromas are associated with Turner syndrome, also referred to as 45X, which is the most common of sex chromosome abnormalities in females.
- Chromosome abnormalities such as trisomies 13, 18, and 21
- Noonan syndrome

The pattern of inheritance for these syndromes varies depending upon the specific syndrome. Isolated cystic hygroma can be inherited as an autosomal recessive disorder for which parents are "silent" carriers. Finally, a cystic hygroma can occur from an unknown cause.

Other imaging findings in Turner syndrome include:

- Increased nuchal thickness
- Increased nuchal translucency
- Coarctation of the aorta
- Bicuspid aortic valve
- Horseshoe kidney/pelvic kidney
- IUGR
- Hydrops fetalis
- Short fetal limbs

Reference: Chen C-P, Chien S-C. Prenatal sonographic features of Turner syndrome. *J Med Ultrasound*. 2007;15:251-257.

13 **Answer B.** A nuchal translucency scan (also called first trimester of pregnancy screening) is carried out during weeks 11 to 13 of a pregnancy. The scan uses ultrasound to screen for Down syndrome or other chromosomal or inherited conditions in the fetus. Other nonchromosomal conditions, such as neural tube defects, abdominal wall defects, limb abnormalities, and some congenital heart diseases, can also be detected at this stage of the pregnancy.

Screening can determine the likelihood or risk of an abnormality but does not diagnose the condition. If screening does identify a possible risk, it does not necessarily mean there is an abnormality present but does mean that further testing is necessary. A nuchal translucency scan is combined with the mother's age and results of a blood test showing the mother's pregnancy hormone levels to provide a "combined risk."

Without the blood test, screening is 75% accurate for predicting Down syndrome. With the blood test, the accuracy increases to 85%. Women who return a high-risk result from the screening will be offered formal genetic testing using other procedures, such as amniocentesis or chorionic villus sampling (CVS).

Reference: ACOG Committee on Practice Bulletins. ACOG Practice Bulletin No. 77: screening for fetal chromosomal abnormalities. *Obstet Gynecol.* 2007;109(1):217-227.

14 **Answer C.** The right and left glenohumeral joints appear subluxed or dislocated. This patient has known Ehlers-Danlos syndrome (EDS), which comprises a heterogeneous group of connective tissue disorders that primarily manifest as hypermobility, elastic or doughy skin, and soft tissue or vascular fragility. According to the 2017 international classification of EDS, there are 13 recognized subtypes of EDS. The most common (80%) EDS subtype is hypermobile EDS. Hypermobile EDS is distinct among EDS subtypes because its genetic loci and impaired protein are unknown, and therefore it cannot be assayed on a molecular basis. Instead, hypermobile EDS is diagnosed clinically, through a combination of family history, physical examination, connective tissue findings, and prior joint dislocations or chronic joint pain. People with hypermobile EDS typically present in late adolescence or early adulthood.

Reference: George MP, Shur NE, Peréz-Rosselló JM. Ehlers-Danlos syndrome: what the radiologist needs to know. *Pediatr Radiol.* 2021;51:1023-1028.

15 **Answer B.** The inheritance pattern of hypermobile EDS is thought to be autosomal dominant. Several other subtypes of EDS also have an autosomal dominant inheritance pattern, although there are also subtypes that have an autosomal recessive pattern.

Reference: George MP, Shur NE, Peréz-Rosselló JM. Ehlers-Danlos syndrome: what the radiologist needs to know. *Pediatr Radiol.* 2021;51:1023-1028.

16 **Answer B.** This patient was treated for tetralogy of Fallot, major aortopulmonary collateral arteries, and hypoplastic pulmonary arteries. A right ventricular outflow track transjugular patch was placed in addition to patch closure of an atrial septal defect (ASD) and ventricular septal defect (VSD). The 22q11.2 deletion syndrome, also known as DiGeorge syndrome (DGS) or velocardiofacial syndrome, is a syndrome where a small portion of chromosome 22 is lost and results in a variable but recognizable pattern of physical and behavioral features. The classic triad of DGS on presentation is conotruncal cardiac anomalies, hypoplastic thymus, and hypocalcemia. The most common cardiac defects that account for two-thirds of the cardiac anomalies seen in patients with DGS include the following:

- Interrupted aortic arch
- Truncus arteriosus
- Tetralogy of Fallot
- ASDs, VSDs
- Vascular rings

References: Alikaşifoğlu M, Malkoç N, Ceviz N, et al. Microdeletion of 22q11 (CATCH 22) in children with conotruncal heart defect and extracardiac malformations. *Turk J Pediatr.* 2000;42(3):215-218.

McDonald-McGinn DM, Sullivan KE. Chromosome 22q11.2 deletion syndrome (DiGeorge syndrome/velocardiofacial syndrome). *Medicine (Baltimore).* 2011;90:1-18.

17   **Answer D.** Chromosome 22 deletion.

18   **Answer A.** MRI demonstrates an extensive venous vascular malformation of the right lower extremity, which extends from the level of the groin to the distal tibiotalar joint and involves both the subcutaneous and intramuscular compartments. Klippel-Trenaunay syndrome (KTS) is a complex congenital disorder characterized by the classic triad of capillary malformation, venous malformation, and limb overgrowth, with or without lymphatic malformation. In KTS, the persistence of embryonic avalvular venous structures, most notably the lateral vein of the thigh (lateral marginal vein of Servelle) and sciatic vein, can result in dilated tortuous varicosities, with superficial varicosities more often located over the anterolateral thigh and leg.

MRI with and without gadolinium contrast is the imaging study of choice to define the nature and extent of vascular anomalies in patients with KTS. MRI provides the highest diagnostic accuracy in the evaluation of the underlying venous and lymphatic abnormalities, as well as soft tissue and bony overgrowth. Venous malformations show uniform enhancement, whereas lymphatic malformations demonstrate rim or septal enhancement of cyst walls. Fluid-fluid levels and high T2 signal intensity are characteristic of lymphatic malformations. The presence of phleboliths as signal voids is characteristic of venous malformations.

Hemihypertrophy or hemihyperplasia describes an asymmetry in size between the right and left side of the body. This can arise sporadically as isolated hemihypertrophy or it can arise as part of the syndromes listed below:

- BWS (Beckwith-Wiedemann syndrome)
- Proteus syndrome
- KTS (Klippel-Trenaunay syndrome)
- NF1 (Neurofibromatosis type 1)
- Hemihyperplasia-multiple lipomatosis (HHML)
- McCune-Albright syndrome
- Langer-Giedion syndrome

BWS is a congenital overgrowth disorder characterized by:

- Macroglossia (most common clinical finding)
- Otic dysplasia
- Omphalocele
- Localized gigantism/macrosomia
- Hemihypertrophy
- Cardiac anomalies
- Pancreatic islet cell hyperplasia
- Organomegaly
- Nephromegaly
- Hepatosplenomegaly

Maffucci syndrome is a congenital nonhereditary mesodermal dysplasia characterized by multiple enchondromas with soft tissue venous malformations. On imaging, it is usually portrayed by a short limb with metaphyseal distortions because of multiple enchondromas, which may appear grotesque, and soft tissue masses with phleboliths depicting venous malformations.

References: Flors L, Leiva-Salinas C, Maged IM, et al. MR imaging of soft-tissue vascular malformations: diagnosis, classification, and therapy follow-up. *Radiographics.* 2011;31:1321-1340; discussion: 1340-1341.

Roebuck DJ, Howlett DC, Frazer CK, et al. Pictorial review: the imaging features of lower limb Klippel-Trenaunay syndrome. *Clin Radiol.* 1994;49(5):346-350.

19 Answer D. Positron emission tomography (PET) imaging demonstrates diffusely increased fluorodeoxyglucose (FDG) uptake identified within the spleen, which is concerning for lymphomatous involvement. Multiple enlarged mesenteric and retroperitoneal lymph nodes are also present and demonstrate increased FDG uptake. Posttransplant lymphoproliferative disorders (PTLDs) are lymphoid and/or plasmacytic proliferations that occur in the setting of solid organ or allogeneic hematopoietic cell transplantation because of immunosuppression. They are among the most serious and potentially fatal complications of transplantation. While the majority appear to be related to the presence of Epstein-Barr virus (EBV), EBV-negative disease does occur.

The range of appearances is large due to the number of possible sites. In general, extranodal involvement is three to four times more common than is nodal involvement and resembles primary lymphoma of those organs:

- Solid organs (liver, spleen, kidney)
  Nodules or diffuse infiltration
- Bowel
  Circumferential wall thickening
  Aneurysmal dilatation
  Ulceration/perforation
- Lung
  Nodules or diffuse infiltration
- Brain
- Nodes
  Nonspecific nodal enlargement, similar to other lymphomas
  Most commonly affecting mediastinum (either lymphadenopathy or anterior mediastinal mass) or retroperitoneum (either as lymphadenopathy or mass)

References: Pickhardt PJ, Siegel MJ, Hayashi RJ, et al. Posttransplantation lymphoproliferative disorder in children: clinical, histopathologic, and imaging features. *Radiology.* 2000;217(1):16-25.

Meador TL, Krebs TL, Cheong JJ, et al. Imaging features of posttransplantation lymphoproliferative disorder in pancreas transplant recipients. *AJR Am J Roentgenol.* 2000;174(1):121-124.

20 Answer A. Left hand radiograph demonstrates polydactyly of the first digit. MRI of the abdomen demonstrates bilateral dysplastic kidneys with multiple cysts, hydronephrosis, and an ectopically located left kidney. Lateral radiograph and MRI image demonstrate segmentation and fusion anomalies in the upper lumbar spine with associated kyphosis.

VACTERL is an acronym that describes a nonrandom constellation of congenital anomalies. It is not a true syndrome as such and is equivalent to the VATER anomaly.

The acronym VACTERL derives from the following:

V: Vertebral anomalies

- Hemivertebrae
- Congenital scoliosis
- Caudal regression
- Spina bifida

A: Anorectal anomalies

• Anal atresia

C: Cardiac anomalies; cleft lip

TE: Tracheoesophageal fistula and/or esophageal atresia

R: Renal anomalies; radial ray anomalies

L: Limb anomalies

• Polydactyly
• Oligodactyly

At least three of the above features (in each category) are considered necessary for the diagnosis of this condition.

Reference: Solomon BD, Baker LA, Bear KA, et al. An approach to the identification of anomalies and etiologies in neonates with identified or suspected VACTERL (vertebral defects, anal atresia, tracheo-esophageal fistula with esophageal atresia, cardiac anomalies, renal anomalies, and limb anomalies) association. *J Pediatr*. 2014;164:451-457.e1.

21 **Answer D.** The coronal image (A) from the patient's CT scan demonstrates interval development of marked ventriculomegaly when compared to the patient's prior MR (B) when the ventricles were not dilated. In addition, there is a small amount of low attenuation in the periventricular white matter surrounding the superior aspect of the right lateral ventricle compatible with transependymal flow of CSF. A high-attenuation structure is seen coursing through the right ventricle, which represents a portion of a shunt catheter. Therefore, these findings raise the concern for shunt malfunction.

Conventional radiography is primarily performed to evaluate for breaks in the shunt, shunt disconnections, or distal catheter migration of the shunt. A typical shunt series includes frontal and lateral radiographs of the head and neck and frontal radiographs of the chest and abdomen and is indicated given the patient's history. The purpose of the shunt series is to image the entire course of the shunt.

Nonaccidental trauma (NAT) can manifest with subdural hematomas. However, there is no evidence of subdural hematomas on the images nor is there anything in the history to suggest the possibility of NAT. Therefore, a skeletal survey consisting of plain radiographs of the axial and appendicular skeleton is not indicated.

The most important clinical application of whole-body MRI in children, as in adults, is the staging of malignant disease and screening for metastatic spread. However, the use of whole-body MRI to evaluate other multisystem disease processes such as chronic recurrent multifocal osteomyelitis is increasing. Nevertheless, a whole-body MRI exam is not indicated in this setting.

References: Chavhan GB, Babyn PS. Whole-body MR imaging in children: principles, technique, current applications, and future directions. *Radiographics*. 2011;31(6):1757-1772.

Guimareas CG. Neuro: genitourinary. In: Donnelly LF, ed. *Fundamentals of Pediatric Imaging*. 3rd ed. Elsevier; 2022:257-360.

Ho ML, Rojas R, Eisenberg RL. Cerebral edema. *AJR Am J Roentgenol*. 2012;199(3):W258-W273.

Lonergan GJ, Baker AM, Morey MK, et al. From the archives of the AFIP. Child abuse: radiologic-pathologic correlation. *Radiographics*. 2003;23(4):811-845.

Wallace AN, McConathy J, Menias CO, et al. Imaging evaluation of CSF shunts. *AJR Am J Roentgenol*. 2014;202(1):38-53.

22 **Answer C.** The image provided from an ultrasound exam surrounding the tip of the ventriculoperitoneal (VP) shunt demonstrates a well-circumscribed anechoic cystic lesion with internal septations (Image B). In a patient with suspected shunt malfunction, the findings are most consistent with a CSF pseudocyst. In addition, the septated nature of the pseudocyst indicates the lesion may be infected.

Pseudocyst formation is a common cause of distal VP shunt catheter obstruction. Pseudocysts are loculated collections of CSF that form around the terminal end of the catheter. In patients with VP shunts, pseudocysts are caused by peritoneal adhesions or migration of the greater omentum over the shunt tip. Pseudocysts can also develop around ventriculopleural shunts because of adhesions caused by chronic pleural irritation. Conventional radiography may show coiling of the distal catheter within an intra-abdominal soft tissue mass in the case of ventricuoperitoneal shunts or loculated pleural effusions in the case of ventriculopleural shunts. Definitive diagnosis can be made by CT or ultrasound showing a loculated fluid collection surrounding the catheter tip. The time from the last shunting procedure to the development of an abdominal pseudocyst ranges from 3 weeks to 5 years and is usually not within the first week.

CSF pseudocysts can sometimes be differentiated from ascites by their characteristic displacement of the bowel gas pattern on abdominal films and by the absence of shifting dullness. Although sonography and CT can accurately localize abdominal fluid collections, differentiation of ascites from pseudocysts sometimes may not be possible. Therefore, fine needle aspiration of the localized CSF collections under sonographic or CT guidance should be performed to increase the diagnostic yield.

If infection is present, the pseudocyst wall should be excised, and the peritoneal shunting catheter removed. The formation of a CSF pseudocyst is a poor prognostic sign for the usefulness of the peritoneal cavity for shunting, but previous abdominal pseudocyst formation and peritonitis are not contraindications to subsequent peritoneal shunting. However, in some reported cases, the CSF had to be diverted to other cavities because of either recurrence of the cysts or failure of the peritoneum to absorb fluid. Culture of the tip of the peritoneal catheter was reported to be more sensitive than culture of the CSF.

References: Chung JJ, Yu JS, Kim JH, et al. Intraabdominal complications secondary to ventriculoperitoneal shunts: CT findings and review of the literature. *AJR Am J Roentgenol.* 2009;193(5):1311-1317.

Wallace AN, McConathy J, Menias CO, et al. Imaging evaluation of CSF shunts. *AJR Am J Roentgenol.* 2014;202(1):38-53.

23 **Answer C.** Interstitial, or hydrocephalic, edema occurs in the setting of increased intraventricular pressures, which cause rupture of the ventricular ependymal lining. This allows transependymal migration of CSF into the extracellular space, most commonly the periventricular white matter. Fluid composition is identical to CSF. Various causes of interstitial edema include obstructing masses, meningitis, subarachnoid hemorrhage, and normal pressure hydrocephalus. In contrast, ependymitis granularis refers to small triangular areas of abnormal signal around the anterolateral frontal horns. This normal anatomic variant results from regionally decreased myelin, increased extracellular fluid, or focal breakdown of the ependymal lining with gliosis. On CT, the combination of ventriculomegaly and increased periventricular hypodensity is suggestive of the diagnosis of interstitial edema. MRI is a more sensitive imaging modality for the detection of transependymal flow of CSF, showing hypointensity on T1-weighted imaging and periventricular hyperintensity on T2-weighted imaging/fluid-attenuated inversion recovery (FLAIR).

In symptomatic patients, decompression with resection of the obstructing lesion (noncommunicating hydrocephalus) or ventriculostomy catheter placement (communicating hydrocephalus) allows normalization of ventricular pressures. In turn, this enables normal antegrade resorption of interstitial fluid across the ependymal lining and back into the ventricular system. Without intervention, the findings ultimately progress to cerebral atrophy and gliosis.

Reference: Ho ML, Rojas R, Eisenberg RL. Cerebral edema. *AJR Am J Roentgenol.* 2012; 199(3):W258-W273.

24 **Answer A.** Flattening of the posterior globes reflects the transmission of elevated perioptic CSF pressure on the compressible posterior sclera. Studies have found it to be one of the most specific indicators of increased intracranial pressure. Low cerebellar tonsils are a finding seen with intracranial hypotension. An empty sella can be seen with increased intracranial pressure but is nonspecific and not the most common finding. Chronically shunted patients with stiff ventricles may not show significant change in ventricular size.

References: Brodsky MC, Vaphiades M. Magnetic resonance imaging in pseudotumor cerebri. *Ophthalmology.* 1998;105(9):1686-1693.

Passi N, Degnan AJ, Levy LM. MR imaging of papilledema and visual pathways: effects of increased intracranial pressure and pathophysiologic mechanisms. *AJNR Am J Neuroradiol.* 2013;34(5):919-924.

25 **Answer C.** The temporal horns of the lateral ventricles dilate sooner than the frontal horns, which may be because they are less resistant to pressure or because of CSF flow dynamics. Papilledema occurs with increased intracranial pressure and is not always present in hydrocephalus. Sutural splaying only occurs with unfused sutures. Venous expansion occurs with intracranial hypotension.

References: Heinz ER, Ward A, Drayer BP, et al. Distinction between obstructive and atrophic dilatation of ventricles in children. *J Comput Assist Tomogr.* 1980;4(3):320-325.

Hosoya T, Yamaguchi K, Adachi M, et al. Dilatation of the temporal horn in subarachnoid haemorrhage. *Neuroradiology.* 1992;34(3):207-209.

Naidich TP, Epstein F, Lin JP, et al. Evaluation of pediatric hydrocephalus by computed tomography. *Radiology.* 1976;119:337-345.

26 **Answer C.** The frontal radiograph demonstrates a cholecystectomy clip in the right upper quadrant and absence of a splenic shadow in the left upper quadrant. The lateral radiograph demonstrates multiple vertebral endplate anomalies in a "Lincoln log" configuration. This constellation of findings is often found in sickle cell disease.

Sickle cell anemia (SCA) is a hemolytic anemia characterized by abnormally shaped (sickled) red blood cells (RBCs), which are removed from the circulation and destroyed at increased rates, leading to anemia. Of greater clinical importance, the sickled RBCs cause vascular occlusion, which leads to tissue ischemia and infarction.

The spleen possesses a slow, tortuous microcirculation that renders it susceptible to congestion, sludging, and polymerization. The result of this process is splenic infarction, which progresses over time to functional autosplenectomy. The infarcted spleen is replaced by fibrosis, with calcium and hemosiderin deposition. By 5 years of age, 94% of patients with SCA are asplenic, which is likely the case with this patient.

Cholelithiasis is one of the common complications of SCA. The treatment of cholelithiasis in patients with SCA is cholecystectomy. Gallstones are usually pigment stones that result from chronic hemolysis leading to increased bilirubin production. A frequency ranging from 5% to 55% has been reported, but an overall 70% of patients with SCA will develop gallstones at one stage of their life.

In the spine, infarction may appear as a central, square-shaped endplate depression, resulting from microvascular endplate occlusion and subsequent overgrowth of the surrounding portions of the endplate. This appearance is seen in approximately 10% of patients, but it is essentially pathognomonic for SCA and has been called the Lincoln log or H-shaped vertebra deformity.

NF1, von Hippel-Lindau disease, and tuberous sclerosis do not typically affect the gallbladder and spleen. In addition, Lincoln log vertebral bodies are not seen in these conditions.

References: Fortman BJ, Kuszyk BS, Urban BA, et al. Neurofibromatosis type 1: a diagnostic mimicker at CT. *Radiographics*. 2001;21(3):601-612.

Leung RS, Biswas SV, Duncan M, et al. Imaging features of von Hippel-Lindau disease. *Radiographics*. 2008;28(1):65-79.

Lonergan GJ, Cline DB, Abbondanzo SL. Sickle cell anemia. *Radiographics*. 2001;21(4):971-994.

Umeoka S, Koyama T, Miki Y, et al. Pictorial review of tuberous sclerosis in various organs. *Radiographics*. 2008;28(7):e32.

27 **Answer D.** The new chest radiograph demonstrates multiple bilateral focal opacities. Although some of these may be related to atelectasis, they may also be due to focal consolidations. In a patient with these findings and the given clinical history, acute chest syndrome (ACS) must be suspected.

ACS describes an acute pulmonary illness, characterized by a new pulmonary consolidation and some combination of fever, chest pain, and signs of pulmonary compromise such as cough, dyspnea, and tachypnea. The cause of ACS is not fully understood, and many causative agents have been identified, including infection and fat emboli; frequently, the underlying cause is not discovered in individual patients. ACS may progress to acute respiratory distress syndrome and death. The severity of the clinical symptoms distinguishes ACS from a clinically milder pneumonia. Because ACS may be caused by pneumonia, the two entities may constitute a continuum.

ACS is the second leading cause of hospitalization in patients with SCA, after painful crises. It accounts for 25% of deaths in patients with SCA and is currently the single leading cause of death in SCA. It occurs most commonly in children between 2 and 4 years of age. Children with sickle cell disease are more prone than adults to develop ACS (50% of all children with sickle cell disease will experience at least one episode of ACS), but adults with sickle cell have a higher mortality rate (4.3%) than do children.

The radiographic findings often show segmental to lobar pulmonary opacities. However, 30% to 60% of patients have no initial radiographic abnormality, often because they are admitted for another reason (usually for pain crises), and subsequently develop ACS. Some people have speculated that pulmonary opacities are due to rib infarction, splinting, and subsequent atelectasis. There can also be associated cardiomegaly on radiographs. Pleural effusions are frequent but do not help differentiate infectious from noninfectious causes of ACS. Patients also may have evidence of rib infarcts on bone scans. The majority (70%) of patients with ACS are hypoxic (oxygen saturation <90%, as measured by pulse oximetry).

Treatment consists of hydration, transfusion, supplemental oxygen, and analgesia. Incentive inspirometry to improve atelectasis, antibiotic therapy for suspected infection, and steroids may also be used. Mechanical ventilation was needed in 13% of patients in one study. In severe cases, extracorporeal membrane oxygenation (ECMO) has been used successfully. The mean hospital stay is 7 days for adults and 4 days for children.

References: Epelman M. Chest. In Donnelly LF, ed. *Fundamentals of Pediatric Imaging*. 3rd ed. Elsevier; 2022:27-70.

Lonergan GJ, Cline DB, Abbondanzo SL. Sickle cell anemia. *Radiographics*. 2001;21(4):971-994.

28 **Answer A.** Stroke, atrophy, and cognitive impairment are major consequences of SCA. Approximately 25% of all patients with SCA will have a neurologic complication over their lifetime; 11% of these complications will occur by age 20 years. Many children experience "silent infarction" (defined as absence of clinical symptoms with MRI findings of infarct). Silent infarction is twice as common as clinical infarction and may occur in up to 22% of children by 12 years of age.

Because of the considerable lifelong cognitive and functional impairments that result from stroke, efforts have been directed toward identifying patients at risk for stroke to institute preventive therapy. Transcranial Doppler US has emerged as a valuable tool for assessing large cerebral artery flow dynamics. Studies show that elevated velocities in the distal internal carotid artery and proximal middle cerebral artery correlate with an increased risk of stroke. Increased velocity in these vessels has been shown to correlate with areas of MRI abnormality and vessel narrowing on both conventional and MR angiography. Preventive therapy (usually monthly maintenance transfusions) is now offered to these patients. Screening transcranial Doppler US should begin by the age of 3 years.

Reports of uncommon colonic abnormalities in SCA include conditions such as acute necrotizing colitis in adults, pseudomembranous colitis (PMC) in a child, ischemic colitis, and life-threatening toxic megacolon. Pathogenesis of these inflammatory complications seems also to be due to intestinal ischemic microvascular occlusion. A barium enema is contraindicated for imaging of these intestinal lesions, if associated with an acute abdomen because of a high risk of perforation. Contrast-enhanced CT with oral water-soluble contrast is the imaging tool of choice and may show long segmental intestinal wall thickening, which is irregular and shaggy, compared to a symmetrical homogeneous pattern that is seen in Crohn disease. Also, CT exams in these patients may show the famous "accordion sign," which represents trapped contrast between thickened edematous colonic haustral folds.

An I-123 metaiodobenzylguanidine (MIBG) scan would be helpful to see if a tumor is MIBG avid as in cases of tumors of neural crest origin such as neuroblastomas, which often originate in the adrenal region. There is no association of SCA and the development of such tumors. In addition, there is no known association between sickle cell disease and the subsequent development of vesicoureteral reflux, so a voiding cystourethrogram (VCUG) would not be of benefit in this patient.

References: Agha M, Eid AF, Sallam M. Sickle cell anemia: imaging from head to toe. *Egypt J Radiol Nucl Med*. 2013;44(3):547-561.

Lonergan GJ, Cline DB, Abbondanzo SL. Sickle cell anemia. *Radiographics*. 2001;21(4):971-994.

29 **Answer C.** Juvenile idiopathic arthritis (JIA) includes all forms of arthritis that develop before the age of 16 years, persist for at least 6 weeks, and have no identifiable cause. JIA is the most common rheumatic disease in children, with a reported prevalence of 16 to 150 per 100,000 children. JIA is a clinical diagnosis with varied manifestations and is influenced by genetic and environmental factors. In the past, imaging evaluation for known or suspected JIA had relied primarily on radiography. However, radiographic findings such as bone erosions, joint space narrowing from cartilage destruction, and growth disturbances are irreversible findings that occur late in the course of the disease. The development of improved therapeutic agents that can prevent joint destruction, especially when treatment is initiated early, highlights the importance of early (preradiographic) detection of inflammation. The potentially serious side effects of these newer therapeutic agents in the pediatric population underscore the importance of accurately assessing disease activity, disease progression, and treatment response. As a result, management of JIA has evolved to include greater utilization of advanced imaging techniques such as contrast-enhanced MRI and Doppler US. Both modalities can help in detecting inflammatory lesions before permanent joint destruction occurs and can monitor disease progression and treatment response to more effectively guide therapy.

Unlike the systematic protocols for monitoring adult patients with rheumatoid arthritis, there are no defined imaging protocols for JIA. The timing and utilization of imaging in JIA must be tailored to the individual patient, with consideration given to the strengths and weaknesses of each available modality in evaluating the joints in question and directing therapeutic decision-making.

Pre-erosive signs of inflammation such as synovitis and osteitis are undetectable on radiographs. Radiographic findings in early-stage JIA are often nonspecific. The most often encountered radiographic findings include soft tissue swelling, joint effusion, and osteopenia. Osteopenia is usually periarticular in the early stages of disease secondary to joint inflammation, whereas in advanced-stage JIA, it can be diffuse due to decreased physical activity or steroid administration.

Because of its multiplanar capability and excellent bone and soft tissue contrast resolution, MRI is ideal for imaging patients with JIA. MRI allows comprehensive evaluation of the synovium, articular cartilage, growth cartilage, bone marrow, cortical bone, and soft tissues. In early JIA, MRI can help detect synovitis before it is apparent at physical examination, a potentially important prognostic indicator. MRI is the only imaging modality that can demonstrate bone marrow edema, although its prognostic significance in JIA has not been clearly defined. In adult rheumatoid arthritis, bone marrow edema is a predictor of future erosions. Therefore, the presence of bone marrow edema in the setting of JIA is considered a pre-erosive abnormality and an indication for initiating therapy to prevent permanent joint damage. MRI has been shown to help detect more than twice as many bone erosions in the wrist as either US or radiography and more than twice as many cases of sacroiliitis as radiography in a pediatric population. It can also help identify radiographically occult extra-articular inflammatory lesions such as tenosynovitis and enthesitis. MRI does not utilize ionizing radiation, which is an important consideration in the pediatric population. However, when a joint is being evaluated with MRI, correlative radiographs should be obtained to document findings and for future reference during treatment monitoring.

The temporomandibular joint (TMJ) can be involved in any of the JIA subtypes and is affected in 17% to 87% of the patient population. Given the morphology and complex anatomy of the TMJ, this joint is at especially high risk for growth disturbances when affected by inflammatory arthritis, and long-term involvement may result in both poor aesthetic and functional outcomes. It is well documented that clinical symptoms, such as pain, may not be present even in the setting of severe erosive TMJ disease, and subjective symptoms may lead to underestimation of the degree of early inflammation.

Reference: Sheybani EF, Khanna G, White AJ, et al. Imaging of juvenile idiopathic arthritis: a multimodality approach. *Radiographics*. 2013;33(5):1253-1273.

30 **Answer C.** Histiocytic disorders are a group of diseases derived from macrophages and dendritic cells. Langerhans cell histiocytosis (LCH) is the most common dendritic cell disorder and is named because of its similarity to the Langerhans cells found in the skin and mucosa. However, it was later discovered that the abnormal cells in LCH are derived from myeloid dendritic cells that exhibit the same antigens (CD1a, S100, and CD207) and exhibit the same unique intracytoplasmic organelles as in Langerhans cells. These intracytoplasmic organelles, known as Birbeck granules, appear racquet shaped at electron microscopy and help differentiate LCH from other histiocytic disorders and xanthogranulomatous diseases. The proliferation and accumulation of LCH cells in various organs result in the clinical disease.

LCH is divided into three groups based on the number of lesions and systems involved. The unifocal (localized) form is seen in approximately 70% of LCH cases, is limited to a single bone or a few bones, and may involve the lung. Patients usually present between 5 and 15 years of age. The multifocal unisystem (chronic recurring) form comprises approximately 20% of cases and involves multiple bones as well as the reticuloendothelial system (liver, spleen, lymph nodes, and skin). It often is accompanied by diabetes insipidus when the pituitary gland is involved. Patients with this form of disease present earlier than those with unifocal disease, typically between 1 and 5 years of age. The multifocal multisystem (fulminant) form constitutes approximately 10% of LCH cases and often is fatal. It typically is diagnosed in the first 2 years of life and is characterized by disseminated involvement of the reticuloendothelial system, anemia, and thrombocytopenia.

The clinical manifestation of LCH depends on its severity and the number of organs involved and ranges from self-limited to fatal disease (in cases where disease has disseminated to multiple systems). The diagnosis of LCH is made by corroborating clinical features, histopathology, immunohistochemistry, and radiologic findings.

The CNS is involved in approximately 16% of LCH cases. If the facial bones or anterior or middle cranial fossa are affected, the incidence of CNS involvement is higher, affecting up to 25% of patients with LCH. The most common clinical CNS manifestation of LCH is diabetes insipidus secondary to infiltration of the posterior pituitary gland, which results in decreased secretion of antidiuretic hormone. T1-weighted MRI demonstrates loss of the normal posterior pituitary bright spot. Approximately 70% of patients will also show thickening of the pituitary stalk, a finding best appreciated on contrast-enhanced MRIs.

Bone lesions are the most common radiographic manifestation of LCH and occur in approximately 80% of patients. Although any bone can be affected, LCH has a predilection for the flat bones. The skull is the most common flat bone involved, followed by the mandible, ribs, pelvis, and spine.

The vertebral body is the most affected part of the spine in LCH. Early lesions appear lytic at radiography and CT. MRI demonstrates decreased T1 signal intensity and increased T2 signal intensity, with areas of enhancement. As the disease progresses, the early lytic lesions can result in symmetric uniform collapse of the vertebral body with preservation of the intervertebral disk spaces. The flattened vertebral body has been termed "vertebra plana" and may result in pain and substantial neurologic defects. The T6 vertebral body on the MR image shown demonstrates this finding. Although vertebra plana can have additional causes in children, such as leukemia, metastatic neuroblastoma, aneurysmal bone cyst, or Ewing sarcoma, the most common cause in children is LCH.

In addition, lung involvement occurs in approximately 10% of LCH cases. It is much more common in adults and is almost always associated with smoking. At CT, LCH is characterized by centrilobular micronodules with a predominantly bilateral symmetric upper- to midlung distribution. The costophrenic angles are usually spared. As the disease progresses, cysts develop and can eventually become the major imaging finding. Cysts vary in size but usually are less than 1 cm. A confluence of cysts may result in bullous formation, which then predisposes the patient to recurrent spontaneous pneumothorax.

Reference: Zaveri J, La Q, Yarmish G, et al. More than just Langerhans cell histiocytosis: a radiologic review of histiocytic disorders. *Radiographics*. 2014;34(7):2008-2024.

31 **Answer D.** The coronal reconstructed image from a contrast-enhanced CT scan is presented in a liver window and shows multiple small foci of low attenuation in the liver parenchyma. In a patient who is status post liver transplantation and presumably immunosuppressed, differential diagnostic considerations include foci of fungal disease, hepatic abscesses, or neoplastic processes including PTLD. A biopsy should be able to differentiate between these etiologies. The gallbladder and kidneys are not included in this study and there is no indication that the patient has gallbladder or renal pathology so a hepatobiliary iminodiacetic acid (HIDA) scan or mercaptoacetyltriglycine (Mag3) scan would not be of benefit. There is also no evidence of concern for gastroparesis or gastric outlet obstruction, so a milk scan would not be of benefit.

Reference: Marie E, Navallas M, Navarro OM, et al. Posttransplant lymphoproliferative disorder in children: a 360-degree perspective. *Radiographics.* 2020;40(1):241-265.

32 **Answer C.** PTLD is the most common malignancy that can occur after organ transplantation in children. PTLD arises because the patient's immune system has been suppressed to protect the graft and may fail to provide an adequate immune check for transformed malignant or premalignant lymphocytes. PTLD risk factors and pathogenesis are not completely understood but EBV is identified in many patients with PTLD and may be a contributing factor. PTLD is a clinical challenge because the biologic behavior and clinical manifestations are diverse, and there is no standardized treatment. Treatment options include reduction in immunosuppression therapy, chemotherapy, radiation therapy, and surgical resection of localized lesions, depending on factors including the type and extent of disease, whether the patient has positive test results for the EBV, and patient comorbidities. Diagnostic imaging modalities such as radiography, US, CT, MRI, and PET are essential in the diagnosis, assessment of therapeutic response, and monitoring of this heterogeneous disease entity. When imaging findings are suggestive of PTLD, prompt tissue biopsy to identify the PTLD subtype is essential for appropriate treatment. PTLD has the potential for reversibility (with reduction of immunosuppression), which distinguishes PTLD from neoplastic lymphoproliferative disorders that occur in immunocompetent patients.

Patients with PTLD present either within 1 year after transplant (early onset) or later than 1 year after transplant (late onset). In one study of 450 pediatric patients, 60% showed early PTLD, with a range of time to presentation between 6 weeks and 7 years after transplant.

The gastrointestinal (GI) tract is the most common extranodal location of PTLD, most likely due to its abundant lymphoid tissue. GI PTLD accounts for 17% to 30% of all patients with PTLD and is seen frequently after lung and multiorgan transplants. PTLD can involve any part of the GI tract. In a report of 34 children with GI PTLD, the sites of involvement were colorectal in 18%, jejunoileal in 12%, gastroduodenal in 9%, and esophageal in 3% of patients. Synchronous multisite GI tract involvement was seen in 47% of patients.

Similar to extranodal non-Hodgkin lymphoma, GI PTLD lesions range from simple nodules to large bulky masses, often containing areas of ulceration where the lymphomatous cells penetrate the mucosa. Ulceration is more common in PTLD than in non-Hodgkin lymphoma. Other findings include diffusely thickened folds or circumferential narrowing, which usually involve a long segment of bowel but show no evidence of obstruction because of a lack of desmoplastic reaction and bowel aneurysmal dilatation. Intestinal obstruction has been described when PTLD masses act as a lead point for intussusception.

Reference: Marie E, Navallas M, Navarro OM, et al. Posttransplant lymphoproliferative disorder in children: a 360-degree perspective. *Radiographics.* 2020;40(1):241-265.

33 **Answer B.** Loeys-Dietz syndrome (LDS) is a recently described genetic connective tissue disorder with a wide spectrum of multisystem involvement. LDS is typically characterized by the triad of hypertelorism, cleft palate or bifid uvula, and arterial aneurysm/tortuosity. The MR images in this case demonstrate marked aneurysmal dilatation of the ascending aorta. Patients with LDS exhibit rapidly progressive aortic and peripheral arterial aneurysmal disease. LDS and the other inherited aortopathies such as Marfan syndrome have overlapping phenotypic features. However, LDS is characterized by a more aggressive vascular course; patient morbidity and mortality occur at an early age, with complications developing at relatively smaller aortic dimensions. In addition, there is more diffuse arterial involvement in LDS, with a large proportion of patients developing aneurysms of the iliac, mesenteric, and intracranial arteries. Furthermore, all vessels can be involved by vascular malformations such as tortuosity, aneurysm, dissection, and stenosis. Because approximately half of all individuals with LDS have an aneurysm distant from the aortic root that would be missed by echocardiography, MR angiography or CT with three-dimensional reconstructions from head to pelvis must be performed. Early diagnosis and careful follow-up are essential for ensuring timely intervention in patients with arterial disease. Cross-sectional angiography has an important role in the baseline assessment, follow-up, and evaluation of acute complications of LDS, the thresholds and considerations of which differ from those of other inherited aortopathies. LDS has autosomal dominant inheritance.

References: Dhouib A, Beghetti M, Didier D. Imaging findings in a child with Loeys-Dietz syndrome. *Circulation*. 2012;126(4):507-508.

Loughborough WW, Minhas KS, Rodrigues JCL, et al. Cardiovascular manifestations and complications of Loeys-Dietz syndrome: CT and MR imaging findings. *Radiographics*. 2018;38(1):275-286.

MacCarrick G, Black JH 3rd, Bowdin S, et al. Loeys-Dietz syndrome: a primer for diagnosis and management. *Genet Med*. 2014;16(8):576-587.

34 **Answer C.** The images demonstrate multiple loops of bowel, many of which demonstrate abnormal thickening and mucosal enhancement along with ascites. In a patient who is status post hematopoietic stem cell transplantation (HSCT), these findings raise concern for graft-versus-host disease (GVHD). HSCT has been used progressively to cure hematopoietic disorders and hematological malignancies. GVHD is one of the most serious complications, with an average incidence of 59% after HSCT. GVHD is an immunological disease that occurs due to the relation between T lymphocytes of the donor and epithelial cells of the recipient. The skin, GI tract, and liver are the most often involved organs. GVHD affecting the GI tract (GI-GVHD) is one of the most common manifestations of acute GVHD with symptoms including abdominal pain, nausea, vomiting, abundant diarrhea, fever, and weight loss.

GVHD is the major reason of morbidity and mortality in patients after HSCT. In one study, acute GI-GVHD developed in 30% of pediatric patients. Acute GVHD characteristically occurs 10 to 40 days after HSCT (generally <100 days), whereas persistent or recurrent acute GVHD may appear after 100 days. Nearly half of the patients with acute GVHD progress to chronic GVHD. Chronic GVHD characteristically develops 100 days after HSCT.

Although endoscopic biopsy is necessary for definitive diagnosis and staging of GI-GVHD, it may be contraindicated in patients with thrombocytopenia and coagulopathy. The prognosis of acute GI-GVHD depends on immediate immunosuppressive treatment. Therefore, a rapid and accurate diagnosis is essential. Abdominopelvic CT is the primary imaging modality to determine abnormal findings in GI-GVHD.

Intestinal CT findings of GI-GVHD may also be seen in neutropenic colitis (typhlitis), pseudomembranous colitis (PMC), drug or radiation-related mucositis, and viral or fungal enterocolitis. Differentiation of GI-GVHD from infectious enterocolitis is essential because GI-GVHD requires immunosuppressive treatment, which is contraindicated in infectious enterocolitis. Neutropenic colitis (typhlitis) mainly involves the cecum, ascending colon, and sometimes the ileum, in contrast to GVHD. It characteristically shows cecal wall thickening with inflammatory stranding on CT. GI-GVHD usually involves both the small bowel and the colon, but the small bowel is more often involved. PMC is related to broad-spectrum antibiotic therapy, which affects the intestinal flora and results in overgrowth of *Clostridium difficile*. It usually manifests as pancolitis with marked wall thickening; small bowel involvement is uncommon. Drug- or radiation-induced mucositis is known as mucosal barrier injury and leads to segmental or diffuse GI tract involvement. Cytomegalovirus (CMV) colitis shows similar findings with typhlitis. Intestinal wall thickening is typically moderate in acute GI-GVHD, whereas it is usually more severe in most cases of infectious enterocolitis. Bowel dilatation and abnormal mucosal enhancement are significantly more common in acute GI-GVHD than the different infectious enterocolitis. Despite these imaging findings, clinical history, time, type of HSCT, laboratory values, and stool studies are crucial for a definitive diagnosis.

Reference: Arpaci T. Computed tomography imaging of acute gastrointestinal graft-versus-host disease after haematopoietic stem cell transplantation in children. *Contemp Oncol (Pozn).* 2018;22(3):178-183.

35 **Answer C.** In one study, extraintestinal CT findings of GI-GVHD were as follows: periportal edema in 9 (26%), ascites in 15 (43%), wall thickening and enhancement of the gall bladder in 13 (37%), pericholecystic fluid in 6 (17%), hepatomegaly in 13 (37%), and splenomegaly in 9 (26%) patients. One patient (3%) demonstrated free intraperitoneal air with a fluid collection owing to intestinal perforation. One patient with GI-GVHD showed multiple splenic abscesses.

Reference: Arpaci T. Computed tomography imaging of acute gastrointestinal graft-versus-host disease after haematopoietic stem cell transplantation in children. *Contemp Oncol (Pozn).* 2018;22(3):178-183.

INDEX